Uroradiology

X-Ray Department
Royal United Hospital
Bath

URORADIOLOGY

THOMAS SHERWOOD
MA MB DCH FRCP FRCR
Professor of Radiology, University of Cambridge

Alan J. Davidson MD
Chief of Radiology,
Mount Zion Hospital
and Medical Center,
San Francisco;
Clinical Professor of Radiology,
University of California,
San Francisco

Lee B. Talner MD
Professor of Radiology,
University of California,
San Diego

BLACKWELL SCIENTIFIC PUBLICATIONS
OXFORD LONDON EDINBURGH MELBOURNE

© 1980 by
Blackwell Scientific Publications
Editorial offices:
Osney Mead, Oxford, OX2 0EL
8 John Street, London, WC1N 2ES
9 Forrest Road, Edinburgh, EH1 2QH
214 Berkeley Street, Carlton
  Victoria 3053, Australia

First published 1980

Set in Monophoto Century Schoolbook

Printed in Great Britain at
The Alden Press, Oxford
and bound by
Mansell (Bookbinders) Ltd.,
Witham, Essex

DISTRIBUTORS

USA
  Blackwell Mosby Book Distributors
  11830 Westline Industrial Drive
  St Louis, Missouri 63141

Canada
  Blackwell Mosby Book Distributors
  86 Northline Road, Toronto
  Ontario, M4B 3E5

Australia
  Blackwell Scientific Book
  Distributors
  214 Berkeley Street, Carlton
  Victoria 3053

British Library
Cataloguing in Publication Data

Sherwood, Thomas
  Uroradiology.
  1. Genito-urinary
  organs—Radiography
  2. Radiology, Medical
  I. Title II. Davidson, Alan J.
  III. Talner, Lee B
  616.6'07'57 RC874
  ISBN 0-632-00493-2

PREFACE

Medical books are now often written by committee. Knowledge is fattening, and one man can no longer hope to have the whole of his subject under his belt, let alone write about it. What reason then for this book? George Orwell (1947) gave plain answers to such pious questions in his essay 'Why I write'. Sheer egoism heads the list, trailing stuff like aesthetic enthusiasm (for medical writers, fun), historical impulse, and political purpose (medical intelligence). As regards medical intelligence, I wanted to give FRCR candidates and others a personal view of what is interesting and important about uroradiology. I have tried to prune or ignore everything else. The defects of the book are therefore entirely mine, but any merits rest on many shoulders. The book is mainly about what I learnt in my 10 years at the Institute of Urology and Royal Postgraduate Medical School. For this I am greatly indebted to many colleagues in clinical, pathological and radiological disciplines. Mr David Innes Williams taught me even more than anybody else. I thank them all very much.

I am especially grateful to my co-authors Alan Davidson and Lee Talner. Contributing to another's book is not particularly enticing. Both are old friends, and on this I traded shamelessly. The book now has at least three good chapters, and I thank them for their generous help.

The last part of my apologia concerns an obsession with the purpose of an investigative discipline in the closing decades of the century. What is scientific radiology about? One view is that the new imaging technology makes key contributions to amassing the evidence on which accurate diagnosis is based. Let us gather all the information we can about our patient, and evaluate the data. This is the apparatus of the diagnostic work-up, the impartial review of evidence leading from observation to conclusion. I think that the diagnostic work-up is unkind, uncritical and—much the worst indictment—deeply unscientific (Sherwood, 1978). Science works by trial-and-error, by generating ideas and testing them. On philosophical, humane and economic grounds, we are much better off if we start with an idea of what may be wrong with our patient, and then use radiological studies to test that hypothesis. In short, by building on the next likely diagnosis. This book therefore deals more with patients' presenting problems than with disease entities. I have not been able to carry this approach consistently through all parts of the book. The organizational muddle is mine, but it is an honest attempt to teach the sort of radiology apposite to our times.

The book has been written in the immediate sense, many times, by my secretary Mary Watts. It would not have come about without her. Peter Saugman commissioned the work, and I also thank David Manson and many other members of the Blackwell Scientific Publications staff.

Thomas Sherwood

REFERENCES

ORWELL G. (1947) Why I write. In *Decline of the English Murder and other Essays,* p. 180. Penguin Books, Harmondsworth, 1965.
SHERWOOD T. (1978) Science in radiology. *Lancet* i, 594.

CONTENTS

PREFACE v
ACKNOWLEDGEMENTS viii

PART I
TOOLS (X-RAY AND ULTRASOUND) 1
A Plain film and intravenous urogram 1
B Micturition cysto-urethrogram and dynamic bladder studies 10
C Urethrogram 13
D Antegrade (percutaneous) pyelogram, nephrostomy and dynamic studies 15
E Retrograde ureterogram/pyelogram 20
F Renal arteriogram and venogram 21
G Ultrasound 29
H Lymphogram 33
I Vasogram and cavernogram 35
J Tools for paediatric work 36

PART II
NUCLEAR MEDICINE AND COMPUTED TOMOGRAPHY 41

A **Nuclear medicine:** *Lee B. Talner* 41

B **Computed tomography in uroradiology:** *Alan J. Davidson* 59

PART III
HYPERTENSION: *Lee B. Talner* 75

PART IV
DIVISIONS 87

Division 1: The kidneys
A Unilateral kidney failure 87
B Renal failure 102
C Hydronephrosis 116
D Urothelial tumours 119
E Stones 124
F Nephrocalcinosis 128
G Hurt calices/papillae 140
H Renal masses 166
J Trauma 199
K Loin pain and haematuria syndrome (renal arteritis) 202

Division 2: The kidney and ureter

A   Duplication   211
B   Dilated ureter: obstruction   222
C   Dilated ureter: reflux   238
D   Dilated ureter: no obstruction or reflux   242
E   Diverted ureter   249

Division 3: The bladder and urethra—adult

A   Obstruction   255
B   Infection   272
C   Incontinence   281
D   Haematuria   291
E   Odd bladder shapes   301
F   Trauma   307

Division 4: The bladder and urethra—child

A   Incontinence/Infection   313
B   Infection/Obstruction   324
C   Double micturition   333
D   Trauma   334
E   Haematuria   334

Division 5: The male genital tract

A   Infertility   338
B   Deformity   341
C   Tumours   342
D   Intersex states   345
E   Scrotum   345

INDEX   347

ACKNOWLEDGEMENTS

We are grateful to several publishers for permission to use illustrations, including the British Institute of Radiology (*British Journal of Radiology*); Williams & Wilkins Co., Baltimore (*Journal of Urology* **99,** 685, Fig. 5); S. Karger AG, Basel (*Contributions to Nephrology* **5,** 20–21, Fig. 10, and 70, Fig. 35); William Heinemann Medical Books Ltd., London (*Scientific Foundations of Urology,* **1,** 127–131, Figs. 2, 3, 5 & 8).

These sections do not aim to provide a comprehensive manual of uroradiological techniques. Most readers will already have worked out their own approaches to common investigations like the IVU. A working knowledge of basic techniques will be taken for granted.

A. PLAIN FILM AND INTRAVENOUS UROGRAM (IVU)

Every radiological text hammers at the good plain film as an essential examination before starting out on contrast medium procedures. However tired, this message is absolutely sound and of pressing everyday importance. It has been said that the sharpest nightmares to haunt clinicians are made up of simple sins of omission or commission. Few patients come to harm for not having the latest laboratory test, but 'why didn't I do a rectal examination on Mr A, or look at the urine of Mrs B,' are the sort of questions that make for discomfiting sweats in the small hours. Inattention to the plain film is the exact counterpart of these sins in uroradiological practice, and many important mistakes still arise in this way.

The worth of the plain film is particularly dependent on good radiographic technique. 'Use a low enough kV and large enough contrast medium dose' is a simple maxim which can improve IVU practice overnight, much more decisively than installing tomographic equipment. Apart from using a low kV, the good radiographer is also keen to cover the whole of the urinary tract on plain films. The standard 35×43 cm film can only do this for perhaps half the usual size adults in this country, and many departments use a routine two-film survey to cope with this difficulty. The added radiation burden is a drawback, and a case can be made for an initial single 30×43 cm film, followed by a further bladder or kidney view if the first film is inadequate in either direction.

CONTRAST MEDIA

Current conventional urographic media are made up of a non-opaque cation (sodium and/or meglumine) and an opaque anion (diatrizoate, iothalamate or metrizoate). Nine combinations are therefore possible, and most are available commercially.

CATION (radiolucent)	*ANION* (radiopaque)
sodium	diatrizoate
meglumine	iothalamate
sodium/meglumine	metrizoate

Sodium agents are preferable for the IVU, since meglumine leads to a more intense diuresis, diluting the pyelogram (Benness, 1970; Dacie & Fry, 1972). Meglumine agents have advantages for angiography, though these do not necessarily apply to the kidney (Talner & Saltzstein, 1975). There is little to

1

choose between the opaque anions: cost per gram of iodine is one good criterion (Saxton, 1969—a key paper).

A jungle of trade names obscures these simple facts. Radiologists are guilty of falling in with the practice of referring to these compounds, some of the main tools of their work, by uninformative and even obscurantist names. Any single manufacturer's trade name for a range of contrast media ('Urografin', 'Conray' or whatever) usually refers to the same anion, but includes different combinations of cations.

Dose

A similar sloppiness extends to the contrast doses used for the IVU, and is taken up by clinical request forms asking for 'high dose urograms'. It is best to state clearly on each X-ray report exactly what and how much contrast medium was given. Most centres now use a minimum dose of 300 mg iodine per kg body weight for the standard adult with normal renal function. In renal failure this dose must be doubled (see Division 1 section B).

Excretion

Glomerular filtration is the only important route of renal excretion (Saxton, 1969). From the point of view of the kidney this is of course a cold, inactive process, the energy being supplied by the heart. The higher the plasma level of contrast medium, the more will be filtered. Plasma level in turn is dependent on the contrast dose and, to a smaller extent, on the speed of injection. The filtered contrast medium produces the *nephrogram,* diffuse opacification of the whole kidney.

The *IVU nephrogram* is therefore an upper nephron event, and can be regarded as a functional window for looking in on the upper nephron. It is dependent only on plasma contrast level, glomerular filtration and the obligatory sodium and water reabsorption occurring in the proximal convoluted tubule. It is *not* affected by the patient's state of hydration, which influences the the pyelogram through distal tubular water reabsorption. The very early nephrogram seen during the IVU is also made up of a vascular component (contrast medium in renal vascular spaces), but its importance is short-lived, lasting seconds rather than minutes.

Extrarenal excretion

In the normal state, renal excretion of contrast medium is dominant, and the existing hepatic and intestinal pathways unimportant. These are of interest, however, in renal failure states. This is not because they are able to take over efficient elimination of the contrast medium—if required, dialysis must be used to this end. The interest lies in explaining otherwise puzzling findings: opacification of the gall-bladder (Fig. I.1) and gut (Fig. I.2). The hepatic route is the most important of the extrarenal excretory pathways, and can lead to an opaque

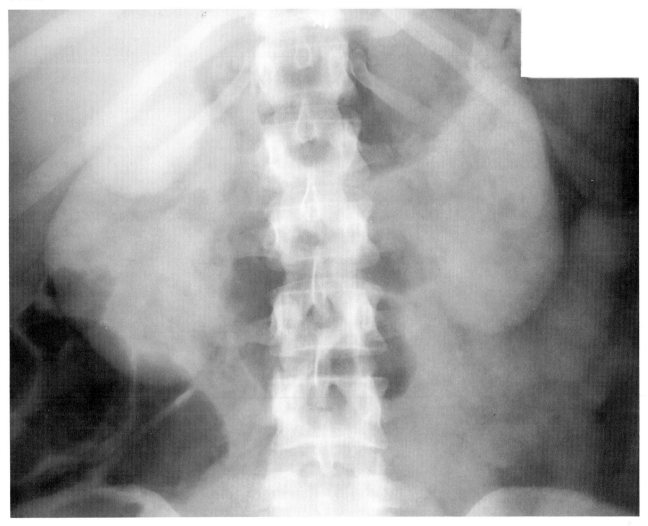

gall-bladder even in the presence of normal renal function. This is seen particularly when one kidney is suddenly obstructed, e.g. in ureteric colic, and Sokoloff and Talner (1973) have elegantly shown that unusually prolonged, high plasma contrast levels are the explanation. There is an impression that this finding is more common when metrizoate is the medium used.

Free iodide—salivary gland enlargement

The iodine in standard contrast media is bound into the organic benzoic acid ring, but a small fraction of free, inorganic iodide is also present (Coel *et al,* 1975). Once injected, there is *in vivo* splitting off of further iodide, and this is

Fig. I.1 Eighteen hours after the start of the IVU in this young woman with acute renal failure, both kidneys are still densely opacified—the long-lasting nephrogram characteristic of acute tubular necrosis. Note that the gallbladder is also opacified.

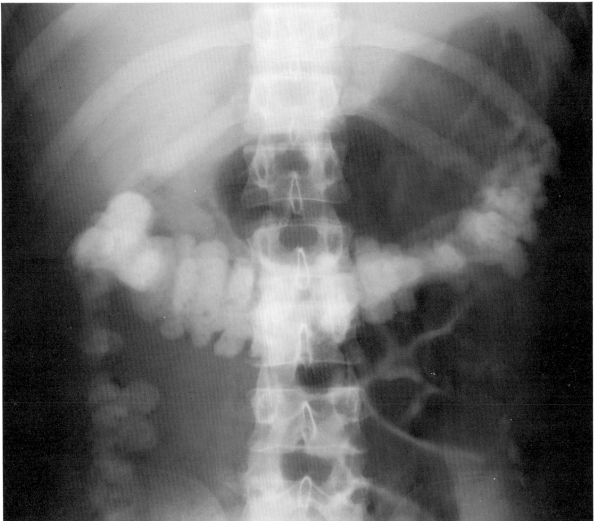

Fig. I.2 Chronic renal failure—6 days after the IVU the colon is seen.

more pronounced in the uraemic patient because contrast medium is retained longer. The salivary glands concentrate iodide, and also secrete the contrast medium intact (Talner *et al*, 1973). For these reasons transient enlargement of the salivary glands ('iodide mumps') may occasionally be seen in uraemic patients several days after the IVU.

Dehydration

By long tradition the patient having an IVU is first deprived of fluid for several hours. This was most necessary when small contrast doses of the order of 50 mg iodine per kg were used: a good pyelogram was not seen without good urine concentration. Even so, overnight dehydration is not a reliable way of ensuring maximal urine concentration—it is a short period in the body's overall water household.

With current IVU techniques of using larger contrast-medium doses, dehydration has become much less important. Opinion is now divided whether it should remain part of the preparation for the standard IVU. Certainly there is no justification for turning down an urgent IVU request 'because the patient hasn't fasted'. This applies with particular force to ureteric colic (Casualty IVU, see Division 2 section B): the important information sought about ureteric obstruction will not be affected by the cups of tea the patient may or may not have had.

The supporters of routine fluid deprivation make several points. On average, somewhat better pyelograms will be seen. No complex, fallible instructions need be given to the patient about keeping to a moderate fluid intake or avoiding diuretics like coffee. If the contrast medium induces nausea, retching on an empty stomach is much safer than vomiting in the supine position

Against this can be ranged serious arguments on the dangers of fluid deprivation. The dehydrated patient with renal impairment (or multiple myeloma) stands to be harmed by the investigation. Most instances of renal failure precipitated or worsened by an IVU can be put down to inappropriate dehydration. Unless there is very close clinical liaison, the radiologist may not always know at the outset of an IVU that his patient does not suffer from renal impairment. Why run these risks when fluid deprivation has only a small influence on IVU quality, is the argument of this school.

The reader of this book will wish to choose his own path between these voices. If he/she works in a unit with excellent clinical rapport, there is still something to be said for fluid deprivation of the patient with assuredly normal renal function. There is no disagreement whatever that dehydration is to be avoided at all costs in three groups of patients who may be *harmed* by it:

1. Renal impairment. For practical purposes this means a raised blood urea or creatinine. Patients in renal failure cannot concentrate their urine, so the attempt at making them do so is silly as well as dangerous.

2. Infants.

3. Myeloma. Diabetes may come to be added to this list.

Newer contrast media

The high osmolality of the conventional urographic media has drawbacks, though distension of the urinary tract by the ensuing osmotic diuresis is helpful. Dimer contrast media, linking together two opaque anions, have been developed, e.g. sodium iocarmate. They have particular advantages in sites where high osmolality is undesirable, e.g. in the subarachnoid space. Six iodine atoms in a dimer molecule have an 'osmolality cost' of only three particles (dimer anion, two cations), as opposed to four particles in the monomer (two anions, two cations). A non-ionic contrast medium, metrizamide, has been developed, with only a third of the osmolality of the monomer per iodine mass.

The high cost of these media militates against their routine use. It might be thought from the armchair that they would have a special place in advanced renal failure, where the kidney is already subject to an osmotic diuresis and reduced glomerular filtration rate. This is not so in experimental practice (Webb *et al,* 1978), and for the IVU their place remains uncertain.

Reactions

Contrast medium reactions are probably the most feared complication in X-ray departments. This is because they occur unheralded, in previously fit patients, and may advance at a frightening pace to death within minutes. Perhaps most worrying of all is that there is as yet no hypothesis which can consistently explain these reactions, and make up a scaffolding for sensible action. Four mechanisms under study are mentioned by Lasser *et al* (1977):

1. An antigen–antibody reaction directed against the contrast medium, which functions as a haptene.

2. Activation of complement and of coagulation systems.

3. Release of histamine from mast cells and basophils.

4. Anxiety.

The unpredictable sequential pattern of contrast medium reactions within the same patient is a particular stumbling block. A patient may have a reaction at one IVU and not at another, using the same contrast compound. There is no crescendo effect of each reaction rather worse than the last, which might be expected on an immunological basis. Reactions are almost unknown under general anaesthesia. It might be argued that most uroradiological examinations under anaesthesia involve retrograde rather than parenteral injections, but contrast medium is in fact absorbed into the circulation in small amounts across the urothelium.

These puzzles lend particular support to the anxiety hypothesis. Thus Lalli (1975) had nine patients with previous life-threatening reactions who suffered no ill effects at their next examination, conducted with calm assurance. I do not think there is any difficulty about accepting that patients may 'die of fright', but I am not yet convinced that all the observed facts can be fitted into this hypothesis. There is no doubt that the personalities and approach of the medical staff are of major importance in this as in most other radiological fields. Reactions may arbitrarily be grouped into three classes of severity.

1. Minimal reactions. Most patients feel uncomfortably warm during the injection because of vasodilatation. Sensations of flushing in face and throat, or of imminent incontinence are common. A few patients develop nausea and retching. These symptoms hardly deserve the title of reactions, and are to be managed with calm explanation.

2. Minor reactions. Patients develop urticaria, at times with very extensive, itchy weals, peri-orbital oedema and stuffy sinuses. These uncomfortable symptoms can be helped by antihistamines, or possibly steroids in severe cases.

3. Major reactions.
(a) *Laryngeal or bronchial obstruction.* Steroids are the traditional stand-by, but subcutaneous adrenaline probably still has a place, arguably more effective.
(b) *Hypotensive collapse or cardiac arrest.* Emergency treatment of these rare complications follows standard resuscitation lines. It is worth remembering to try to obtain a quick abdominal radiograph during the recovery phase: it is probably the only IVU ever advisable in that patient.

Prophylaxis

Various manoeuvres have been tried, often without success.

Pre-testing. This has involved applying contrast medium to various sites like the cornea, or injecting a small bolus intravenously. There is now general nihilism about the value of such testing. Certainly a negative result does not preclude a major reaction. However, those with a positive intravenous pre-test perhaps run a greater risk of serious reaction if the full dose is then given (Lasser *et al*, 1977). The rarity of a positive pre-test result makes this rather unimportant.

Change of contrast medium. There is no convincing evidence that this is an important consideration in dealing with the patient who has already suffered a reaction. Meglumine compounds appear more likely to be associated with bronchospasm (Ansell, 1976), so a change to a sodium compound might be sensible for a subsequent examination in a patient with such a reaction.

Pre-treatment. The place of intravenous steroids in the treatment of the acute incident is accepted rather uncritically. However, Lasser *et al* (1977), authoritative voices, support steroid pre-treatment of patients who have already had a reaction (or those 'thought specifically at risk') for two days before the new examination.

Summary comment

Any department carrying out IVUs must clearly be prepared to deal with contrast medium reactions. Because the life-threatening occasion is rare, arises unannounced and progresses quickly, the doctor first on the scene may never have met one before. He can guard against disasters by remaining easily within call of the IVU room for the first 10 minutes following injection—most reactions arise early. There is everything to be said for having a wall chart or booklet on diagnosis and treatment of reactions in every IVU room (e.g. Ansell's *Notes on Radiological Emergencies,* Blackwell Scientific Publications).

The tentative evidence on the importance of anxiety in reactions is cheering: the kind, considerate radiologist can look forward to fewer reactions than his surly colleague.

TECHNIQUE POINTS

Compression

The best pyelograms for demonstrating caliceal detail will need compression. It is therefore a good manoeuvre, providing it is well done (Saxton & Strickland, 1972). Compression must be used with common sense and discretion, e.g. avoided in those with abdominal masses, tenderness, or urinary tract obstruction. Rarely, compression has led to renal rupture. Since acute ureteric obstruction alone can rupture a kidney (Fig. I.3), it is not sensible or necessary to add this insult to patients having an IVU for ureteric colic. For many patients having follow-up IVUs the questions posed do not bear on caliceal detail, but on ureteric drainage. Compression is then clearly inappropriate.

Effective compression is uncomfortable and tends to be remembered with particular aversion by many patients. There is no point in using it in any half-cocked way. There are also instances when it is best forgotten altogether, e.g. in frightened children.

Tomography

This is an essential technique for the renal failure IVU: the nephrogram which is the key to the investigation may not be seen properly without it. A control pre-injection tomogram should be done first, so that comparison is possible for the doubtful nephrogram. Many centres now use tomograms as part of their standard initial IVU. Providing this does not become a radiation extravaganza, the pay-off in avoiding ambiguous examinations is probably justified.

Follow-up IVUs

Most second or further IVUs can be severely curtailed. It should be a point of honour for the radiologist to use the bare minimum of films. The questions asked of the examination are usually sharply limited at this stage, and can often be answered by two radiographs, plain film and ten-minute full-length film.

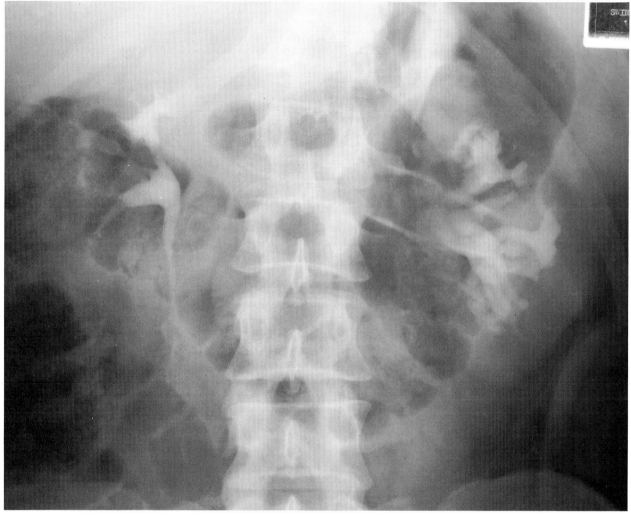

Fig. I.3 Left ureteric colic and stone causing renal rupture—note contrast medium in the left renal sinus.

Injection speed

Remember the worries about patients with known heart disease—see Division 1 section B under 'Contrast medium and dose'.

Children

Children are not small scale adults. Their IVU needs are different—see section J p. 36.

B. MICTURITION CYSTO-URETHROGRAM (MCU) AND DYNAMIC BLADDER STUDIES

MCU

This is an uncomfortable, undignified examination for adults as well as children. This high price is usually well worth while for the information gained about the lower urinary tract. It does mean that there is no room at all for frivolous or 'let's-just-see-if-there-is-anything-wrong' requests for MCUs. The investigation is splendid at answering properly framed questions, for instance in children's urinary tract infections (see Division 4 section B). It is very nearly useless as a general survey examination for adults with common bladder symptoms like frequency, urgency or dysuria (see Division 3 sections A & B).

Catheterization is the usual method for introducing contrast medium into the bladder. There are three alternatives for performing MCUs if necessary without catheters:

1. IVU. The patient can be screened during voiding at the end of the IVU. Contrast medium in the bladder is often too poor to give accurate pictures of the urethra, and reflux will not be caught. However, the method has obvious advantages for answering limited questions, for instance in the 6-year-old boy who has suffered a urinary infection and is now having a normal IVU. If he is screened at its end it should be possible to exclude urethral obstruction during the one examination. What matter to careful clinical management if a little vesico-ureteric reflux is missed? If the IVU cystogram is inadequate, a formal MCU will of course have to be done.

2. Suprapubic bladder puncture is of obvious attraction in infants. It is splendidly clean in the bacteriological sense. The fact that it allows looking in on repeated bladder filling and voiding is a considerable boon—infant MCUs can be difficult, and it is easy to mess up the study of the one episode granted by catheterization.

3. Urethral stricture and urethrogram. If an impassable stricture is shown by the retrograde examination, cystographic contrast medium can be instilled through the device already in position for the urethrogram (Knutsson clamp or whatever). This will have to be done under pressure and therefore with care: hand syringes can readily generate enormously high pressures of several hundred millimetres of mercury.

Technique points

1. Catheterization

The quickest and simplest but also clean method is generally best, and will vary between departments and individuals. A theatre technique with gowns and gloves is not essential with present-day doubly-packed catheters: they can be introduced by a rigorous no-touch technique without the expense (and perhaps false security) of gloves.

Local anaesthetic is usually used, especially in the male, by squeezing a tube of jelly down the urethra. Arguably this is very nearly as uncomfortable as the later passage of the catheter, and of variable effectiveness. There is something to be said for carrying out the whole unpleasant manoeuvre of catheterization briskly and gently in one stage, the tip of the catheter being well lubricated with anaesthetic jelly.

2. Contrast medium

Water-soluble contrast medium is mandatory. Barium is no longer usable because of the dangers of barium reflux into the kidney (granuloma formation). The concentration of the medium should not be as high as for intravenous urography, since all bladder detail will then be quickly blotted out by the large iodine mass: 15–25% contrast-medium solutions are suitable.

3. The bladder must be adequately filled

Voiding on an X-ray table in front of an audience is a *tour de force* for most patients. The standing posture imposes an additional burden on women. The chances of a successful examination are not good if the bladder stimulus to micturition is less than maximal. In practice this means filling the bladder uncomfortably full. Most adults will understand this readily enough, and explanation, chat and banter will help to tide the subject over these discomforts. It is misplaced kindness to stop bladder filling the moment the patient complains, perhaps after only a few hundred millilitres. A prolonged, unsuccessful examination is then likely to follow. The promise 'you won't burst' is reassuring to many individuals, and true for the conscious patient.

4. Screening and filming

Spot films taken during the examination answer most needs, and are cheaper in radiation terms than cine. Some routines use rather too many films during the filling stage: the look-out here is for major bladder disarrays like diverticula, and for ureteric reflux.

During voiding 'best stream' pictures are important, so that the urethra is seen at its functional best. The oblique posture is generally entirely adequate for this stage—the lateral position is at least twice as radiation-expensive, for no great gain.

5. The patient who cannot void

With adequate bladder filling, and with tact and persuasion, this should not be a frequent problem. Women sometimes have great difficulty with this part of the examination. It is positively counter-productive to ask them to strain: the sphincters will be tighter than ever. The message should be 'relax'. It can be helpful to ask the patient to visit the lavatory in private just to start off, and then to hurry back to the X-ray table for a second performance.

Quite often, immediate post-micturition rather than voiding views will answer all the remaining clinical questions, particularly on important reflux. There is then little point in persisting with the fruitless voiding attempts. The unlikelihood of urethral obstruction in the female makes this an especially apt abbreviation of the investigation. However, when voiding views are essential, e.g. in boys, it is usually better to give the patient a rest rather than to work up sphincter tension by a crescendo dialogue of 'no I can't'—'yes, you can'. The next patient can be seen, and 15 minutes later the first patient can have a new, confident start.

DOUBLE CONTRAST CYSTOGRAMS

Outlining mucosal lesions in the bladder by double contrast, using an opaque medium and gas, appeared promising at one time, but is now very little used. The cystoscope is more reliable for the diagnosis of such lesions. Bladder wall mobility can be assessed by the double-contrast cystogram, and this may be of value in judging tumour invasion. The technique probably still has a place where a tumour is suspected in a bladder diverticulum, whose inside is beyond the reach of the cystoscope.

DYNAMIC BLADDER STUDIES (pressure/flow video cystography)

The basic technique is shown in Fig. I.4 (Whiteside & Turner Warwick, 1976).

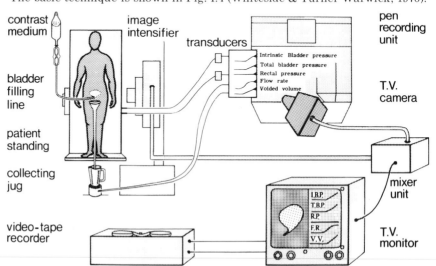

Fig. I.4 Dynamic cystogram.

The purpose of the examination is to see, side by side and at the same time, how the bladder works (pressure/flow traces) and what it looks like (MCU image). To this end a small perurethral catheter is placed in the bladder, and another in the rectum. These just measure pressure, and are small enough not to interfere with urine flow rate through the urethra. Total bladder pressure is made up of the activity of the bladder muscle (detrusor), and also of intra-abdominal pressure. Measuring total bladder pressure on its own, as in the conventional cystometrogram, therefore gives a compound picture: pressure will rise not only when the bladder contracts, but each time the patient coughs. The rectal line, monitoring intra-abdominal pressure, is used to tease these activities apart. By continuously subtracting intra-abdominal from total bladder pressure, a third pressure trace is derived which reflects bladder activity alone—intrinsic bladder or detrusor pressure.

The bladder is filled in the usual way through a large catheter lying alongside the tiny pressure line. An eye is kept on the traces at this stage for unwanted detrusor contractions—evidence of an unstable bladder (see Division 3 section A). In the normal subject, detrusor pressure hardly rises during filling, even when there is an urgent call to micturition near the end. After removal of the filling catheter, the patient is asked to void under fluoroscopy in the usual upright position, and voiding flow rate is recorded.

The technique is obviously more cumbersome than a straightforward cystogram, but with practice it need not take very much longer. Careful selection of patients for the study is essential, but given such care the examination can be very rewarding in the investigation of bladder symptoms (see Division 3 sections A, B, C). By recording onto video-tape, the examination can be played back later at leisure for joint study between clinician and radiologist. In general, the dynamic data point to the functional diagnosis (e.g. obstruction), and synchronous fluoroscopy to the site of the lesion (e.g. the bladder neck).

C. URETHROGRAM

There is a range of methods available for ascending urethrography. My preference is for injecting viscous, jelly-like contrast medium by the Knutsson clamp. Good distension of the urethra is obtained with the jelly, readily lighting up strictures. Warming the contrast medium to comfortable body heat before injection is essential—it is too viscous otherwise. The Knutsson clamp perhaps looks forbiddingly like a mediaeval torture instrument, but is in practice one of the kindest devices for this examination. The mechanical prerequisite for urethrography is to establish a firm anchor point from which the urethra can be injected. It is less unpleasant if an external surface like keratinized skin can be used for this, as in the Knutsson clamp, rather than an internal delicate mucous membrane, as in catheter-balloon techniques. Note that the foreskin must be retracted for the Knutsson clamp so that the arms are applied behind the corona glandis—they will slip off otherwise. The nozzle of the device is then pressed gently but firmly into the urethral meatus and locked in position.

Because considerable pressures are needed for injecting, the procedure is best monitored under fluoroscopy. *Intravasation,* i.e. dissection of the contrast medium into vascular spaces, can be detected at once in this way, and the examination stopped. This is not a frequent or serious complication, but very alarming for the patient. Once the injecting device is removed, there may well be copious bleeding from the penis. The patient should be assured that this will stop spontaneously, and then sat down comfortably with a good supply of absorbent material. He will probably be able to leave the department shortly, without further bleeding.

Intravasation usually occurs with severe strictures. To avoid it, injection pressures should not be excessive, and urethrograms avoided altogether for 2–3 weeks after urethral instrumentation. If an earlier urethrogram becomes essential, then simple urographic contrast medium should be used rather than jelly. Intravasation of the simpler compound is less likely to set up an inflammatory reaction.

Projections. Films in both oblique positions are usually adequate. There is a large difference in the tissue density the X-ray beam has to traverse as between the anterior and posterior urethra. It is often advantageous to record each part separately, therefore, with differing exposures.

Multiple sites of obstruction. Once a severe stricture has been shown by the technique, say in the bulbar urethra, chances of pinpointing an additional higher obstruction, e.g. at the bladder neck, are not good. A voiding study (MCU) is best done at the end if there is suspicion of further proximal lesions. The bladder can be filled with urographic contrast medium immediately by the Knutsson clamp already in position (see section B p. 10).

Catheter-balloon techniques

Blowing up a small balloon catheter in the anterior urethra can be used as an alternative and excellent urethrogram technique. Ordinary urographic contrast medium is then infused. This can be done by gravity from a drip bottle, splendidly simplifying the whole procedure. No screening is needed, standard high-quality radiographs can be obtained with an overhead X-ray tube, and at the end of the urethrogram the patient is ready for an immediate MCU (de Lacy & Wignall, 1977).

Summary comment

By design, the urethrogram sets out to give excellent structural information about the urethra. It cannot say anything about the functional importance of the lesions which may be found. An MCU or dynamic study would be needed to this end. However, most patients with a urethral stricture can be managed satisfactorily using urethrogram, symptoms and voiding flow rate as guides.

D. ANTEGRADE (PERCUTANEOUS) PYELOGRAM, NEPHROS-TOMY AND DYNAMIC STUDIES

Needling the kidney in order to obtain a pyelogram is an old technique which has enjoyed a rebirth in recent years (Sherwood & Stevenson, 1972). Two developments have sprung from it: (1) leaving a drainage device behind to make a radiologist's nephrostomy; (2) measuring upper urinary tract pressure for diagnosing obstruction.

ANTEGRADE PYELOGRAM

The accepted indication for this technique is where the necessary information about the patient has not been obtained by other means, i.e. inadequate IVU and failed retrograde pyelogram. In practice this last ditch indication is too narrow, and it may be proper to move straight from the inadequate IVU to the antegrade study. However, patients should always be selected with care, after joint consultation between clinician and radiologist.

Obstruction is the common indication, and the antegrade pyelogram is then usually easy. Puncturing the pelvi-caliceal system of an unobstructed, undistended kidney is more difficult, but not forbiddingly so (Fig. I.5). The needle can be a lumbar puncture needle, but must be long enough (15 cm). The bore should

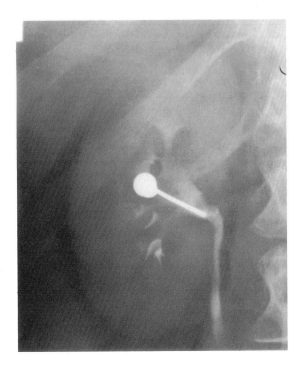

Fig. I.5 Puncture of an undistended right renal pelvis for collecting cells near a urothelial carcinoma. Confirmation of the diagnosis in this way was needed in this patient with recurrent tumours in order to plan conservative surgery.

not be too large for fear of causing a retroperitoneal urine leak—20 gauge is a good compromise. Very fine needles of the order 22 or 23 gauge have disadvantages: they are too flexible for a very accurate aim, and urine cannot be aspirated readily through them. It is attractive to puncture a renal calix rather than the pelvis (Fig. I.6). In this way a better seal is made round the needle track (by renal parenchyma), and any vessels which may be hit will be smaller. However, the renal pelvis is often the large, obvious, and therefore preferable target.

Technique

The procedure is done under local anaesthesia, except in young children, with the patient prone on a fluorosocopy table. An intravenous contrast medium injection is helpful for outlining a target, but often the examination is done just because an IVU is too poor. 'Blind' puncture can then be entirely successful, but a blind radiologist is of course a nonsense. Careful inspection of the plain film will almost always show something of the renal outline, so that a sensible target can be selected in relation to bony landmarks. Fluoroscopy is used for checking on this mental map at puncture.

Once the pelvi-caliceal system has been entered, contrast medium is injected to outline the whole upper urinary tract (Fig. I.7). In the obstructed state, the tract will be full of stagnant urine. Proper mixing of the contrast medium with this pool is essential in order not to be deceived about the level of the responsible lesion. Gravity must be called in to help here, and upright views on a tilting table are important. It is probably good practice to empty the system as much as possible at the end of the procedure.

Complications are remarkably few. Arteries and veins are sometimes hit, usually without ill effect. The most worrying hazard is a urine leak through the needle track from the obstructed kidney. Providing fine needles are used, this is not of any great moment in practice. From this point of view it is comforting that chronic obstruction is a low pressure state. However, if an acutely obstructed kidney is diagnosed on clinico-radiological grounds, it may well be advisable to leave a draining device in position (see below).

NEPHROSTOMY

A number of techniques are available for draining the kidney at antegrade pyelography.

1. Catheter through large needle

The simplest method uses a needle big enough for introducing a catheter

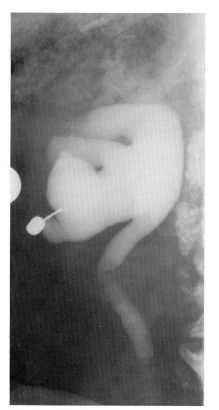

Fig. I.6 The tip of the puncturing needle is entering a distended calix.

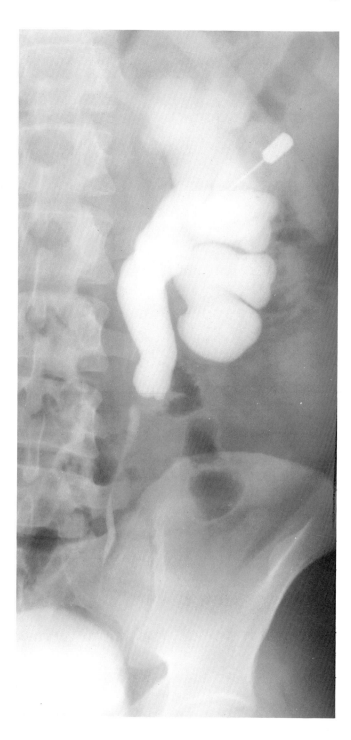

Fig. I.7 Ureteric stricture (carcinoma) on antegrade pyelography.

through it, e.g. a renal biopsy needle (Fig. I.8). Against the attraction of simplicity must be put the fact that a larger than necessary hole is made, with the possibility of urine seepage around the catheter.

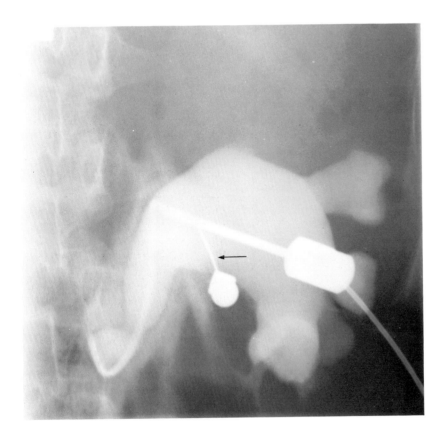

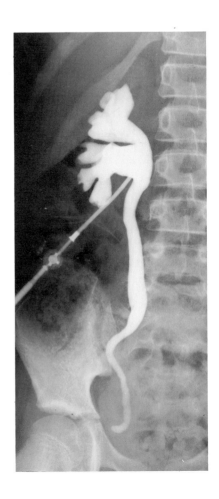

Fig. I.8   *(left)* A ureteric catheter has been advanced through a large renal biopsy needle entering the renal pelvis. Note that a smaller needle (arrow) is still in position, having been used first to outline the target.

Fig. I.9   *(right)* A Teflon sheath has been left behind for drainage after withdrawal of the needle puncturing the right kidney. This child's right lower ureter is obstructed following reimplantation surgery.

2. Sheath over needle

A Teflon or other sheath/needle system can be used to puncture the kidney, withdrawing the needle to leave the sheath behind (Fig. I.9). This too is splendidly simple, but has drawbacks. The length of sheath that can be introduced down the upper urinary tract is determined by needle length, in turn severely limited by the geometry of the screening table. The method is particularly useful where attempts at the more desirable technique no. 3 below have failed. The sheath is then left as a temporary device, to be exchanged a day or two later when a track has formed.

3. Guide wire methods

A J-shaped guide wire is introduced into the upper urinary tract through a small puncturing needle as for any Seldinger technique (Fig. I.10). The needle is withdrawn, and a catheter with side holes put in over the wire. This sounds very straightforward, and works well enough in experienced hands. Problems can be encountered, however. They are mainly determined by the fact that the object for attack by the Seldinger exchange technique, the renal calix, is inches away from the surface, rather than beneath the skin like a femoral artery. The common difficulty is for the catheter to kink in the peri-renal space rather than enter the kidney. Preparing a good track for the catheter through the retroperitoneal tissues is necessary, and for this a Teflon vessel dilator is best used first over the guide wire. It can be jiggled up and down with careful vigour. Successively larger dilators can also be used at this stage (Burnett *et al*, 1976). The size of catheter introduced will depend on these preparations—it need not be very large.

During the next few weeks exchanges for larger and softer catheters can be done via guide wires. A good track will have formed after a month or so, and intermediate guide wires need no longer be used then. A self-retaining catheter like a balloon catheter can be left, to be changed occasionally (Fig. I.11). Long-term drainage can be arranged in this way (Harris *et al*, 1976).

Point of puncture. The patient will be much more comfortable if the catheter is placed postero-laterally rather than directly posteriorly. An oblique approach is therefore desirable for drainage procedures. This is only a little more difficult than standard posterior puncture. The patient is either turned into the desired oblique position and the needle inserted vertically downwards, or biplane screening is used with the needle oblique and the patient straight.

Summary comment

Percutaneous nephrostomy is so straightforward and attractive a technique that there is sometimes a temptation to use it indiscriminately. The method is splendid for short-term renal drainage, buying time for making a proper diagnosis, and for doing a calm, considered operation later. This approach implies close clinico-radiological consultation at all times. Similar care is needed for the often vexed question of long-term drainage. Whether a patient with inoperable urinary obstruction by malignant disease really stands to benefit from the manoeuvre is a moot point. The interested radiologist should insist on being a member of the team which discusses these problems jointly. If he is just the technician who sticks catheters into people as directed, he may do his patients more harm than good.

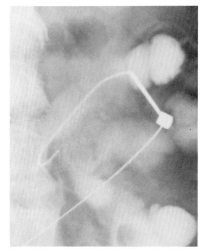

Fig. I.10 A curved guidewire has been introduced into the left renal pelvis through a thin puncturing needle.

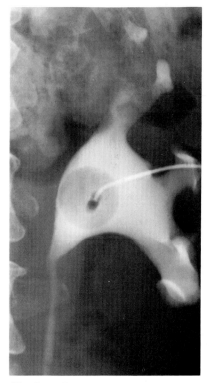

Fig. I.11 Long-standing percutaneous nephrostomy, using a Foley balloon catheter.

DYNAMIC UPPER TRACT STUDIES

Because chronic obstruction is a low pressure state, simple measurement of renal pelvis pressure will not solve any questions about it. Measuring pressure during perfusion of the upper urinary tract at a known flow rate has therefore been developed for patients with doubtful obstruction (Whitaker, 1973). The technique is essentially that of a complex antegrade pyelogram (Fig. I.12), and considered further in Division 2 section D.

E. RETROGRADE URETEROGRAM/PYELOGRAM

As IVUs have improved, the need for retrograde studies has decreased sharply. It has been said that the IVU quality of a radiology department can be judged by the number of retrogrades that have to be done. It is therefore especially important that the few retrogrades now required are performed well.

The indication for a retrograde study is simply inadequate information from the IVU. With ureteric diversion the study may not be possible. This is only one instance where the antegrade pyelogram can usefully bypass the need for retrogrades. A severe IVU contrast medium reaction is sometimes advanced as indication for a retrograde when follow-up examinations are needed. This is a debatable topic—the incidental general anaesthetic is perhaps the only decisive difference (see section A p. 16).

The technique is now best performed under fluoroscopy. This is because:

1. Contrast medium injection can be monitored, and the hazard of over-filling and dissection largely avoided.

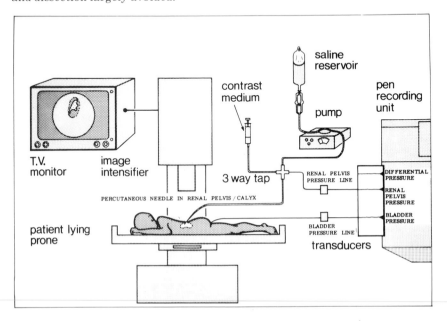

Fig. I.12 Dynamic antegrade pyelogram.

2. Precisely aimed, tailored radiographs can be taken to solve the patient's particular problem.

These reasons are so compelling that there is now very little place for the operating theatre retrograde, where a single blind film is taken with inadequate X-ray apparatus. The chances that the patient will leave the theatre with the correct diagnosis are not good.

Dissection. A voluminous literature documents the various sorts of 'backflow' that may be produced by overfilling of the pelvi-caliceal system. Pyelo-sinous, pyelo-tubular, pyelo-venous and pyelo-lymphatic dissection may occur, all illustrated in Fig. I.13. They are now of little importance.

Technique

Two alternatives exist:

1. Ureterogram. A bulb catheter is gently wedged in the lower ureter. Contrast medium is injected so that a continuous contrast column comes to opacify the whole upper urinary tract on that side. The method does away with many interpretative difficulties, arising from incomplete filling of the system, and there is little doubt that it is the best technique. However, the catheter has to be held in position during the procedure, so that surgeon and radiologist, working together on a fluoroscopy table, are needed at the same time for a joint effort.

2. Pyelogram. A catheter is introduced into the upper urinary tract, and films taken on subsequent contrast injection. The catheter placement can be done in theatre, and the patient returned to the X-ray department for spot films. These logistic attractions are balanced by various drawbacks: the catheter may not stay where it ought to in the interval, and contrast filling of the required structures is uncertain. Depending on local circumstances, it may have to be the method used, and is still better than the blind theatre retrograde.

If interpretative difficulties arise, such as air bubbles or incomplete filling, it is worth remembering the help offered by gravity, particularly prone views for suspected tumours (see Division 1 section D).

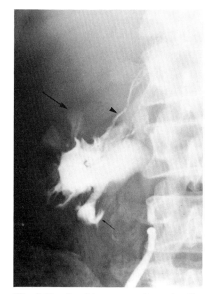

Fig. I.13 On this retrograde study all forms of dissection are shown. The irregular calix in the lower renal pelvis points to a tear into the renal sinus (small arrow). In the upper renal pole two renal lobes are delicately outlined (large arrow) by backflow into the nephron (pyelo-tubular). The renal vein is filling with contrast medium shed into the renal parenchyma, and the delicate strands near it are lymphatics (arrowhead).

F. RENAL ARTERIOGRAM AND VENOGRAM

ARTERIOGRAPHY

The renal arteriogram adds up to a beautiful study of normal and abnormal kidney structure. Renal architecture can be seen in exquisite detail, including lobar arrays (Fig. I.14). This very attractiveness can beguile clinicians and radiologists into overemphasizing the place of angiography in diagnosis. 'Well, let's do an angiogram' is often used as a final cry of appeal when there seems to be a diagnostic cul-de-sac. The indication for the study in any particular patient should always be soundly defensible, particularly in hypertension (see Part III).

Technique

This will vary between schools and differing indications. There is probably general agreement that the investigation should be done briskly with catheters which are not overlarge. The risk of femoral artery thromboembolism is particularly related to catheter size (Jacobsson & Schlossman, 1969). See Part III for the importance of magnification arteriograms.

Fig. I.14a & b Note the lobar structure of the kidney on these two frames from an arteriogram. The septa of Bertin (arrowheads) are clearly seen, but note that the arcuate arteries (small arrow) run between the cortex and medulla of each lobe, not in the middle of the septa.

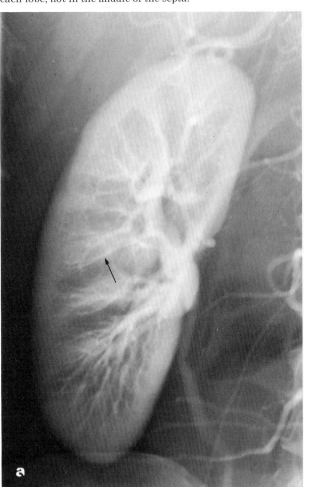

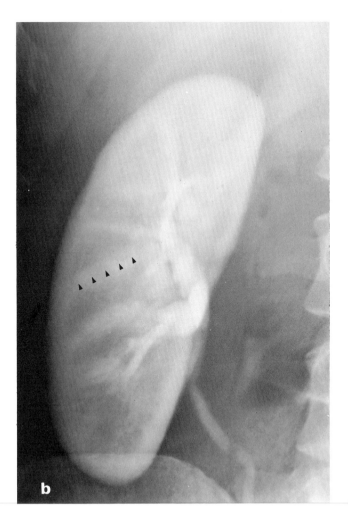

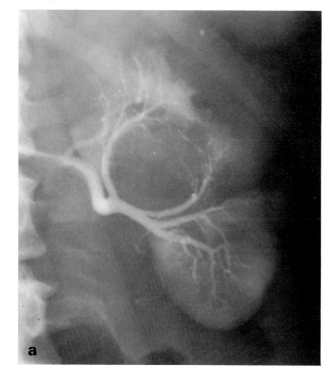

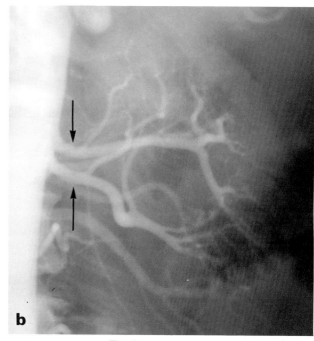

Fig. I.15a Selective left renal arteriogram with a raggedly avascular upper pole, and smooth central avascular lesion.

Fig. I.15b The aortogram makes clear that this is a cyst in a kidney supplied by two main renal arteries (arrows).

Aortogram vs immediate selective arteriogram

The tyro is well advised to begin with an aortogram. This general survey will show him where exactly the renal arteries arise, how many there are on each side, and the likely nature of the renal lesion he is investigating. These are valuable basic diagnostic building blocks, especially if selective catheterization manoeuvres should prove difficult or impossible.

The expert will reply that there is really no difficulty in selective catheterization of the renal arteries. He will wish to do this first in order to obtain the clearest possible pictures, before an excretion pyelogram begins to overshadow some parts. Even he, however, might on occasion be foxed by the multiple renal vessel problem. Where the vascular territory of only one of several arteries to a kidney is outlined by selective catheterization, bizarre pictures result (Fig. I.15). Although this is a very well recognized subject, diagnostic mistakes are still frequently made. They can be avoided with the help of an aortogram.

The multiple renal artery problem is of special importance when healthy kidney donors have arteriograms to test their suitability. We have found a 35% prevalence of multiple renal arteries in such 'patients', some missed at angiography (Sherwood *et al,* 1978). The important mistakes occurred because of inadequate interpretation of the aortogram, not because of failure to find tiny additional vessels at selective angiography.

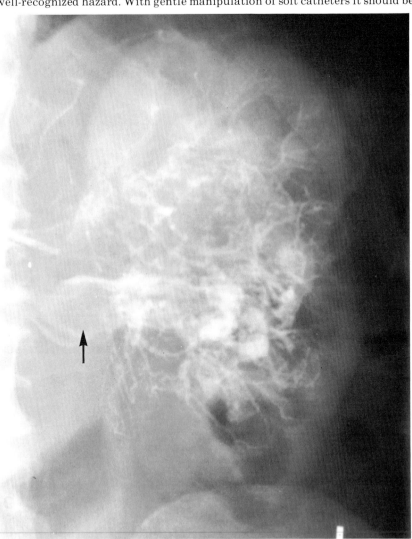

Selective arteriography

The selective renal arteriogram gives a splendidly detailed demonstration of the renal vasculature. It is generally right to press on with this technique after the aortogram for complete diagnosis of kidney lesions, unless the proximal renal arteries are diseased, or very small. If a carcinoma has already been shown on the aortogram, a very large, perhaps nephrotoxic bolus of contrast medium can be injected. This is not only to show the carcinoma at its most beautiful/ugly, but also to see the renal vein (Fig. I.16).

Complications. Dissection of the renal artery during selective manoeuvres is a well-recognized hazard. With gentle manipulation of soft catheters it should be

Fig. I.16 Selective left renal arteriogram in a patient with a renal carcinoma. Note a large filling defect in the renal vein—tumour extension (arrow).

very uncommon indeed. It is essential to recognize the disaster once it has occurred (Fig. I.17). An immediate aortogram can be done to assess the blood flow impairment, which may call for urgent surgical disobliteration.

Careful test injections are important for guarding against improper positioning of the catheter tip, for instance in the mouth of a capsular vessel (Fig. I.18).

Contrast medium. The conventional teaching that the more concentrated contrast media are unsuitable appears out of date (Talner & Saltzstein, 1975). If indicated for obtaining good radiographs in any individual patient, it is worth considering their use. Renal overdosage should of course be avoided, except for a carcinoma. A case is on record of an apparently innocuous injection of a massive contrast dose into one renal segment (Pepper *et al*, 1974).

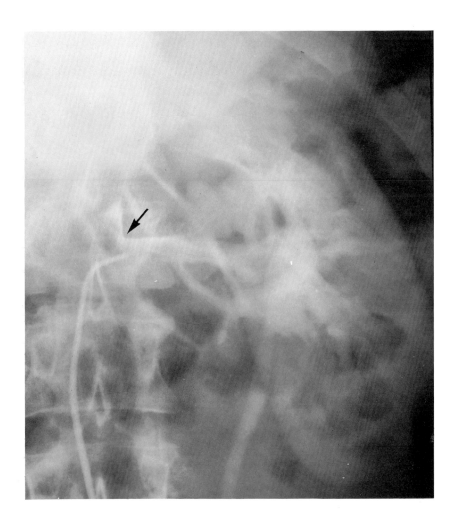

Fig. I.17 At the end of this selective left renal arteriogram, a pencil-sharp sliver of contrast medium remains behind—the sign of a dissection (arrow). The left renal artery was pulseless at exploration.

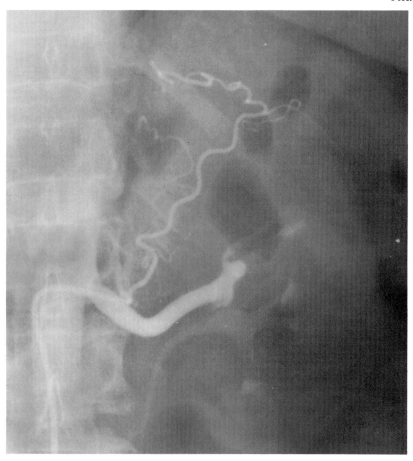

Fig. I.18 The selective catheter tip has hitched in the origin of a capsular artery.

Adrenalin (epinephrine). Normal renal vessels respond to a small intra-arterial adrenalin injection by sharp, transient vasoconstriction—tumour vessels do not. The hope that hidden carcinoma vessels could thus be lit up in a critical way during the examination has been largely dashed (see Division 1 section H). If the method is used at all, small enough amounts must be given, of the order of 5 μg., to prevent shut-down of the arteries supplying the lesion.

Embolization. This technique is advancing by leaps and bounds, and anything now written will be out of date by publication. It is briefly considered in the section on renal carcinoma (Division 1 section H).

VENOGRAPHY

Demonstrating tumour extension in the renal vein is the most common indication. Preferably this follows on an arteriogram where the renal vein has failed to

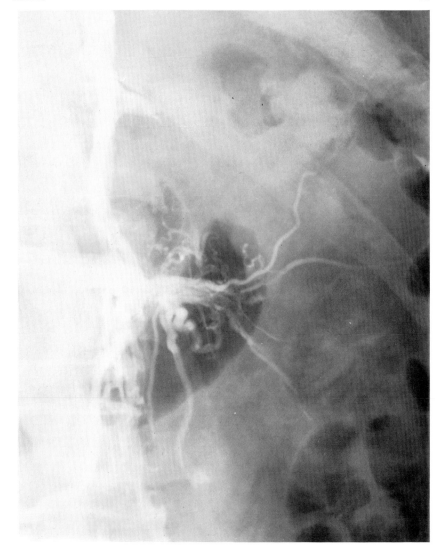

Fig. I.19 Selective left renal venogram —there is clot in the main renal vein and hemiazygous collaterals are shown.

opacify (see above). The patient with unilateral or bilateral kidney failure suspected of renal vein thrombosis also needs a venogram to confirm or refute the diagnosis (Fig. I.19). Selective catheterization is usually required for such studies, but care must be taken not to dislodge tumour or thrombus. To this end, studying the inferior vena cava is advisable first, either by fluoroscopy or by formal serial films. This is of especial importance when tumour has already invaded the cava, possibly extending into the right atrium.

Multiple renal veins are at least as frequent as multiple arteries. However, there are often intra-renal communications between the systems, so that one selective catheter injection may outline the whole venous tree (Fig. I.20). More complex anomalies of renal venous drainage are not uncommon (Fig. I.21).

The best renal venograms are obtained when renal blood flow is temporarily arrested (Fig. I.22). This can be done most conveniently by injecting a small amount of adrenalin by selective catheter into the renal artery (see above), followed immediately by the venogram.

Fig. I.21 *(right)* On this late frame from a normal left renal arteriogram, the main renal vein passes downwards, and splits into two before joining the iliac venous tree.

Fig. I.20 *(below left)* The selective catheter enters one of two main right renal veins, but the whole tree is filled by peripheral communications.

Fig. I.22 *(below right)* Right renal venogram—depressed renal blood flow because of parenchymal disease makes for good venous demonstration.

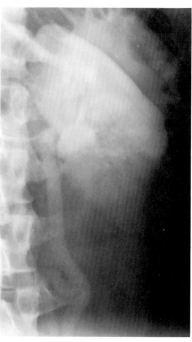

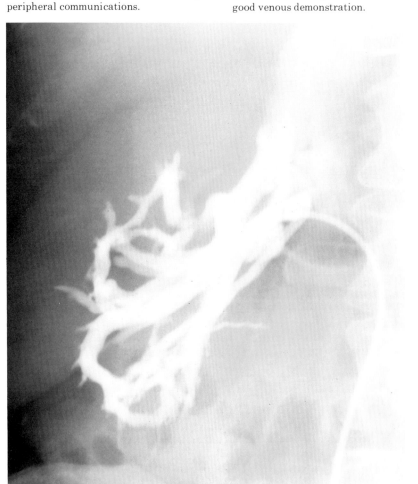

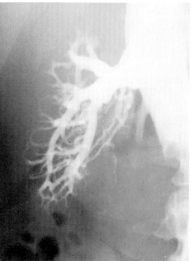

It is worth remembering that veins are thin-walled, feeble structures. They can be readily perforated, or deformed by the Venturi effect during injection (Fig. I.23).

G. ULTRASOUND

The placing and length of this section has nothing to do with the importance of the subject in uroradiology—a long introductory chapter would then have been needed. Ultrasound has proved enormously useful in investigation of the kidney. This was the proving ground where the method first established its clinical value outside obstetrics. The indications for arteriography in the renal mass problem were cut down sharply as an immediate outcome (see Division 1 section H). It is a very great attraction that this is a non-invasive technique in the true sense: safe and painless. It is also quite cheap.

Fig. I.23a Iliac venogram by pressure injection—note how the walls of the vein are sucked in toward the catheter tip.
Fig. I.23b At the end of injection the normal structure of the vein is restored.

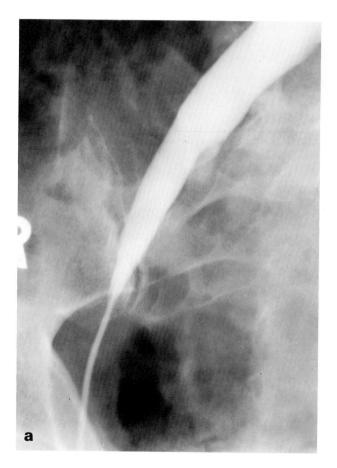

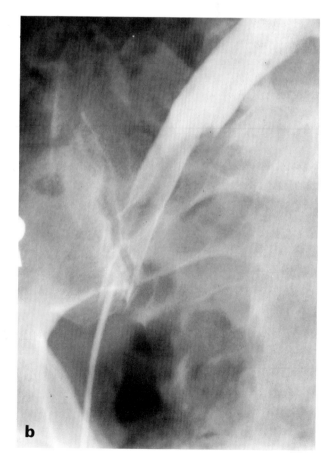

Indications

Kidney

Ultrasound is still developing new skills, for instance in studying structural detail like the renal pyramids (Cook *et al*, 1977).

Kidney length can be determined accurately. Even more important, renal parenchyma can be distinguished from urine collecting spaces by the echoes

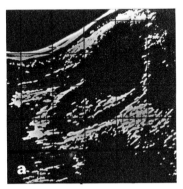

Fig. I.24a & b Renal cyst—the prone longitudinal ultrasound scan shows a large echo-free space at the upper renal pole, confirmed by cyst puncture.

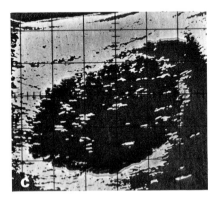

Fig. I.24c By contrast this prone longitudinal ultrasound scan shows a kidney diffusely enlarged with multiple abnormal echo patterns—the picture of an infiltrating carcinoma.

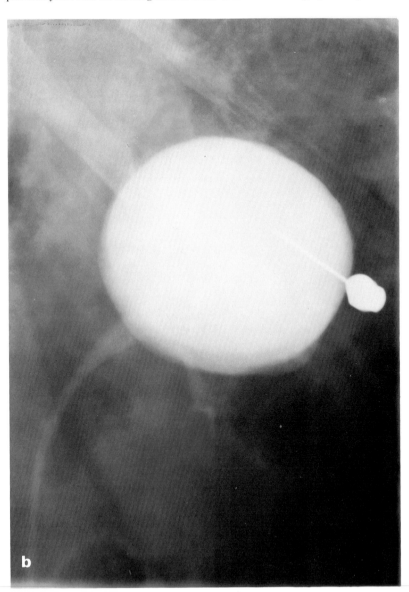

arising in the renal sinus. In this way a composite picture of *parenchymal mass* can be built up by multiple cross-sections of the kidney, though ideally this needs computer help. This method could lead to safe, radiation-free monitoring of the growing kidney of the child, with important clinical messages (see 'Renal Size' at start of Division 1).

Space-occupying lesions can be characterized as to their acoustic nature, distinguishing simple cysts from complex lesions like carcinomas (Fig. 1.24). Polycystic disease shows a unique ultrasound pattern of distorted parenchymal structure, with multiple echoes from the innumerable cysts (see Division 1 section H).

Obstruction can be inferred from finding a dilated pelvi-caliceal system (Sanders & Conrad, 1977). There are hazards to this inference (see Division 2 section D), but in the appropriate clinical setting the ultrasound pointer to dilatation/possible obstruction can be a vital first clue. Even more intriguing is the important question whether a normal ultrasound scan in renal failure can be taken to exclude obstruction. The evidence so far supports the idea that it can (Ellenbogen *et al*, 1978).

The diagnosis of an *absent kidney* generally needs cystoscopic proof, but an ultrasound scan showing an empty loin on one side is valuable preliminary support. More valuable, it may be noted, than angiography (see Division 1A).

Retroperitoneum

Suspected pararenal lesions, e.g. adrenal tumours, are well worth ultrasound investigation. In skilled hands the method rivals computed tomography in this territory (but note Dr Davidson's comments in Part II section B on the primacy of CT).

Bladder

Residual urine after voiding can be estimated. Without a computer this cannot easily be translated into volume measurements, but the pictorial estimate, as in the IVU, is usually quite sufficient for clinical management. The method is particularly valuable for serial, radiation-free monitoring of the badly emptying bladder, for instance in children with a neuropathic bladder.

Accurate staging of *bladder tumours* as to depth of invasion is difficult by the clinico-pathological approach of bimanual examination and biopsy. It is a vital matter for correct management, and ultrasound would seem to offer splendid opportunities for help here. In the very best, skilled hands this is indeed so (Barnett & Morley, 1976). This field is one of the few ultrasound indications in the urinary tract where grey-scale techniques are absolutely essential. It is not an easy ultrasound territory, and the experience of the operator counts for much. For these reasons computed tomography will probably come to take over this task.

Prostate

Per rectum scanning of the prostate perhaps sounds rather unattractive, but has apparently given good results, judging by innovative Japanese reports (Watanabe *et al,* 1974). It is said that reliable diagnoses on the nature of prostatic disease can be made in this way.

Testis

Enlarged testes have inevitably been scanned. Whether the method can usefully contribute in a field where the clinician and pathologist are already established princes must be in doubt.

Technique points on the kidney

Machine settings are generally chosen so as to make the renal parenchyma transonic (Fig. I.25). Renal outlines can then be well seen, and the internal border of kidney parenchyma is delineated by the renal sinus echoes. It looks as if these normally arise from collagen or fat in pelvi-caliceal walls rather than parenchyma/urine interfaces.

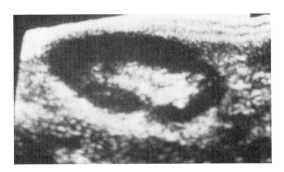

Fig. I.25 Normal kidney ultrasound scan, with densely packed renal sinus echoes, and transonic parenchyma.

The prone position is usually the most helpful for renal scans, but there are exceptions. The right kidney can often be well seen by the ultrasound beam entering through the hepatic window, i.e. with the patient in the supine position. This posture is also preferable for checking on a suspected horseshoe kidney.

Renal masses

1. Lesions deforming the renal outline are usually much more straightforward ultrasound problems than those which are deeply placed within the kidney. Distinguishing a small solid central lesion among renal sinus echoes can be very difficult or impossible. This limitation should be recognized, so that an abnormal IVU suggesting such a lesion is not dismissed because of unremarkable ultrasound findings.

2. It is always worth exploring a supposed cyst with altered machine settings, attempting to raise echoes within it by high gain. Obvious cystic structures like the bladder can be helpful for gauging the appropriate machine settings. The diagnosis of a cyst always depends on more than its echo-free nature: the sharp distal interface with normal parenchyma, and ready sound transmission through the fluid.

3. Cysts can of course be punctured under ultrasound guidance, most easily with the help of a hollow transducer through which a needle can be passed.

4. Grey-scale technique has made very little difference to the accuracy of ultrasound diagnosis in renal masses, compared to bistable (black-white) images. There need be no fear that the patient is having a poor deal if grey-scale is not available in this field.

5. Individual scanning techniques vary very widely. In the effort to build up a composite three-dimensional picture from multiple two-dimensional sections, the operator doing the scan has very considerable advantages over any later observer shown a few representative cuts. At present renal ultrasound scanning is best done personally by the radiologist who has to shoulder the responsibility for advice on the outcome. Does any further diagnostic step need to be taken, like cyst puncture or arteriography, or is everything so clear cut in the clinical context that a final management decision can be made with confidence (see Division I section H)? This will require careful review of all the findings, including the IVU, together with clinico-radiological consultation. I doubt whether the radiologist who is not directly involved in ultrasound is well placed to play his full part here. This dependence on the operator in ultrasound could change as more standard section techniques are developed on the computed tomography model.

Summary comment

Ultrasound has impressed many welcome changes on uroradiology over a quite short time span (*British Medical Journal,* 1976). This has been a delightful take-over, not following the usual depressing path of investigative innovation, which tends to run 'this important method, whilst not replacing existing tests, adds vital new information'. Ultrasound can now tackle subtle and difficult problems, for instance differentiating multicystic disease from hydronephrosis in the non-excreting kidney of the infant.

Leopold and Talner (1977), in *Urological Ultrasonography,* provide valuable further reading on this subject.

H. LYMPHOGRAM

Death knells were rung for this technique soon after the arrival of ultrasound, and then of computed tomography. It now looks as if lymphography will be needed for quite some time yet. Whilst the staging of lymphomas is the most pressing reason, uroradiology accounts for the next best indication: *testicular tumours*. Lymphograms are important in these fields because they have a decisive impact on clinical management.

The enthusiast will say the same about the importance of detecting metastases in *carcinoma* of the bladder, the kidney, or the prostate. The realist will have some reservations about the value of a hunt-the-deposits strategy in these diseases. There is no doubt that, for instance, carcinoma of the kidney is frequently already in the lymph node metastasis stage when diagnosed (Macdonald & Paxton, 1976). The real doubt concerns the sensitivity of detecting carcinoma deposits on the lymphogram, and what critical clinical management changes should sensibly be based on such evidence. The question of *accuracy* has been investigated particularly in carcinoma of the prostate by Spellman *et al.* (1977) and by our own group. In these studies node-by-node comparisons were made between the lymphogram and the histologist's examination (biopsy). Such detailed assessments are essential, on the lines 'is this node in the left external iliac group normal?'. Blanket statements like 'lymph nodes involved' will not do. There is good agreement in these studies that sensitivity (true positive ratio) is poor. Correspondingly the false negative ratio is so high that a normal lymphogram means very little. However, the specificity (true negative ratio) is less depressing, with a correspondingly low false positive ratio. (For a good primer on sensitivity and specificity, essential terms for the investigative radiologist, see McNeil *et al*, 1975). An abnormal lymphogram is therefore more likely to be modestly reliable in the carcinoma deposit question.

Complications and contraindications

Blue dye, local anaesthetic and contrast media reactions may occur—they are rare. A few patients experience a transient fever within 24 hours of the examination, which is generally of no moment. The central worry concerns the oil emboli inevitably sent to the lungs. All patients suffer temporary impairment of lung function after lymphography (White *et al*, 1973). This is of no importance to fit individuals, but can be lethal for those with already existing respiratory impairment. Any patient who is too breathless to climb a flight of stairs to the radiology department, to lie flat, or to blow out a match at arm's length, needs full lung function studies and joint consultation before a lymphogram is ever begun. Lymphograms can kill—a fact impossible to overemphasize.

Technique points

1. Radiographic monitoring of the progress of the examination is very helpful. Even in the best hands small veins can sometimes be mistaken for lymphatics at dissection, and early radiographs of the lower leg will check on this (Fig. I.26). The safety of the examination also depends on not giving too much contrast medium (oil emboli), and it is better to look at how much is needed than to work by rule-of-thumb dosage. Avoid particularly dosages based on body weight: the

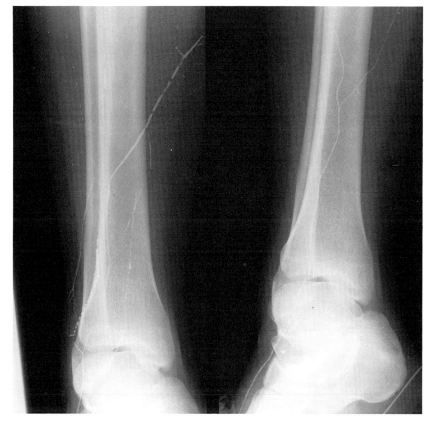

Fig. I.26 Two ankles, illustrating proper and improper lymphatic cannulation. The venous injection is characterized by discontinuous columns of contrast medium—blobs of oil not mixing with a watery stream.

fat patient does not have larger lymph spaces. Once the common iliac chains are well filled during the injection, enough will usually have been given to see the para-aortic nodes the next day. The individual with already irradiated nodes will need less than the normal.

2. *Follow-up films* 3–4 weeks after the examination can help to resolve questionable filling defects. Are these growing (deposits), shrinking after irradiation (deposits), or static (possible fat replacement or scars)?

3. *Oblique films* are always essential: most deposits are spherical, most unimportant filling defects asymmetric.

I. VASOGRAM AND CAVERNOGRAM

VASOGRAM (see Division 5A)

The usual method involves small bilateral skin incisions, and injection of the vasa under direct vision. This can be done under local or general anaesthesia. A few millilitres of water-soluble (urographic) contrast medium are used, till the vasa, vesicles and ejaculatory ducts are filled.

The alternative method of retrograde injection of the ejaculatory ducts at urethroscopy sounds attractive enough, and is mentioned as a matter of form in many textbooks. It must be very difficult in practice, and I have not found it easy to pin down anyone actually using this approach.

CAVERNOGRAM (see Division 5 section B)

Very simple technically, rather painful, and of limited clinical usefulness. A small needle (say 21 gauge butterfly) is thrust into one side of the shaft of the penis dorso-laterally. Local anaesthesia of the skin means two stabs instead of one, and is not recommended. Water-soluble (urographic) contrast medium is injected under fluoroscopy till both corpora cavernosa and the draining veins are filled. An initial tourniquet round the base of the penis is a helpful manoeuvre toward this. Saline is used to flush out the contrast medium at the end of this short examination as in any venogram. A painful erection is usual by this stage—the patient can be told that it should subside. However, *priapism* with impotence has been reported as a complication. Cavernography is therefore not to be undertaken lightly.

J. TOOLS FOR PAEDIATRIC WORK

Children are sometimes seen as rather a nuisance in radiology departments—noisy, difficult, time-consuming patients. This is particularly so in large departments where children are occasional passengers in a traffic scheme designed for adults. There is then little chance of staff gaining confidence and expertise in paediatric work. Calm, competent radiographers and radiologists grow uneasy when a child is announced, and premonitions of trouble and likely failure hang gloomily in the air. This section is to help such departments doing paediatric IVUs and MCUs—it will not teach the expert anything.

A treacly 'knack with little ones' can be overdone. Children in radiology departments have special needs in matters like organization, instruments and radiography. They have much the same needs as adults for tact and understanding during frightening experiences.

Organization

Particular care is needed in appointment procedures in order to avoid overbooking and long waiting periods, making for fractious, overwrought, hungry patients. Adults and children will benefit from a special waiting area with toys and books.

Instruments and technique points

The right tools are essential. Butterfly needles have made IVUs much easier, and there is no point in even starting an MCU if small enough catheters have not been made ready.

IVU

Dehydration is undesirable in young children, and contraindicated in infants. Contrast medium doses should be chosen with particular care on a body weight basis (see section A p. 2).

Immobilization of a peripheral part (hands or feet) is much easier than a more central one. A child can be allowed to thrash around a hand held still, and good veins can usually be found there. Immobilization of the elbow, the traditional adult venepuncture site, is considerably more difficult.

Follow-up IVUs. The second examination should almost always be much shorter than the first (see section A p. 8). A one or two film IVU is generally entirely adequate for following children with reflux problems. If an MCU is also needed, it can be done immediately before the IVU in one appointment.

MCU

A good light is essential for catheterizing girls. The 'heels together, let your knees flop apart' position is generally best here. It is helpful to have support for head and shoulders so that the child is not tempted to wriggle upwards.

A small jug or potty is needed for voiding, rather than the usual adult devices.

Radiography

High output apparatus for short exposures is particularly important. Small children may not keep still long enough for tomograms, and pointless attempts at this technique should not be part of a routine ritual. Remember to shield the gonads.

The parents

Practices vary widely between excluding the parent from the examination, often with the best intentions of saving distress, and encouraging parental help. It would be foolish to lay down rules, and indeed the very rigidity of the schools of thought at either extreme is unattractive. I find parents very helpful, and usually ask them to be with me for the examination if they want to. I do this for the sake of the child, the parents, and myself.

The child has a trusted person to see him through a frightening experience. The familiar physical presence of the parent can be put to good use for restraint—the father or mother sits at the head of the X-ray table, grasps both hands for catheterization or just one for venepuncture, holds the potty for voiding etc.

Parents are not made to feel they have abandoned their children at times of stress. They learn something of the blood, sweat and tears of hospital medicine, importantly different from the glossy television image of the biological repair shop where you park your body or child for overhaul and maintenance.

The doctor benefits because the presence of the parent makes clear that the unpleasant things are being done, and seen to be done, not as punishment, but with the consent of the people the child trusts most.

The child

Like any adult, the child needs calm, tactful explanation appropriate to his intelligence and years. 'Don't worry' is a phrase for the gallows. Trust can be built up if the patient senses that possibly unpleasant things are going to be done inevitably, confidently and briskly. This trust is broken at once if the doctor jabs a needle or catheter having just said 'it won't hurt'—he is exposed as an incompetent and, therefore, frightening liar. Parents and staff often need tactful reminders not to go in for this sort of preliminary lying which is badly counter-productive for the successful IVU or MCU.

Speed and success at the first attempt count for much. Fear should not be allowed to build up unnecessarily. Thus for an IVU a hand is first inspected carefully to choose the best vein ('I'm going to have a look at your arm'). Parents and helpers are arranged for the set piece, and the doctor by now has the butterfly needle in his hand but out of sight. A brief optimistic explanation is followed at once by the venepuncture. Loud protest at this moment is of course the healthy, expected reaction.

Sedation. Natural but ill-informed kindness is responsible for the idea that all children need sedation for unpleasant investigations. Doing the examination in a half-cocked, inconclusive way is the real unkindness, rendering the worst possible service to the patient. Drowsy, half-awake children will not void either normally or at all, cannot be talked to, and tend to thrash around for IVU venepuncture and radiographs. There are of course individual instances where sedation is helpful. They are very few.

REFERENCES

ANSELL G. (1976) *Complications in Diagnostic Radiology,* Chapter 1. Blackwell Scientific Publications, Oxford.
BARNETT E. & MORLEY P. (1976) Ultrasound. In *Scientific Foundations of Urology,* Vol. II, Chapter 58, eds G.D.Chisholm & D.I.Williams, William Heinemann Medical Books, London.

BENNESS G.T. (1970) Urographic contrast agents: a comparison of sodium and methylglu-
    camine salts. *Clinical Radiology* **21**, 150–156.

BRITISH MEDICAL JOURNAL (1976) Ultrasound and the kidney. **1**, 1489–1490.

BURNETT L.L., CORREA R.J. & BUSH W.H. (1976) A new method for percutaneous nephros-
    tomy. *Radiology* **120**, 557–561.

COEL M.N., TALNER L.B. & LANG J.H. (1975) Mechanism of radioactive iodine uptake
    depression following intravenous urography. *British Journal of Radiology* **48**,
    146–147.

COOK J.H., ROSENFELD A.T. & TAYLOR K.J.W. (1977) Ultrasonic demonstration of intra-
    renal anatomy. *American Journal of Roentgenology* **129**, 831–835.

DACIE J.E. & FRY I.K. (1972) Comparison of sodium and methylglucamine diatrizoate in
    high dose urography. *British Journal of Radiology* **45**, 385–387.

ELLENBOGEN P.H., SCHEIBLE F.W., TALNER L.B. & LEOPOLD G.R. (1978) Sensitivity of gray
    scale ultrasound in detecting urinary tract obstruction. *American Journal of Roent-
    genology* **130**, 731–733.

HARRIS R.D., MCCULLOUGH D.L. & TALNER L.B. (1976) Percutaneous nephrostomy. *Jour-
    nal of Urology* **115**, 628–631.

JACOBSSON B. & SCHLOSSMAN D. (1969) Thromboembolism of leg following percutaneous
    catheterization of femoral artery for angiography. *Acta Radiologica Diagnosis* **8**,
    109–118.

DE LACEY G.J. & WIGNALL B.K. (1977) Urethrography simplified: the drip infusion tech-
    nique. *British Journal of Radiology* **50**, 138–140.

LALLI A.F. (1975) Urography, shock reaction and repeated urography. *American Journal
    of Roentgenology* **125**, 264–268.

LASSER E.C. *et al.* (1977) Steroids: theoretical and experimental basis for utilization in
    prevention of contrast media reactions. *Radiology* **125**, 1–9.

LEOPOLD G.R. & TALNER L.B. (1977) *Urological Ultrasonography. Diagnostic Radiology*,
    supplement V/I of *Encyclopedia of Urology*. Springer, Berlin.

MACDONALD J.S. & PAXTON R.M. (1976) Lymphography. In *Scientific Foundations of
    Urology*, Vol. II, Chapter 27, eds G.D.Chisholm & D.I.Williams, William Heinemann
    Medical Books, London.

MCNEIL B.J., KEELER E. & ADELSTEIN S.J. (1975) Primer on certain elements of medical
    decision making. *New England Journal of Medicine* **293**, 211–215.

PEPPER H.W., KOROBKIN M. & PALUBINSKAS A.J. (1974) Massive injection of contrast
    medium into a renal artery segment. *Radiology* **112**, 273–274.

SANDERS R.C. & CONRAD M.R. (1977) The ultrasound characteristics of the renal pelvica-
    lyceal echo complex. *Journal of Clinical Ultrasound* **5**, 372–377.

SAXTON H.M. (1969) Urography. *British Journal of Radiology* **42**, 321–346.

SAXTON H.M. & STRICKLAND B. (1972) *Practical Procedures in Diagnostic Radiology*, 2nd
    edn, chapter 5. H.K.Lewis, London.

SHERWOOD T., RUUTU M. & CHISHOLM G.D. (1978) Renal angiography problems in live
    kidney donors. *British Journal of Radiology* **51**, 99–105.

SHERWOOD T. & STEVENSON J.J. (1972) Antegrade pyelography. *British Journal of Radio-
    logy* **45**, 812–820.

SOKOLOFF J. & TALNER L.B. (1973) The heterotopic excretion of sodium iothalamate.
    British Journal of Radiology **46**, 571–577.

SPELLMAN M.C., CASTELLINO R.A., RAY G.R., PISTENMA D.A. & BAGSHAW M.A. (1977) An
    evaluation of lymphography in localized carcinoma of the prostate. *Radiology* **125**,
    637–644.

TALNER L.B., COEL M.N. & LANG J.H. (1973) Salivary secretion of iodine after urography.
    Radiology **106**, 263–268.

TALNER L.B. & SALTZSTEIN, S. (1975) Renal arteriography: the choice of contrast material.
    Investigative Radiology **10**, 91–99.

WATANABE H., IGARI D., TANAHASI Y., HARADA K. & SAITOH M. (1974) Development and application of new equipment for transrectal ultrasonography. *Journal of Clinical Ultrasound* **2**, 91–98.

WEBB J.A.W., FRY I.K., CATTELL W.R., CUMMACK B. & JEWELL S.E. (1978) The effect of osmotic diuresis on urinary iodine concentration using contrast media of differing osmolality. *British Journal of Radiology* **51**, 106–110.

WHITAKER R.H. (1973) Methods of assessing obstruction in dilated ureters. *British Journal of Urology* **45**, 15–22.

WHITE R.J., WEBB J.A.W., TUCKER A.K. & FOSTER K.M. (1973) Pulmonary function after lymphography. *British Medical Journal* **4**, 775–777.

WHITESIDE C.G. & TURNER WARWICK R. (1976) Urodynamic studies: the unstable bladder. *Scientific Foundations of Urology*, Vol. II, Chapter 12, eds D.I.Williams & G.D. Chisholm, William Heinemann Medical Books, London.

A. NUCLEAR MEDICINE

Lee B. Talner

Physicians dealing with urinary tract disease are often uncertain about what information to expect from nuclear-medicine studies on their patients. One common misconception is that nuclear studies are superfluous to or competitive with traditional laboratory and radiological tests, and that little is to be gained by sending the patient for these sometimes mysterious examinations. Paradoxically, much of the apparent mystery surrounding nuclear medicine is explained by the rapid rate of progress in the field; today's renogram or scan method is 'old hat' tomorrow. Equipment improves, computers abound, and radionuclides come and go with predictable regularity. Forward-looking nuclear-medicine departments seem to take great pride in creating their own variations on standard nuclear procedures. Understandably, the referring physician or general radiologist finds it difficult to keep up with the state of the art. It must also be said that nuclear technology and expertise in the evaluation of the urinary tract has reached a level of extreme sophistication in relatively few medical centres. What is routine and easily accomplished in these clinical laboratories may not even be available in general nuclear-medicine divisions elsewhere.

Does all this mean we should ignore a discussion of what is achievable (though perhaps beyond easy reach today) and concentrate only on what is available in the average hospital? Obviously the answer is no. The yield of functional and anatomic information possible from nuclear techniques is so impressive that its actual and potential role in the management of urinary tract disease should not be understated.

The purposes of this section are twofold: (1) to describe briefly nuclear techniques for evaluating the urinary tract, and (2) to point out the clinical situations in which they offer information unique and important to patient management. Radionuclide studies can be divided into those which test function only, those which offer anatomic information only, and those which combine the two. While in specific clinical situations anatomic information is needed to complement uroradiographic examinations, the impact of nuclear medicine is definitely greatest in providing functional information.

Measurements of total renal function

Traditionally, glomerular filtration rate (GFR) has been determined by measuring the clearance of inulin, and effective renal plasma flow (ERPF) has been determined by measurement of PAH clearance. While these methods are

41

accurate, they suffer from the need for constant intravenous infusion, multiple, timed blood and urine collections, and laborious chemical determinations. Endogenous creatinine clearance is easier to measure but is much less accurate than inulin clearance. Using radionuclides, approximations of GFR and ERPF can be obtained which suffice for clinical care and obviate the annoying disadvantages associated with traditional clearance techniques, especially in children (Barratt & Chantler, 1975).

A variety of radionuclides have been used to estimate GFR: ^{51}Cr-inulin, ^{57}Co-vitamin B_{12}, ^{51}Cr-EDTA, ^{169}Yb-DTPA, ^{131}I-diatrizoate, and ^{125}I-iothalamate (Blaufox & Freeman, 1975). The radiopharmaceutical is given by bolus injection and one or more blood samples are taken. Gamma counting of each sample enables one to construct a plasma radioactivity disappearance curve which is subjected to mathematical analysis using a single or double exponential model. Alternatively, a probe or gamma camera over the heart is used to generate the plasma disappearance curve. Technetium-99m-DTPA and ^{125}I-iothalamate are now the most popular agents for measuring GFR clinically.

Iodine-131 ortho-iodohippuric acid, or hippuran, is the radioactive agent of choice to measure ERPF, and values with hippuran are only slightly less than those derived by PAH clearance. Effective renal plasma flow can be derived mathematically from plasma disappearance curves based on blood samples or from surface detectors over the heart. Each nuclear medicine laboratory has its favourite way of obtaining total GFR and ERPF. It is important that each laboratory tests its method against a standard, especially when the technique is simplified by taking fewer blood samples.

Measurements of renal function have been especially helpful when used serially to monitor progress of disease or response to treatment. For example, in renal transplant patients a decline in ERPF occurs early in rejection, one or more days before serum creatinine begins to rise. Serial GFR or ERPF values in children with vesicoureteric reflux or in patients with previous urologic surgery permit early detection of deterioration.

Renography

Radiorenography, or more simply, renography, was the first nuclear technique applied to the diagnosis of unilateral renal disorders. As originally devised more than 20 years ago, radiation detectors (probes) were placed posteriorly over each kidney and a gamma-emitting radionuclide excreted by glomerular filtration and tubular secretion was injected intravenously. Iodine-131 Diodrast was used initially but has since been replaced by ^{131}I-hippuran. From each detector a graph of radioactivity versus time was generated, reflecting the kidney's handling of the radioisotope during a 20–30 minute period. Lack of symmetry between the two curves indicated unilateral renal dysfunction.

There was a great deal of early enthusiasm for renography, especially as a screening test for renal artery stenosis, but the test had problems. Abnormal curves were non-specific. Standards of normal varied from one laboratory to the next, and attempts at quantitation were unreliable and unreproducible. The shape and amplitude of the curves were affected by posture, distance of the kidneys from the probes, the patient's state of hydration, and the type of equipment used. Moreover, there was no agreement about exactly what information was contained in the curves, and there was certainly no agreement how best to extract that information. More recently, probe-type detectors have been replaced by gamma-scintillation cameras, permitting the recording of sequential images (scans) of the kidneys and renogram curves generated either from whole kidney or retrospectively chosen regions of interest.

Renogram curves, whether obtained from older probes or gamma cameras, summate a complex series of functional events, all occurring with overlap in time within the field of view of the detector. After bolus injection of hippuran there is a 30-45 second initial upswing as the relatively intact bolus of radiopharmaceutical passes from the aorta into the renal arteries and through the kidney. Much of this upstroke reflects vascular supply to the kidney and to a much lesser extent to the splanchnic bed, but immediately radionuclide begins to enter tubular fluid by glomerular filtration and tubular secretion. After 30-45 seconds there is an inflection point after which the curve rises less steeply to a peak within 3-5 minutes. In this phase the amount of hippuran being extracted from the blood exceeds that moving towards the bladder. Subsequently the curve declines as the plasma level falls, relatively less hippuran is extracted and the already excreted radionuclide is transported towards the bladder (Fig. IIA.1).

Since the determinants of each portion of the renogram are complex, it is no wonder that abnormal curves are non-specific. This remains a major drawback. For example renal artery stenosis causes a slower upstroke, a lower, flatter and usually later peak, and a delayed decline. But similar renograms are seen with post-obstructive atrophy, partial obstruction, venous obstruction, or severe acute infection. Sequential gamma-camera images of the kidney obtained during hippuran renography aid interpretation of the curve, as obstruction causes enough accumulation of radioactivity to make the dilated collecting system and/or ureter visible (Fig. IIA.1). However, the hippuran images of renal *parenchyma* are too indistinct to be of much clinical value.

Mathematicians have had a field-day analysing the renogram. Many different techniques have been proposed ranging from qualitative inspection to measuring the time from maximum peak to time of disappearance of half the activity, to sophisticated, computer assisted 'deconvolution' analyses. No one method is universally accepted (Farmelant & Burrows, 1974; Britton & Brown, 1971). Several laboratories derive split function data from the renogram. The 1-2 minute portion of the renogram has been used to estimate percentage ERPF going to each kidney (Bueschen *et al*, 1974), and newer computer programs even permit the estimation of absolute ERPF for each kidney. Unfortunately, the techniques require special purpose computers, a method for blood background subtraction, or both (Schlegel & Hamway, 1976; Bueschen *et al*, 1978; Fowler, 1978; Britton & Brown, 1971). So far these drawbacks have prevented wide use of

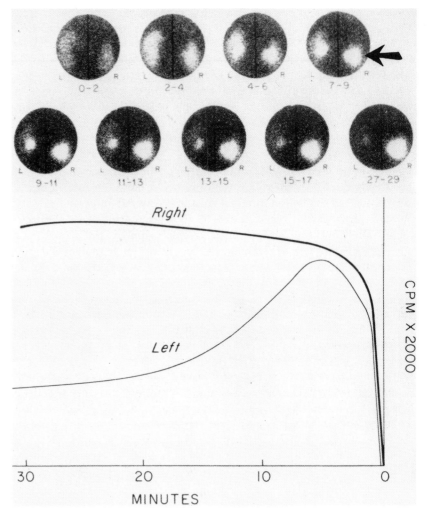

Fig. IIA.1 Iodine-131 hippuran renogram in patient with right pelviureteric junction obstruction. Scintiphotos at two-minute intervals and corresponding curves below. Scintiphotos show prompt appearance of radionuclide in both kidneys, but the right kidney is smaller and accumulates increasing amounts of radioactivity in the dilated renal pelvis (arrow). Left scintiphotos and renogram curve are normal. Upstroke for right kidney is normal, but delayed downstroke suggests outflow obstruction (CPM = counts per minute).

renogram quantitation, but this will probably improve. Quantitation of renal uptake using 99mTc-labelled, cortex-seeking radionuclides is a simpler method of estimating relative split function and will be discussed later.

In hypertensive patients renography is not terribly effective as a screening test. The curves show asymmetry in about 85% of those with subsequently proved renal artery stenosis, but positive studies occur in at least 10% of patients with essential hypertension as well as in those with asymmetric renal parenchymal disease. With the current trend away from early use of expensive screening tests, renography will be used even less frequently as a primary screening technique (McAfee *et al,* 1977).

Renography has been recommended in patients with renal failure to gain information about cause. In general its lack of specificity limits its usefulness. The presence or absence of obstruction is better determined by either urography or ultrasound, with retrograde or antegrade pyelography performed subsequently for localization of the obstructing lesion. When decent urography and ultrasound are at hand, there is no reason to perform renography in patients with renal failure.

Renogram curves can be generated from ^{99m}Tc-DTPA just as well as from hippuran. Since DTPA is excreted solely by glomerular filtration, the corresponding 'glomerulogram' curves are different in shape from the hippuran curves, but renographic asymmetry will still be evident when unilateral renal dysfunction is present. More importantly, modern gamma cameras record renal parenchymal and collecting system images from ^{99m}Tc-DTPA which are far superior to those obtained from ^{131}I-hippuran. For this reason, DTPA is gradually replacing hippuran in many centres.

In summary, renography is sensitive in detecting unilateral renal abnormalities, but is not specific enough to compete with contrast studies for diagnostic accuracy. It is most effective when used serially to follow problems already defined by uroradiologic methods, or when used to quantitate individual function.

Some clinical settings well suited to renography follow: (1) Children with vesicoureteric reflux treated non-operatively can be followed serially with renographic split-function measurements to detect deterioration long before it is reflected in the serum creatinine. (2) Patients with partial obstruction can be followed in a similar fashion. (3) Serial renograms can be used for follow-up evaluation of patients who have had surgery to relieve obstruction. (4) Serial split function measurements may be the best way to follow patients with neuropathic bladder for upper tract deterioration. They certainly complement urography and cystography. (5) The decision to perform nephrectomy or lithotomy in patients with calculus disease causing unilateral renal damage can be based upon function measurements made from the renogram. Urographic studies are not accurate enough. (6) Serial renograms, either with or without simultaneous ERPF measurements, are key evaluations in transplant patients at many centres (Fig. IIA.2). Despite claims to the contrary, the ^{131}I-hippuran renogram is not reliable for distinguishing acute tubular necrosis from rejection in the early transplant period.

Dynamic perfusion studies

Rapid, sequential gamma camera images obtained during the first 20–30 seconds after bolus intravenous injection of ^{99m}Tc-DTPA provide a radionuclide arteriogram or 'dynamic study'. This is a visual display of both renal blood flow and early glomerular filtration of DTPA. Qualitative perfusion information is easily gleaned by 'eye balling' the scintiphotos. Marked discrepancies in renal arterial flow are readily apparent. Severe renal artery stenosis, acute venous obstruction, severe trauma with vascular spasm, and advanced rejection show markedly reduced perfusion. Renal artery thrombosis, embolism, or dissection with

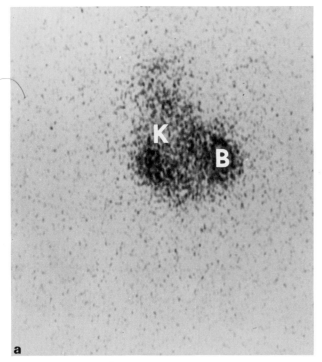

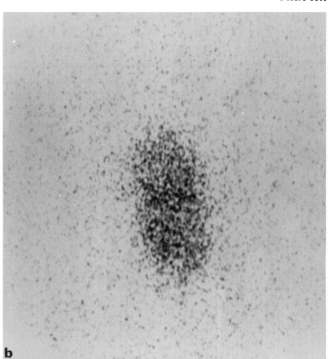

Fig. IIA.2. Serial ^{131}I-hippuran renography in right iliac fossa renal transplant. Each scintiphoto taken 6–8 minutes after injection.

a. Post-transplant day three. Patient doing well. Radioactivity in kidney (K) and bladder (B).

b. Post-transplant day six. Fever and decreased urine output. Radioactivity in kidney only. Diagnosis: Rejection.

c. Post-transplant day eight: Afebrile, urine output improved after steroids increased. Radioactivity in both kidney and bladder indicates improving function.

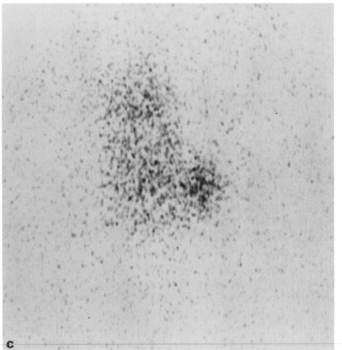

complete arterial obstruction show absent flow to the kidney. Large arterio-venous fistulae are demonstrated and some vascular tumours 'light up' with radioactivity for several seconds. Dynamic studies are perhaps most important in the early post-transplant period to look for arterial occlusions (Fig. IIA.3). Computer analysis is still in its infancy, but appears promising for both relative and absolute quantitation of flow by 'external' detectors alone.

Measurement of residual urine

A simple radionuclide method exists for non-invasively measuring post-micturi-tion bladder volume. Following renography or at the time of radionuclide cystography (see below), count rate is measured over the bladder area, the patient is asked to void, and a repeat count rate is taken over the bladder area. If there is no residual count rate, there is no residual urine. If there are residual counts, residual volume can be calculated once the voided volume is measured. In practice, residual volume is estimated closely enough from urography on post-void films, but if follow-up radionuclide studies are being done in children with lower tract problems, the added information about residual urine is certainly worthwhile at no extra radiation cost (Blaufox & Freeman, 1975).

Renal scintillation scanning

While gamma-camera images can be recorded during ^{131}I-hippuran renography,

Fig. IIA.3 Dynamic ^{99m}Tc-DTPA study in renal transplant patient shown in Fig. IIA.2. Patient clinically well. Scintiphotos taken every two seconds show progression of radioactive bolus through abdominal aorta, iliac, and femoral arteries. Simultaneous appearance of radionuclide in kidney and iliac artery indicates patent anastomosis and satisfactory flow.

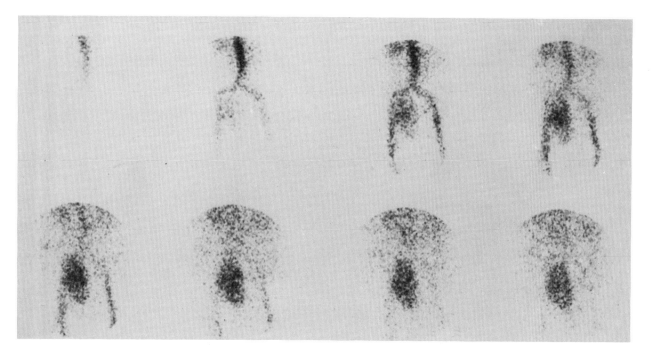

the amount of radioactivity trapped within the renal substance at any instant is relatively small because this agent is excreted rapidly into the collecting system. The scans do not show the renal parenchyma well. On the other hand, renal scintiphotos taken 1–3 minutes after ^{99m}Tc-DTPA injection display the renal parenchyma quite nicely. While the renal images are short-lived compared with those obtained with cortex-seeking radiopharmaceuticals, they are comparable in quality and usually suffice to tell whether a renal mass is present or not. Later scintiphotos are useful for evaluating collecting system size. Because only a single injection of ^{99m}Tc-DTPA need be used to obtain dynamic, renographic and anatomic information, this agent is becoming increasingly popular in many medical centres.

Several gamma-emitting radionuclides have great affinity for proximal or distal renal tubule cells and are excreted only very slowly into the urine. Their intrarenal distribution depends upon blood flow in the presence of functioning tubule cells. High concentrations of radioactivity in the renal cortex with virtually none in the medulla or collecting system make for impressive scintillation scans obtainable for several hours, and show peripheral cortex and columns of Bertin as discrete structures (Fig. IIA.4).

The earlier radionuclides for cortical renal scanning were ^{197}Hg or ^{203}Hg as chlormerodrin or mercuric chloride. Image quality was acceptable and split function could be estimated, but the radiation cost was high. Today a variety of ^{99m}Tc-labelled compounds are used, the most popular being dimercaptosuccinate (DMSA), glucoheptonate, penicillamine, and the newer thiomalic acid. All have the tremendous advantage of short physical half life (6 hours) and excellent photon energy (140 keV) for scintillation imaging. *Both* flow studies and anatomic scans can be obtained easily after bolus intravenous injection of any of these ^{99m}Tc-labelled agents.

Scanning for anatomy

Even with the excellent renal scans obtained regularly with ^{99m}Tc-labelled radionuclides, the display of anatomy cannot match the urographic image. In practice this means there are only a few clinical indications for purely anatomic renal scans. The most obvious is a patient with haematuria who has a history of severe reaction to urographic contrast material. In such a patient plain radiographs and retrograde pyelograms performed without overdistension of the collecting system will often suffice. Grey-scale ultrasound can be done to look for obstruction or large calculi, but the renal scan is probably more sensitive in detecting small, solid renal tumours. Any kidney mass not composed of normal cortical tissue will show as a 'cold' spot on the scan, devoid of radioactivity. Solid renal tumour, renal cyst, abscess, haematoma or infarct are therefore indistinguishable from one another by scanning (see Fig. IIA.7b). In the non-allergic patient with a known renal mass, radionuclide studies are almost never indicated. The path to follow is ultrasound, often succeeded by puncture, angiography, or computed tomography in some combination.

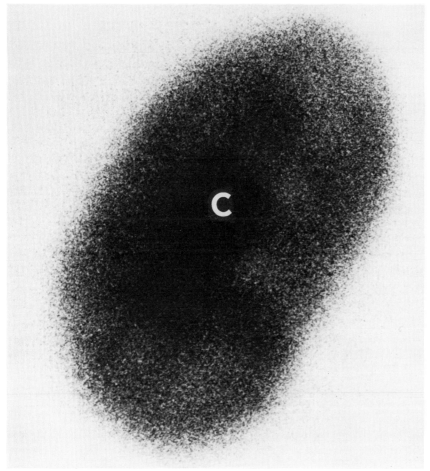

Fig. IIA.4 Renal pseudotumour (prominent column of Bertin). Technetium-99m-DMSA scintiphoto at 45 minutes shows region of increased radioactivity (C) corresponding to central 'mass' seen on urography. Only abundant cortical tissue can create such a 'hot' spot.

On the other hand, some renal 'masses', the so-called pseudotumours, are in fact best evaluated by nuclear imaging when the diagnosis is not clear either from urography or nephrotomography. A pseudotumour is normal parenchyma formed into a lump, bump, or nodule. They occur as prominent supra- or infrahilar lips, dromedary or splenic bumps, roundish columns of Bertin usually in association with partial duplication, and focal hypertrophy adjacent to deep scars. In most cases they are readily diagnosed on good quality nephrotomograms (see Figs IV.1.H2–H5). In all cases, the nephrographic or nephrotomographic density of the pseudotumour is the same as or greater than the neighbouring renal parenchyma. When this is recognized, no further diagnostic studies are indicated. Rarely, a deformity of a nearby calix or a suspicion of nephrographic inhomogeneity requires more information to exclude a true lesion. The renal scan is diagnostic of pseudotumour when the region in question accumulates cortical radiopharmaceutical either normally or in excess, showing as a 'hot' spot (Feldman *et al,* 1978) (Fig. IIA.4).

Renal trauma

Renal scanning is more sensitive than urography in evaluating patients with renal trauma. With a radionuclide dynamic study followed by static scinti-photos, asymmetric kidney perfusion and regions of contusion, laceration, or infarction will be shown if present. Contusions improve over a period of several weeks while infarction remains unchanged on serial scans. From a practical standpoint, the need to know whether there is contusion or laceration is not very great. At most centres dealing with renal trauma, patient management is accomplished on the basis of clinical and urographic findings. If there is uro-graphic non-visualization of a kidney, angiography should be done immediately to look for a major vascular injury. If urographic visualization is only moder-ately impaired, management is generally conservative unless the patient's clinical status deteriorates.

Split function measurements from renal scans

Animal and human studies have shown that the per cent distribution of either ^{99m}Tc-DMSA or penicillamine to each kidney is a reasonably accurate measure of individual kidney glomerular filtration rate, expressed as percentage of total filtration rate. Consequently, renal scanning with either of these two agents allows one to examine function as well as anatomy (Taylor & Talner, 1978). Technology for estimating split function from these renal scans is far less sophisticated than that required to quantitate hippuran renograms. Techne-tium-99m DMSA or penicillamine scans are especially useful in candidates for renal surgery when the major question is whether the kidney is contributing enough function to warrant salvage (Fig IIA.5).

There is one major limitation of both quantitative renal scanning and quantitative renography as predictors of functional potential. In the presence of high grade obstruction or acute renal infection, ischaemia, or renal oedema from other causes, the uptake of radionuclide may be severely impaired because of temporary tubule cell dysfunction. To rely on quantitative data obtained at this stage would underestimate maximum recoverable function. Of course, this limitation applies as well to any clinical or laboratory test of function done in the face of an acute renal insult. After the renal insult has cleared, tubule cell function often improves markedly and is reflected in the quantitative scans (Fig. IIA.6).

Gallium scanning

Gallium-67 citrate is an interesting radionuclide which has been used with variable success in a wide variety of clinical problems. It accumulates unpre-dictably in many tumours, especially lymphoma, and has been used to assess mediastinal involvement in patients with lung cancer. It is also useful in the diagnosis of inflammatory conditions because of avid uptake by neutrophils,

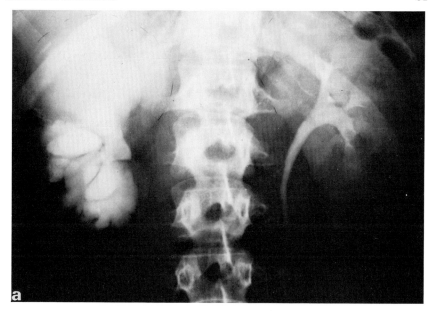

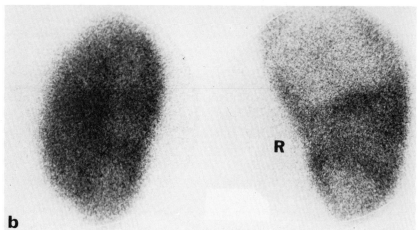

Fig. IIA.5   Right hydronephrosis and obstructive atrophy due to calculus in renal pelvis. Use of quantitative scanning to estimate function.

a   Urography shows severe caliceal dilatation and apparent marked parenchymal thinning. Is right kidney worth saving?

b   Technetium-99m-penicillamine scans at 45 minutes. Very little radionuclide in dilated right upper and lower pole calyces (R). Nevertheless, radioactivity in right kidney measured 44% of combined renal activity indicating that right kidney is worth saving. Post-operatively, split function measurements via nephrostomy tube and bladder catheter confirmed surprisingly high GFR in right kidney.

cellular debris, and bacteria. The exact mechanism of uptake is not known, but gallium has been shown to complex with intracellular metal-binding proteins in the lysosomes of white blood cells.

Faint gallium uptake may be seen in *normal* kidneys up to 72 hours after injection. Strong uptake occurs in kidneys with acute pyelonephritis, renal abscess, and perirenal abscess. Experimental studies have shown that gallium continues to accumulate as long as active inflammation is present.

In the presence of back pain, fever, pyuria, bacteriuria, and cylindruria, renal infection is certainly present and gallium is not indicated. But when clinical signs point to renal infection and urinalysis is negative, or when the

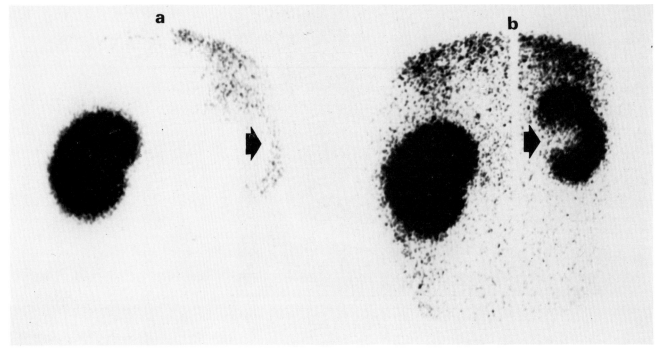

Fig. IIA.6 Limitation of quantitative scanning in predicting functional recovery (dog experiment).
a Technetium-99m penicillamine scan two weeks after ligation of right ureter and just before drainage was established with transureteroureterostomy (TUU). Only 12% of total renal counts are in right kidney (arrow).
b Scan 15 days after TUU shows increase in right renal activity compared to earlier scan. Twenty three percent of renal counts are now in right kidney (arrow). Split inulin clearances showed right kidney contributing 21% of total GFR. Quantitative scans in presence of high-grade obstruction underestimate recoverable function.

source of a patient's infection is an enigma, strong uptake in or around the kidney is virtually diagnostic of abscess. Perirenal abscesses occasionally defy the usual uroradiological attempts at localization, even including inspiration–expiration films and nephrotomography. If nephrotomography, ultrasonography, or computed tomography show a focal renal or perirenal abnormality in a patient with occult infection, diagnostic puncture can be done straight away, or gallium scanning may be interposed to assure that the lesion is inflammatory.

There are several drawbacks to gallium scanning which prevent its assuming a fundamental role in the diagnosis of urinary tract infection. (1) Kidney images are fuzzy and weak compared with standard renal scans with technetium-labelled agents. Even with positive gallium uptake it is a challenge to distinguish renal from perirenal processes, and often the two coexist. (2) While most active renal and perirenal infections are 'hot' within 2–6 hours after injection, occasionally it takes up to 72 hours before inflammatory processes accumulate enough radioactivity to be clearly differentiated from background. (3) Overcalls should not be made when a small amount of gallium is seen symmetrically in the kidneys up to 72 hours after injection. (4) Normal gallium uptake in the colon may be mistaken for uptake in the renal bed. (5) Uptake of gallium is not specific for infection.

Any lesion characterized by an acute inflammatory response will trap gallium (Fig. IIA.7). Positive scans have been described with renal infarction, acute

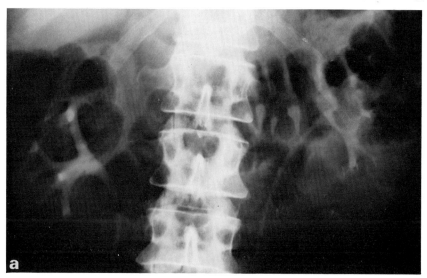

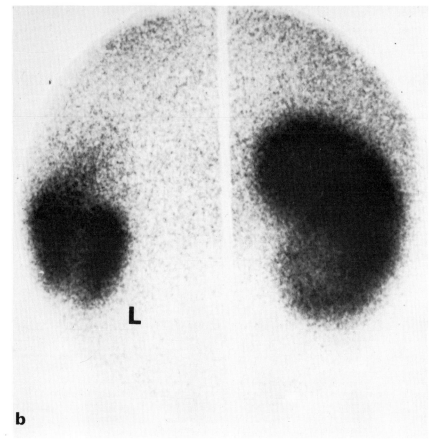

Fig. IIA.7 Renal infarction.
Forty-eight-year-old man with
polycythaemia, fever, severe left loin
pain, normal urinalysis, and high serum
LDH.
a Urography: Poor filling of left upper
pole calices and diminished contrast
material density in calices and ureter.
Upper pole mass was questioned.
b Technetium-99m penicillamine scan:
'Cold' region in left upper pole; also focal
decreased activity in right lower pole.
Picture compatible with left upper pole
tumour, abscess, cyst, haematoma,
infarct, etc., i.e., non-specific.
c *(overpage)* Gallium-67 scan at 24 hours
(left) and seven days *(right)*: Left upper
kidney 'hot' on both scans. Liver (H) and
spine uptake is normal. Picture
compatible with tumour, abscess,
infarction; i.e., non-specific.
d *(overpage)* Left renal arteriogram:
Multiple emboli and occluded arteries
(arrows) to upper pole. Source was aortic
thrombus (arrowheads) adherent to
ulcerated atherosclerotic plaque.

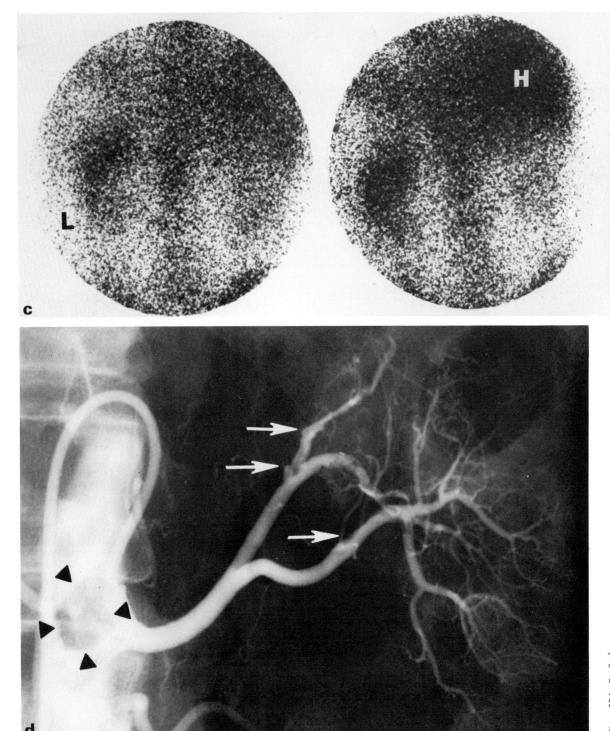

Figs. IIA. 7c & d

interstitial nephritis with negative urine cultures, renal vein thrombosis with infarction, vasculitis, acute tubular necrosis, nephrotic syndrome, and after renal surgery. Approximately one-third of renal neoplasms also pick up gallium. Early focal uptake of gallium in high concentration strongly favours an acute infection over tumour. In spite of its lack of specificity, gallium scanning is sometimes the only examination to detect an occult abnormality in the renal bed.

Radionuclide cystography

Vesicoureteric reflux can be demonstrated by radionuclide cystography (Fig IIA.8). The technique is straightforward, involving catheterization of the bladder, instillation of ^{99m}Tc-pertechnetate, filling the bladder with fluid, and taking sequential scintiphotos during filling, voiding, and after voiding. Reflux to the kidneys is easily demonstrated at the expense of very little radiation, of particular importance in children.

Radionuclide cystography should not be used as the initial evaluation of children suspected of having reflux. Rather, it should be used for follow-up once the presence or absence of reflux is established by X-ray cystography. It can also be used after ureteroneocystostomy to detect persistence or recurrence of reflux.

Because many nuclear medicine laboratories do not see enough children to make the examination routine, and because contamination with radioactivity can be a problem during voiding in toddlers, the technique has not become widespread at this time. However, in several centres seeing large numbers of such children the technique has indeed become routine and is a welcome substitute for the high radiation dose associated with repeated X-ray cysto-urethrograms (Conway *et al*, 1972; Blaufox *et al*, 1971).

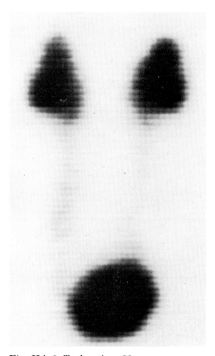

Fig. IIA.8. Technetium-99m pertechnetate cystogram. Severe, bilateral vesico-ureteric reflux. An excellent way to follow children with reflux at expense of little radiation.

Bone scanning

Bone scanning with ^{99m}Tc-labelled phosphate compounds plays an important role in staging patients with carcinoma of the bladder and prostate. As in other malignancies, bone scanning in urinary tract cancer is the most sensitive way to demonstrate metastatic disease to bone. 'Hot' spots on the scan indicate regions of increased osteoblastic activity, thought to be a hyperplastic response of normal bone adjacent to a focus of tumour. Bone scanning should be done first, and if positive, appropriate radiographs should be obtained to determine whether radionuclide uptake is related to an underlying benign condition such as osteoarthritis or healed fracture. Osteolytic and osteoblastic lesions appear similar on scans.

Since the pyrophosphate, polyphosphate, and diphosphonate compounds are excreted by the kidneys, one expects to see the kidneys faintly on bone scans. When ureteric obstruction is present, the bone scan shows retention of

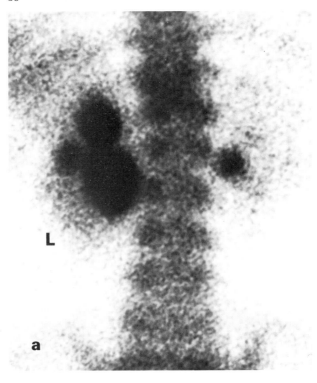

L

a

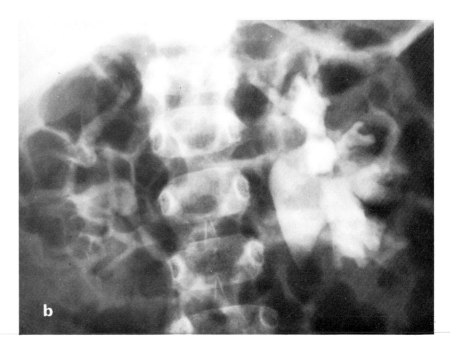

b

Fig. IIA.9a Technetium-99m
pyrophosphate bone scan showing left
hydronephrosis. Scan done to evaluate
T12 L1 interspace for symptoms of
diskitis. Surprise finding was retention of
radionuclide in dilated left renal pelvis
and calices, clinically silent. Small
amount of radioactivity in right renal
pelvis is normal.
b Subsequent intravenous urogram
shows left pelviureteric obstruction
causing mild hydronephrosis.

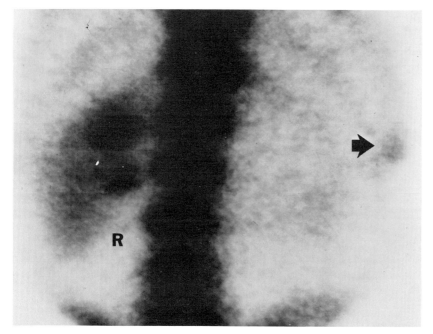

Fig. IIA.10 Technetium-99m pyrophosphate bone scan in patient with left lower rib pain and weight loss. Localized uptake in distal left tenth rib (arrow). Rib X-ray showed osteolytic metastasis. Note absence of radionuclide in left renal area. Intravenous urography showed non-visualization of left kidney, subsequently shown to be due to extensive transitional cell carcinoma. Radionuclide in right upper calices suspicious of localized hydronephrosis, but right kidney was urographically normal.

radionuclide in the dilated collecting system (Fig. IIA.9). In the case of a large renal mass, the involved portion of the kidney will be devoid of radioactivity (Fig. IIA.10).

Patients with a variety of malignancies will not have had intravenous urography prior to bone scans. The incidental detection of a renal abnormality on the bone scan should make one consider urography if the results will influence patient management. In some patients, retention of bone scanning radionuclide in the dependent upper pole calices or renal pelvis is a normal finding easily confused with partial obstruction (Figs IIA.9 and IIA.10).

REFERENCES

BARRATT T.M. & CHANTLER C. (1975) Clinical assessment of renal function. In *Pediatric Nephrology*, eds M.I.Rubin & T.M. Barratt, Williams and Wilkins Company, Baltimore.

BLAUFOX M.D. & FREEMAN L.M. (1975) *Radionuclide Studies of the Genitourinary System*. Grune and Stratton, New York.

BLAUFOX M.D., GRUSKIN A., SANDLER P. *et al.* (1971) Radionuclide scintiphotography for the detection of vesicoureteral reflux in children. *Journal of Pediatrics* **79**, 239–246.

BRITTON K.E. & BROWN N.J.G. (1971) *Clinical Renography*. Lloyd-Luke, London.

BUESCHEN A.J., EVANS B.B. & SCHLEGEL J.U. (1974) Renal scintillation camera studies in children. *Journal of Urology* **111**, 821–824.

BUESCHEN A.J., LLOYD L.K., DUBOVSKY E.V. *et al.* (1978) Radionuclide kidney function evaluation in the management of urolithiasis. *Journal of Urology* **120**, 16–20.

CONWAY J., KING L., BELMAN A. *et al.* (1972) Detection of vesical ureteral reflux with radionuclide cystography. *American Journal of Roentgenology* **115,** 720–727.

FARMELANT M.H. & BURROWS B.A. (1974) The renogram: physiologic basis and current clinical use. *Seminars in Nuclear Medicine* **4,** 61–73.

FELDMAN A.E., POLLACK H.M., PERRI A.J., JR. *et al.* (1978) Renal pseudotumors: an anatomic-radiologic classification. *Journal of Urology* **120,** 133–139.

FOWLER J.E., JR. (1978) The renal perfusion/excretion determination renogram: a new method of individual renal function determination in obstructive renal disease. *Journal of Urology* **119,** 449–452.

MCAFEE J.G., THOMAS F.D., GROSSMAN Z. *et al.* (1977) Diagnosis of angiotensinogenic hypertension: the complementary roles of renal scintigraphy and the saralasin infusion test. *Journal of Nuclear Medicine* **18,** 669–675.

SCHLEGEL J.U. & HAMWAY S.A. (1976) Individual renal plasma flow determination in 2 minutes. *Journal of Urology* **116,** 282–285.

TAYLOR A. & TALNER L.B. (1978) Relative renal accumulation of Tc-99m penicillamine as an index of differential renal function: concise communication. *Journal of Nuclear Medicine* **19,** 178–179.

B. COMPUTED TOMOGRAPHY IN URORADIOLOGY

Alan J. Davidson

Computed tomography (CT) has had a major impact on uroradiological diagnosis. Diagnostic capability has been extended into previously obscure areas. Traditional ways of perceiving anatomy have had to be reorganized. Radiologists already possessing many complementary uroradiological techniques of established accuracy and safety have been forced to define the role and value of this new method with precision and reason.

This chapter is a survey of the use of computed tomography in the diagnosis of diseases of the urinary tract and related structures. The first section discusses a few selected technical considerations. The sections that follow present the applications of CT to the kidney, perirenal and pararenal spaces, retroperitoneum, and the structures within the bony pelvis. Each section includes illustrations of the capability of CT to display accurately normal and pathological anatomy, reviews data on diagnostic accuracy where available, and compares the practicality of computed tomography in relation to other available diagnostic techniques.

Technical considerations

Since the CT image represents differential attenuation of transmitted X-rays by the electron density and mean atomic number of the tissue examined, it has the same physical determinants as do traditional radiographs. This is unlike other newly introduced or developing imaging systems such as ultrasound, heavy particle radiography, or nuclear magnetic resonance, in which different physical or biological characteristics determine the nature of the diagnostic information. The advantage of computed tomography over traditional radiography, then, lies not in a difference in the nature of the information generated, but in the former's greater contrast resolution (0.5%) and its useful display of anatomy in a tomographic cross-sectional representation uninfluenced by overlying high-X-ray-absorbing tissue, such as bone. While future technical advances may enhance these advantages, the fact that both methods rely on identical physical factors for their image will not change. It is not surprising, then, that the principles of interpreting computed tomographic images are the same as those used for radiographs, namely, analysis of organ contours, inherent tissue density, and alterations in tissue density produced by exogenous contrast material.

Contiguous structures in the area of uroradiological interest often have similar attenuation values. Therefore, computed tomography usually requires intravenous contrast material to distinguish normal from abnormal renal tissue and to identify the kidney collecting structures, ureters, or bladder. Usually, this is administered as an infusion of 10–15 grams of iodine over a 10–15-minute period. It is possible that images generated by fast scanners (scanning time under 5 seconds) immediately after a bolus injection of contrast material might yield information regarding renal perfusion or extravascular distribution of contrast material not obtained with slow infusion and delayed scans. This has not been fully explored, however. In the examination of the kidney for masses, both pre-contrast and post-contrast scans are necessary (Kirkpatrick *et al*, 1978). In retroperitoneal and pelvic examinations, on the other hand, contrast material is given prior to the examination to mark the ureters and bladder. In these examinations, only a small amount of iodine (3–6 grams) should be used to avoid high density artefacts and obscuring of detail in the bladder.

Respiratory motion of the kidney and peristaltic movement of intestinal gas are two sources of image degradation in CT uroradiology. These problems are infrequent with fast scanners (less than 5 seconds). With longer scan time, administration of 1 mg of intramuscular glucagon or atropine-like agents and prolonged suspension of respiration are necessary to minimize motion artefacts.

Computed tomography of the kidney (Abrams & McNeil, 1978; Hattery *et al*, 1977; Sagel *et al*, 1977)

Normal anatomy

The renal outline is sharply defined by surrounding perirenal fat (Fig. IIB.1).

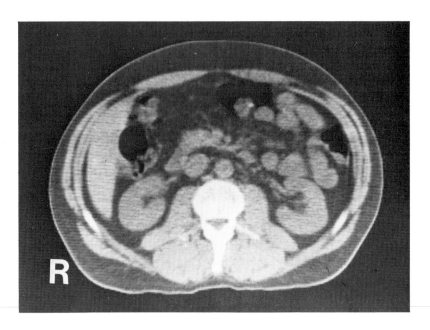

Fig. IIB.1 Normal scan through level of kidneys. Segments of the left renal vein anterior to the left renal artery are seen. The aorta is prevertebral and near midline, and the inferior vena cava lies to its right and slightly anterior. A portion of the diaphragmatic crura is seen anterior to the vertebral body between the aorta and inferior vena cava. Note symmetry of the psoas, quadratus lumborum and paraspinous muscles.

The hilus is situated anteromedially and contains low density fat. The renal artery and vein are identified on sequential sections, and their course to the aorta and inferior vena cava noted. Renal tissue is of homogeneous density, usually equal to filled loops of intestine, muscle, pancreas and spleen, and less than that of liver. Cortex cannot be distinguished from medulla except fortuitously immediately after a bolus of contrast material is injected. Later on, there is uniform enhancement of the parenchyma. The pelvicaliceal system is not well seen except with contrast enhancement.

Solid mass (Fig. IIB.2)

The criteria for the CT diagnosis of renal adenocarcinoma are similar to those of excretory urography. If the mass is border forming, contour deformity results. In the absence of exogenous contrast material, adenocarcinomas are isodense with normal kidney tissue, or nearly so. Some may have a mixture of densities due to areas of necrosis or haemorrhage. The interface between an adenocarcinoma and surrounding normal tissue is irregular and usually not defined precisely. The density of an adenocarcinoma characteristically is enhanced by intravenous contrast material, but to a lesser degree than normal parenchyma. Enhancement is influenced by duration of injection and the amount of iodine injected in relation to scanning time. The vascularity of the tumour itself also affects the degree of contrast enhancement.

Metastases to the kidney, primary neoplasms other than adenocarcinoma, abscesses, and the tumefactive form of xanthogranulomatous pyelonephritis have a CT appearance similar to adenocarcinoma, although the process may be

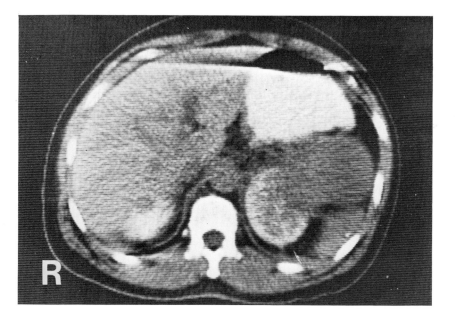

Fig. IIB.2 Adenocarcinoma of left kidney. Post-contrast material enhancement. A large mass distorts the left renal contour. The central low density of the left kidney is probably due to renal vein occlusion and is of uncertain basis (see Fig. IIB.4). A low density metastatic deposit is present in the posterior liver just anterior to the enhanced density of the upper pole of the right kidney.

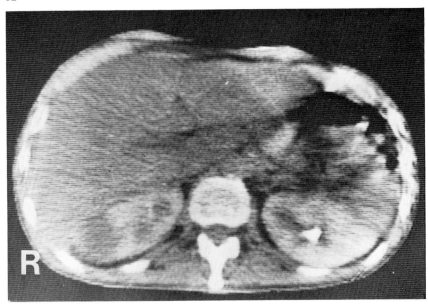

Fig. IIB.3 Metastases to both kidneys from lung primary. Post-contrast material enhancement. There are multiple low density, poorly defined masses in each kidney.

multifocal (Fig. IIB.3). When a hamartoma has large fat deposits, corresponding focal areas of negative attenuation values will allow precise diagnosis. A liquefied abscess may have lower attenuation values than a solid tumour; other features, especially a thick wall, simulate tumour rather than simple cyst.

One useful application of computed tomography is in the determination of whether or not a pelvicaliceal or renal contour deformity is due to lobar dysmorphism, prominent fetal lobulation, excessive peripelvic fat, or a true neoplasm. In all but the latter, the area in question will have attenuation values identical to normal tissue before and after contrast enhancement.

Computed tomography can demonstrate tumour extending outside the renal capsule, involvement of hilar or peri-aortic nodes, extension of tumour into the renal vein or inferior vena cava, or distant metastases (Figs IIB.2 and IIB.4). Information of this nature may permit a more informed surgical approach or, under some clinical circumstances, stay the surgeon's hand.

Simple cyst

The CT image of a simple cyst is that of a rounded mass sharply circumscribed from surrounding renal tissue (Fig. IIB.5). The free wall is 1–2 mm thick. Cysts as small as 1 cm are detectable. Cyst fluid is imaged as a homogeneous density with attenuation values close to those of water, i.e., less than surrounding unenhanced renal tissue. These values do not change following intravenous contrast material.

The CT appearance of a simple cyst may be altered by infection or haemorrhage. The free wall thickens (greater than 2 mm), and the attenuation values of the cyst contents increase. Fluid–pus or fluid–blood levels may be seen. In this

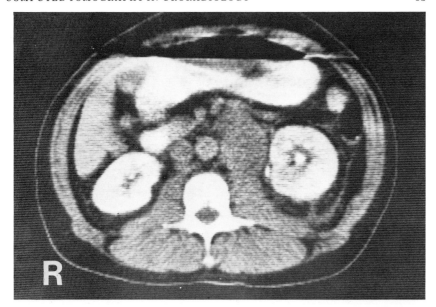

Fig. IIB.4 Adenocarcinoma of left kidney. Same patient illustrated in Fig. IIB.2. Post-contrast material enhancement. A large mass medial to the kidney represents hilar node proven to involve and occlude renal vein.

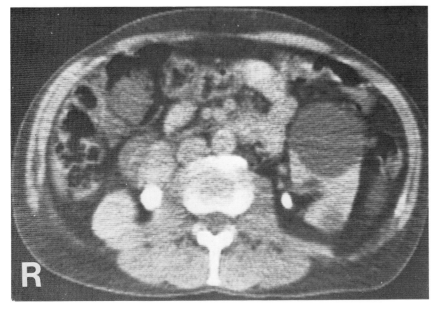

Fig. IIB.5 Simple cysts (two), left kidney. The large anterior cyst demonstrates classic findings. A smaller, posterior cyst is of higher attenuation values because of 'partial volume artefact'.

circumstance, differentiation from tumour or primary abscess is not possible by CT criteria alone.

The CT diagnosis of a small simple cyst presents special problems based on the following considerations. Each point in the CT scan represents an average of the attenuation values in the thickness of the section. When a structure, such as a cyst, occupies the full thickness of the section, the attenuation value for that structure truly represents its contents. If the section is at the margin of the cyst, or through a very small cyst, the numerical value assigned to the cyst will be an average of both the cyst and adjacent non-cyst tissue included in the section. This is known as the 'partial volume artefact', a potential source of error in the CT diagnosis of renal cysts (Fig. II.B5). Partial volume effect varies inversely with the size of the cyst. When a cyst is less than 3 cm in diameter, it is important to evaluate the tomographic slice that is through the centre of the cyst to avoid falsely high attenuation values. In cysts below 1·5 cm in diameter, partial volume artefact is unavoidable in most equipment unless special collimators are used to obtain thinner sections.

Accuracy of CT in diagnosis of renal masses (Abrams & McNeil, 1978).

There are few reports on the sensitivity of CT in the diagnosis of renal adenocarcinoma and none on its overall accuracy in the investigation of renal masses. Those series that have been published suggest a true positive rate of 88–95% for the diagnosis of adenocarcinoma (Hattery *et al*, 1977; Sagel *et al*, 1977). However, these reports have a separate category of 'indeterminate' applied to patients whose renal masses produced CT images that did not fully satisfy strict criteria, or whose examinations were suboptimal because of image degradation by motion, partial volume effect, or the failure to examine the patient both before and after intravenous contrast material. The exclusion of these patients in calculating sensitivity produces a falsely high accuracy rate. As for the diagnosis of renal cyst, no report based on substantial numbers of patients with verification by cyst puncture, ultrasound, or surgery is available. The sensitivity of CT in the diagnosis of simple cyst is probably quite high, but directly related to the size of the cyst.

In the diagnosis of renal masses the overall accuracy of excretory urography, ultrasound, cyst puncture and angiography applied in a logical and carefully chosen sequence approaches 100%. Is there a need, then, for yet another test? The generally negative answer to this question is reinforced by consideration of the high cost and lack of widespread availability of CT. On the other hand, there are some occasions when CT can be gainfully employed, as when ultrasound fails due to patient obesity, the small size of a mass, or interference in ultrasonic imaging detail by overlying ribs. CT does provide information regarding local spread, and regional or distant metastases that might be valuable in formulating therapeutic plans in patients with adenocarcinoma. It does not replace angiography, however, in evaluating arterial supply and venous drainage of a solid mass. When hamartoma is suspected, the CT image may prove diagnostic. Finally, this method can be useful in following patients after nephrectomy for evidence of recurrence of tumour in the renal fossa. In these patients, dilute oral contrast material must be used to distinguish loops of bowel lying in the renal fossa from tumour regrowth.

The failed kidney(s)

Computed tomography has been proposed as a valuable method for determining the cause of failure of one or both kidneys (Sagel *et al*, 1977). CT clearly can demonstrate hydronephrosis of moderate to marked degree with or without the use of exogenous contrast material (Fig. IIB.6). No data are available, however, regarding the limitations of CT in identifying minimal hydronephrosis. Classification of renal failure as acute or chronic can be based on the CT demonstration of renal parenchymal thickness. Polycystic disease has a unique CT presentation of multiple, bilateral, sharply defined low density masses of varying size in enlarged kidneys.

As with renal masses, CT competes directly with excretory urography and ultrasound in assessing the failed kidney(s). These tests maintain their superiority over CT by virtue of their established accuracy, lower cost, wider availability and absent to minimal hazards. In addition, excretory urography provides more detail of caliceal and papillary architecture than does CT. Ultrasound applied to the problem of renal failure is very efficacious and often obviates the need for excretory urography in the diagnosis of hydronephrosis, polycystic kidney disease, or determining renal size.

Limited, unpublished experience with CT in renal-vein thrombosis suggests that unusual alterations may occur in the renal image (Figs IIB.2 and IIB.4). These include variations in parenchymal attenuation values and linear densities radiating into perirenal fat. The possibility that abnormalities of perfusion or nephron function may be detected by temporal variation in CT attenuation values following contrast material injection has not been fully studied.

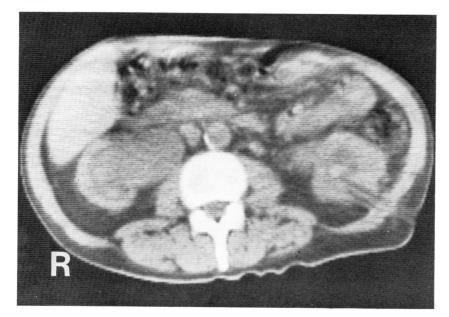

Fig. IIB.6 Right hydronephrosis due to retroperitoneal spread of carcinoma of the bladder. Post-contrast material enhancement. The markedly dilated right renal pelvis and thinned parenchyma are easily seen. A nephrostomy tube can be seen draining the previously obstructed left kidney.

Perirenal, pararenal and retroperitoneal spaces (Abrams & McNeil, 1978; Stephens *et al*, 1977).

Computed tomography comes into its own as a primary diagnostic method in the investigation of the retroperitoneum, perirenal and pararenal spaces. These areas are ideal for CT imaging because they normally contain abundant fat and lack motion artefact producing components. This advantage is reinforced by the notorious insensitivity of traditional radiographic techniques in detecting abnormalities in these regions. Likewise, ultrasound examination of these spaces often is hampered by the sound-reflective properties of fat, or acoustical shadows caused by ribs, spine, or bowel gas.

Normal anatomy

The muscles, fat planes and fascia that are within the retroperitoneum or form its borders are remarkably symmetrical (Fig. IIB.1). Asymmetry of these structures often signifies tumour. This applies particularly to the psoas, iliacus, iliopsoas and quadratus lumborum muscle groups. The margins of normal blood vessels are defined sharply by surrounding fat. In lower lumbar sections, both the aorta and inferior vena cava lie anterior to the spine on either side of the midline; at more cephalic levels, the inferior vena cava courses laterally to the right. The diaphragmatic crura have a characteristic curvilinear shape in the upper abdomen and become more rounded in their caudal attachments where they can be confused with lymph nodes (Fig. IIB.1). Normal lymph nodes are identifiable as small round structures in a peri-aortic or pericaval location. The range of size of normal lymph nodes has not been established. Portions of the fascia that separates the perirenal and pararenal components of the retroperitoneum frequently are distinguishable. The right and left anterior pararenal spaces are limited anteriorly by peritoneum and posteriorly by the anterior renal fascia. These spaces contain ascending and descending colon, duodenum and pancreas. The perirenal space is enclosed by Gerota's fascia and contains kidney and fat. The posterior pararenal fascia is defined anteriorly by the posterior renal fascia and posteriorly by the transversalis fascia. Loops of bowel may be confused with retroperitoneal masses unless dilute, water-soluble contrast material given orally is used.

Perirenal and pararenal spaces

The bulk of a primary tumour of the kidney can be assessed easily by CT. However, invasion of the capsule and beyond cannot be inferred from tumour size alone. Strands of density emanating from a tumour into perinephric fat are sometimes seen. The exact significance of this finding is unknown. Extension of tumour beyond the capsule, oedema due to renal vein thrombosis, or hilar lymphatic obstruction with perinephric collaterals are possible explanations.

Haematoma formation, either subcapsular or perirenal, is demonstrated well by CT. The use of intravenous contrast material serves to distinguish a subcapsular collection of blood from subjacent renal parenchyma. Other processes in the perirenal or pararenal space that are detectable by CT include abscess, urinoma, tumours of the capsule, fascia or fat, and metastases (Fig. IIB.7). These present as mass lesions without specific characteristics that permit distinction of one from another. Frequently, fascial thickening is present in these disorders.

CT can be useful in evaluating patients with axis deviation of the kidney noted on excretory urography. Tumour is easily detected as a cause. Usually though, abundant but otherwise normal fat deposition is found.

Retroperitoneum

Computed tomography detects disease in lymph nodes by virtue of their enlargement. A large, continuous mass of tissue that obliterates the aortic and inferior vena caval silhouette usually is due to malignant lymphoma or Hodgkin's disease (Fig. IIB.8). Lymph node metastases from primary epithelial tumours appear as a distinct mass in the lymph node-bearing area of the retroperitoneum (Fig. IIB.9). Overlapping of these patterns occurs frequently, however.

CT is especially useful in evaluating areas normally not opacified during pedal lymphangiography, particularly the right paravertebral/pericaval chain of lymph nodes, and nodes at the level of, or cephalic to, the renal hila and cisterna chyli. This is of particular value in staging patients with testicular tumours, which often metastasize first to renal hilar nodes. Metastases from renal tumours to retrocrural and inferior mediastinal nodes may be detected.

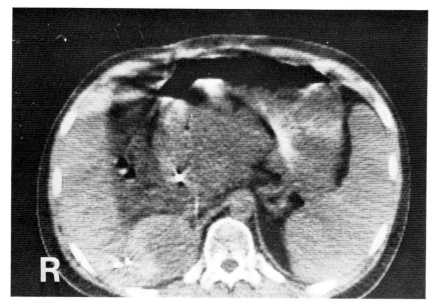

Fig. IIB.7 Liposarcoma in the right pararenal-perirenal space and in the root of mesentery. Two large masses are present. Attenuation value does not suggest fatty nature of tumours. Structure of mixed attenuation values medial to spleen is the stomach.

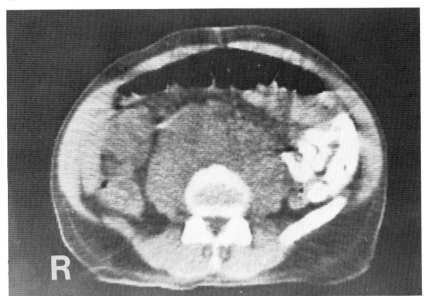

Fig. IIB.8 Retroperitoneal lymphoma. An extensive mantle of tissue surrounds and obliterates the aorta, inferior vena cava and paravertebral muscles.

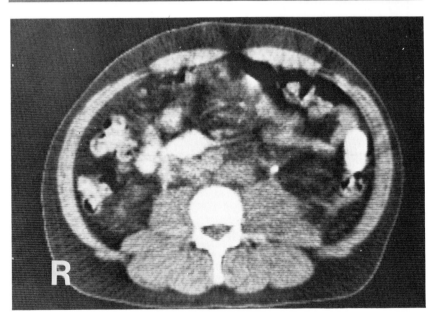

Fig. IIB.9 Malignant melanoma. Multiple metastatic deposits distort the symmetry of the psoas muscle on the left and produce soft tissue masses adjacent to the aorta and inferior vena cava.

Computed tomography accurately defines the extent of a nodal mass, but, unlike lymphangiography, provides no information regarding internal architecture of the node. The two techniques, therefore, are complementary, particularly in diseases that cause disordered nodal architecture before enlargement occurs. CT demonstration of lymph node enlargement, on the other hand, obviates the need for lymphangiography, as illustrated in Fig. IIB.8.

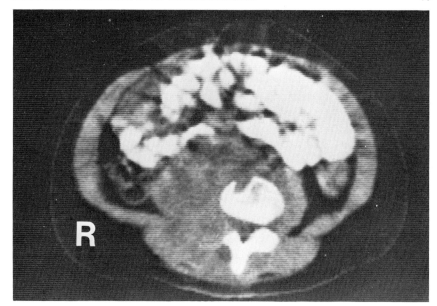

Fig. IIB.10 Retroperitoneal leiomyosarcoma. Tissue necrosis and cystic degeneration cause focal areas of decreased attenuation. This finding is considered more characteristic of leiomyosarcoma than of other primary retroperitoneal tumours.

Retroperitoneal tumour masses other than those of lymph node origin can be precisely identified by CT. Leiomyosarcoma, malignant histiocytoma, and liposarcoma were the commonest of these in a series of patients reported from the Mayo Clinic. None have features that specifically indicate tissue type. It has been suggested that tissue necrosis and cystic degeneration causing low attenuation values may be more characteristic of leiomyosarcoma than other types of retroperitoneal tumours (Fig. IIB.10). The attenuation values of tumours derived from fat cells vary according to their fat content; many have the same value as non-fatty tumours (Fig. IIB.7).

CT is useful in establishing radiation ports for therapy of tumours. Similarly, serial CT examination permits monitoring of the response of a tumour to radiation or chemotherapy, or the detection of recurrence following surgery.

Retroperitoneal fibrosis appears on a computed tomogram as a paravertebral pre-aortic mantle of tissue. This is indistinguishable from lymphoma or other forms of extensive lymph node tumour. The relation of the ureters to the fibrotic mass is easily determined after contrast material injection. Occasionally, retroperitoneal fibrosis may cause thickening of normal structures, such as the aortic wall, rather than a mantle of obscuring tissue. This appearance, particularly if accompanied by evidence of ureteric obstruction, allows confident diagnosis of retroperitoneal fibrosis.

Haemorrhage, aneurysm, lymphocoele and abscess are additional retroperitoneal abnormalities that present as masses. The attenuation value of an abscess may decrease as it becomes purulent, while that of a lymphocoele will approximate that of water. Gas in a mass indicates an abscess. Aneurysms are identified by their relation to the aorta or iliac artery. Contrast material may be used to identify the residual lumen and demonstrate intraluminal thrombus.

Often, CT is used in a patient suspected of retroperitoneal disease in whom other diagnostic studies have given negative or indefinite results. It is likely that the specificity and sensitivity of CT applied to retroperitoneal disease is superior to excretory urography, lymphangiography, radionuclide scans, and ultrasound, although conclusive data have not yet been published. The absence of fat in children and in cachectic or lean patients is a potential source of error, leading to the false impression of tumour causing obliteration of fat planes. The use of dilute contrast material to distinguish bowel from retroperitoneal tissue and intravenous contrast to opacify ureters, vena cava and aorta will aid diagnostic accuracy.

The pelvis (Abrams & McNeil, 1978; Redman, 1977; Schapiro & Chiu, 1977).

Like the retroperitoneum, the quality of pelvic CT images is favoured by the abundant fat deposits around blood vessels, lymph nodes and the viscera of this region, and the absence of image-degrading physiologic motion. The bladder, prostate, seminal vesicles, corpus spongiosum, uterus, rectum, and bony structures are identified routinely (Fig. IIB.11). The urethra is localized when a catheter is in place. A tampon can be used to mark the vagina. Gas or water-soluble contrast material can be used to distend the rectum, if necessary. The obturator internus and levator ani muscles are sharply defined by surrounding fat and characteristically are symmetrical. These muscles are seen on the caudal sections through the pelvis while the iliacus, psoas and iliopsoas muscles identify cephalic sections. The many muscle groups of the proximal thigh, gluteal regions and the anterior abdominal wall are included in sections of the

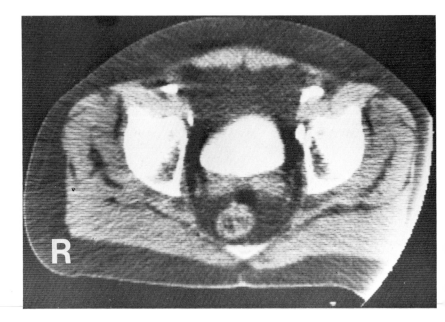

Fig. IIB.11 Normal male pelvis above level of prostate. The bladder is opacified by injected contrast material. Note the seminal vesicles extending posterolaterally between bladder and rectum. Inguinal lymph nodes are opacified following lymphangiography.

pelvis as well. Normal pelvic lymph nodes, iliac arteries and veins and ovaries are not always identified.

Pelvic scans are performed with the patient in a supine position. Urine has a lower attenuation value than the bladder wall, thus permitting definition of the inner aspect of the bladder wall. Contrast enhancement of the bladder requires a small amount of iodine (3–6 g) given intravenously. Larger amounts will produce excessive density that obscures bladder detail and produces artefacts. Intravenous contrast material allows identification of the pelvic portions of the ureters (Fig. IIB.12). Dilute oral water-soluble contrast material is a useful adjunct that aids in the differentiation of loops of bowel in the pelvis from masses.

Pelvic CT scanning has been applied to the diagnosis and/or staging of tumours of the prostate, bladder, ovaries, uterus, rectum or lymph nodes (Fig. IIB.12 and IIB.13). The technique for staging of bladder cancer requires gas distension of the bladder, and its overall accuracy is not yet established (Seidelmann et al, 1977). CT has not been proven efficacious in the detection of a primary tumour still confined to the organ of origin. Spread beyond the margins of the primary organ may produce an irregularity of contour. Nodular prostatic contours have been noted only in prostatic carcinoma and not in benign prostatic hypertrophy in one small series (Price & Davidson, 1979). With further extension of tumour, masses in the pelvic fat and along the lateral side walls develop. These correspond to the lymphatic drainage along hypogastric, obturator and iliac lymph nodes. Since the hypogastric/obturator chain of lymph nodes usually is bypassed or incompletely filled by pedal lymphography, the use of CT is valuable in this area. Lymphomatous disease of the pelvic lymph nodes

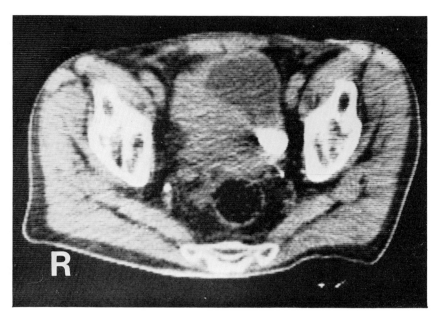

Fig. IIB.12 Sarcoma of bladder. The lumen of the displaced bladder is filled by unopacified urine of low attenuation value and high density contrast material that has layered posteriorly. The ureters are opacified. Tumour can be seen extending posterior to the bladder on the right side.

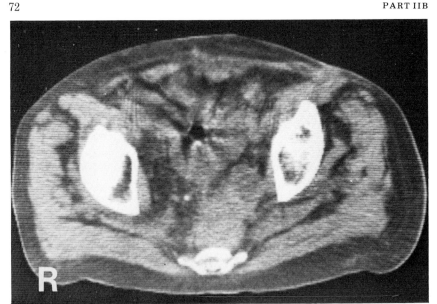

Fig. IIB.13 Recurrent cloacogenic carcinoma presenting as soft tissue mass contiguous with and anterolateral to the rectum.

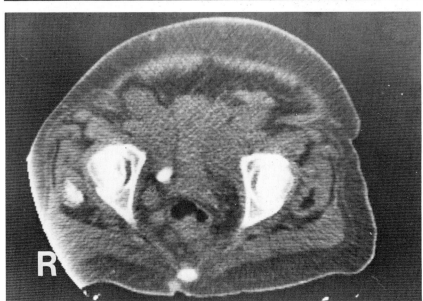

Fig. IIB.14 Lymphoma involving pelvic lymph nodes. The midline structure impressed by the enlarged nodes is the bladder. Contrast is seen in dilated right ureter.

is detected easily by CT once the lymph nodes become enlarged (Fig. IIB.14). However, as noted previously, architectural deformities within a normal sized node are not defined by CT.

Pelvic lipomatosis produces bladder and rectal deformities identical to those caused by some pelvic tumours. This diagnosis can be readily established by CT demonstration of pelvic fat encroaching on these structures (Fig. IIB.15).

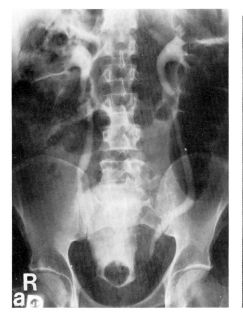

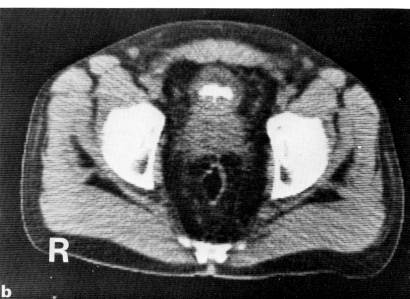

Compared with the many other diagnostic tests used to evaluate disease of the pelvic organs, computed tomography is most efficacious in the evaluation of tumour along the pelvic sidewalls, in the hypogastric/obturator lymph node chains that normally are not visualized during lymphangiography, in detecting early spread beyond the limits of the organ of origin, and in pelvic abscess (Fig. IIB.16). CT has not proved a substitute for endoscopy of the urethra and bladder.

Fig. IIB.15a & b   Pelvic lipomatosis. Excretory urogram (a) raises possibility of pelvic mass deforming bladder. CT (b) demonstrates abundant pelvic fat, no mass and an enlarged prostate between the rectum posteriorly and a collapsed, thick walled bladder containing a small amount of high density contrast material.

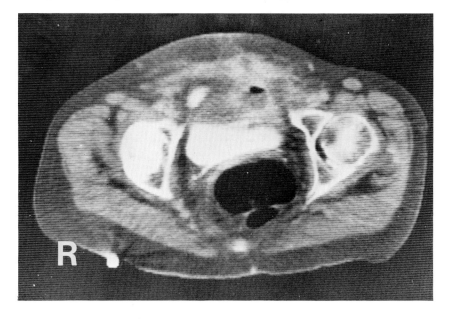

Fig. IIB.16   Abscess of space of Retzius. An air-fluid level is present at site of abscess. Abscess developed after radiation therapy for pelvic malignancy.

Ultrasound is generally more applicable than CT in evaluating diseases of the uterus, adnexae and ovaries. Successful pelvic ultrasound requires a fully distended bladder. When this is not possible because of previous radiation, surgery or tumour bulk, CT is an excellent alternative.

Summary

Computed tomography produces cross-sectional anatomic representations with exquisite accuracy. Anatomic accuracy, however, is only one factor in assessing the overall value of a new diagnostic procedure. The ability of the test to detect disease correctly (true positive rate, or sensitivity) and to establish normalcy (true negative, or specificity) are of equal importance. The extent to which a new test replaces other diagnostic procedures, its impact on patient management and its ultimate effect on patient morbidity and mortality must be taken into account. Cost and availability of equipment are additional important factors. Many of these considerations are yet to be determined in assessing the overall application of computed tomography to uroradiological problems.

Computed tomography in uroradiology has generally been most useful where existing diagnostic techniques are least sensitive, namely in the detection, staging or exclusion of disease, usually tumours, in the perirenal, pararenal or retroperitoneal spaces and in the pelvis. Computed tomography used for disease of the kidney and collecting structures usually duplicates information normally obtained from simpler, less costly, and more readily available techniques, such as excretory urography and ultrasound. Its use in this area is best reserved for situations in which these tests fail and for those occasional, unusual, isolated problems for which no generalized principle seems valid.

REFERENCES

ABRAMS H.L. & McNEIL B.J. (1978) Medical implications of computed tomography ('CAT Scanning'), (second of two parts). *New England Journal of Medicine* **298**, 310–318.

HATTERY R.R. *et al.* (1977) Computed tomography of renal abnormalities. *Radiologic Clinics of North America* **15**, 401–418.

KIRKPATRICK R.H. *et al.* (1978) Scanning techniques in computed body tomography. *American Journal of Roentgenology* **130**, 1069–1075.

PRICE J.M. & DAVIDSON A.J. (1979) Computed tomography in the evaluation of the suspected carcinomatous prostate. *Urologic Radiology* **1**, 39–42.

REDMAN H.C. (1977) Computed tomography of the pelvis. *Radiologic Clinics of North America* **15**, 377–390.

SAGEL S.S. *et al.* (1977) Computed tomography of the kidney. *Radiology* **124**, 359–370.

SCHAPIRO R.L. & CHIU L.C. (1977) A primer in computed axial tomographic anatomy. III. The male pelvis. *Computed Axial Tomography* **1**, 213–218.

SEIDELMANN F.E., COHEN W.N. & BRYAN P.J. (1977) Computed tomographic staging of bladder neoplasms. *Radiologica Clinics of North America* **15**, 419–440.

STEPHENS D.H. *et al.* (1977) Computed tomography of the retroperitoneal space. *Radiologic Clinics of North America* **15**, 377–390.

Urography

The role of urography in hypertensive patients is continually changing as we become smarter about hypertension. Several years ago it was common practice, at least in the United States, to request rapid sequence urography on many newly discovered hypertensive patients, regardless of age, severity of hypertension, ease of control of blood pressure by medicines, or even commitment to perform surgery if a surgical lesion was discovered. This approach fattened uroradiology schedules, cost a great deal of money, and was frustratingly unrewarding. With the justified and belated increasing concern with cost effectiveness of what we do in medicine, improvements in drugs available to treat hypertension, and more realistic expectations from surgery, urography in hypertensives has slowed from a torrent to a trickle.

To understand why we do urography at all in hypertensive patients, several bits of background information are required. (1) High blood pressure is a well-established risk factor for strokes, coronary artery disease, congestive heart failure, and renal damage. In general, the wear and tear effects on target organs can be minimized if the blood pressure is kept normal. Of course, controlling blood pressure can do little to offset one's genetic tendency to diffuse atherosclerotic cardiovascular disease. (2) Elevated blood pressure can be lowered by judicious use of antihypertensive drugs in most patients. One might ask, why not treat all hypertensives with drugs, and forget about finding the cause? In fact this appealing approach is being adopted more and more in middle-aged and older hypertensive patients once the standard battery of blood and urine tests has excluded glomerular disease, renal insufficiency, phaeochromocytoma, hyperaldosteronism, and the rare renin producing tumour, diseases which merit recognition because of therapeutic implications. What difference does it make if an older patient has renal artery stenosis as long as renal function is satisfactory and blood pressure can be controlled medically? (3) Results of surgery for renal artery stenosis in older patients (atherosclerosis) are not nearly as impressive as in the young (fibromuscular dysplasia). Surgical morbidity and mortality is higher, the cure or improvement rate from technically successful surgery is less, and the likelihood of achieving longevity is reduced because atherosclerosis characteristically is a generalized disease, affecting coronary and cerebral arteries as well as the renals. (4) In children, renal or renovascular lesions account for hypertension in 40–70% of the cases (Korobkin et al, 1976). While surgical cure appears more appealing than a lifetime of antihypertensive drugs, no study has yet evaluated the long-term results of surgical versus medical therapy in children. In practice, surgery is almost always carried out when a suitable lesion is discovered in a child. With these facts in mind we should be aggressive in the search for renal or renovascular causes in all young patients, but only in those older patients with moderate or severe hypertension unresponsive to medical therapy, or responsive to drugs but with too bothersome side effects.

Now what do I mean by aggressive? I mean we should perform the examina-

PART III
Hypertension

Lee B. Talner

tion that will detect all correctable lesions, i.e. arteriography. Rapid sequence urography does not suffice in younger patients because the incidence of false negatives is too high—at least 30–40%. This in part reflects the higher incidence of fibromuscular dysplasia in the young with its tendency to affect segmental arteries. Even in adults with proven renal artery stenosis causing hypertension, rapid sequency urography will miss one in five patients; so the test, even with all its enthusiastic modifications, is not sensitive enough for these high risk patients. Let me reiterate that this 'pull out all the stops' philosophy holds for all the young patients but only for the older ones refractory to medical treatment. Just where to draw the 'young' age line is a difficult philosophical issue which has no simple answer. But by considering the history, presence or absence of an abdominal bruit, response to drugs, and perhaps the results of urography, the decision to proceed with arteriography is made somewhat less than arbitrary in the middle age group, say age 30–40 years.

Having decided *a priori*, based upon youth or poor response to medication to 'go for broke' with an arteriogram, should the urogram be bypassed? Unfortunately, the answer is no. Rather than doing urography to fish out patients who might benefit from arteriography as in the old days, paradoxically we should now be asking for urography in these patients preselected for arteriography in order to find something which would *preclude* the vascular study. A kidney atrophied from obstruction, reflux, trauma, or radiation would do this. So would polycystic disease. Cysts or tumours are usually unrelated to hypertension, but once in a while hypertension has been cured after a cyst was emptied or a cancer-bearing kidney was removed.

Only in the middle-aged group might urography still be thought of as a screening aid for *detecting* renovascular hypertension. Here the superiority of surgery versus long-term medical treatment is not known and a negative rapid-sequence urogram lowers the odds of renovascular hypertension sufficiently to stop the search.

Despite having demoted rapid-sequence urography to a position of relatively minor importance, the technique still deserves description. A bolus of 50 ml of any modern urographic agent is injected within 15–20 seconds, and films coned to the kidneys are taken at 1, 2, 3, 5, and 10 minutes. The three early films at least can be done with 10 degree arc tomograms to maximize nephrographic information. Any one of the following is grounds for calling the study positive: (1) discrepancy of renal length more than 1.5 cm (2 cm if left longer than right); (2) discrepancy of 1 minute or more in caliceal appearance time; (3) difference in estimated concentration of contrast material in urine (due allowance being made for volume differences); and (4) ureteric notching. Approximately four out of five patients cured or improved by surgery show one or more of these findings (Fig. III.1). For a more complete discussion of rapid-sequence urography in renovascular hypertension, see Bookstein *et al* (1972). Modifications of urography for hypertension, including furosemide-augmented and urea washout urography are not believed to improve things sufficiently to recommend their adoption (Talner *et al*, 1978).

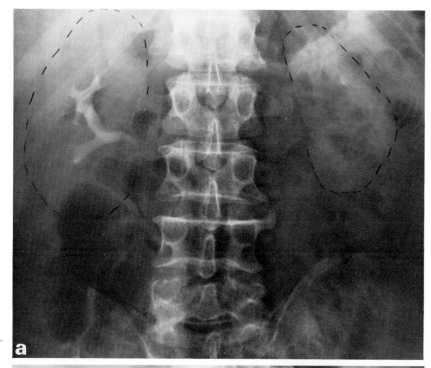

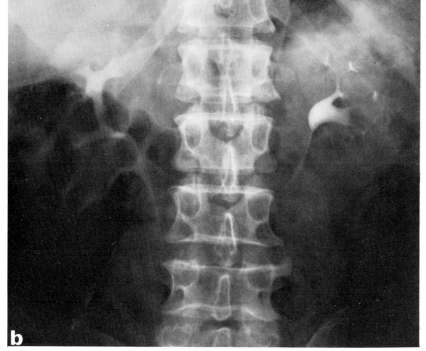

Fig. III.1 Renovascular hypertension.
a Two-minute film from rapid-sequence urogram suggests left renal artery stenosis. Left kidney is 1.9 cm shorter than right, and contrast material appearance is delayed in left calices.
b Ten-minute film shows increased pyelogram density left kidney, suggesting hyperconcentration.

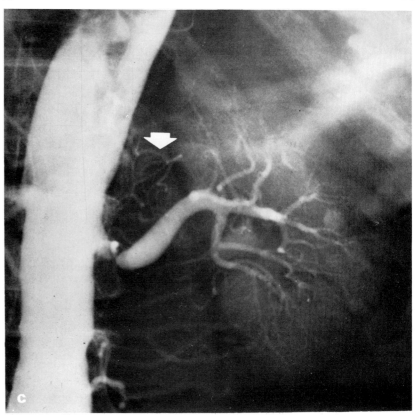

Fig. III.1 c Aortogram shows focal, atherosclerotic stenosis of left renal artery. Presence of lumbar collaterals (arrow) indicates haemodynamic significance of stenosis.

Renography

Renography with either ^{131}I-hippuran or [99m]technetium-DTPA detects approximately 85% of renal artery stenoses, but there are 10% false positive studies in patients with essential hypertension (see Part IIA Nuclear Medicine). Moreover, renography has considerable difficulty distinguishing between unilateral renovascular lesions and unilateral renal lesions. Because of these problems, renography is rarely used as a primary screening test for renovascular hypertension, but it can be used occasionally in a supplementary screening role (McAfee *et al* 1977).

Arteriography

The first task of arteriography is to demonstrate an anatomic abnormality which *could* cause hypertension. Renal artery stenosis heads the list, but renal artery aneurysm, embolism, dissection, arteriovenous fistula, post-traumatic renal infarction-ischaemia, Page kidney, renal carcinoma, Wilms' tumour, renal cyst, and the rare juxtaglomerular tumour (reninoma) must be sought when no stenosis is uncovered. Regrettably, finding any one of these lesions in a patient with hypertension is no guarantee of causality. Current thinking holds that all unilateral renovascular lesions causing hypertension do so via hypersecretion of renin. Therefore, to prove cause, angiographers are asked to look for evidence of increased renin secretion by sampling renal venous blood for renin activity. More about this later.

Renal artery stenosis

Reviews of the subject detail the location of stenotic lesions, their incidence, radiographic appearance, histology, and natural history (Abrams *et al.,* 1967; Stewart *et al,* 1970). None of this has changed much in recent years, so a repeat is not in order here. Several issues are worth emphasizing, however.

Fibromuscular dysplasia (FMD) has been subgrouped according to the cross-sectional histologic involvement as primarily intimal, medial, perimedial, or adventitial. In our experience the histologic abnormality is rarely confined to just one of these sites, commonly affecting both intima and media, or other combinations. Intimal and medial involvement predispose to spontaneous renal artery dissection and thrombosis, and definitely increase the risk of catheter induced dissection at selective arteriography. Of all fibromuscular stenoses the most common (60–70%) is medial fibroplasia with aneurysm, causing the familiar 'string of beads' appearance on the arteriogram (Fig. III.2). FMD is bilateral in 30–60% of cases, has at least a 4:1 female predominance, and frequently either extends into or involves solely segmental branches of the renal artery. For this reason selective arteriography, preferably with twofold direct magnification, is very important if one is not to miss the more subtle lesions (see Fig. III.5). Oblique views of the aorta may be needed to show renal artery origins, and oblique selective arteriograms have been especially valuable in detecting extension of disease into and sometimes distal to the bifurcation or trifurcation of the main renal artery. For the vascular surgeon this is information essential for proper choice of surgical technique.

Fibromuscular disease progresses (Fig. III.3). Just how frequently is hard to say because several of the histopathological classes progress more consistently than others, and series of cases differ in their classification. Lumping all subgroups together, it appears that progression occurs in at least 30–40% of patients. It is especially common with predominant intimal fibroplasia, medial hyperplasia, and perimedial fibroplasia. Progression occurs less commonly with medial fibroplasia (string of beads) (Stewart *et al,* 1970). Improved accuracy in predicting disease progression would aid patient management considerably. FMD occurs in extrarenal arteries and may be symptomatic when the carotid artery is affected. Patients with renal artery FMD may be normotensive just like patients with atherosclerotic stenosis of the renal artery (Youngberg *et al,* 1977).

Atherosclerotic plaques account for most renal artery stenoses in patients over 50. Characteristically plaques narrow the proximal 1–2 cm of the renal artery and usually, but not always, are associated with quite advanced aortic disease (see Fig. III.1c). Obviously, selective catheterization can become a risky business in these well-worn, craggy aortas, and the enthusiasm to push on with selective catheterization after the aortogram has shown a clear-cut narrowing of the renal artery must be tempered by good judgment (Talner, 1976). Remember that renal vein renins may give quite enough information for the surgeon once aortography has demonstrated a stenosis.

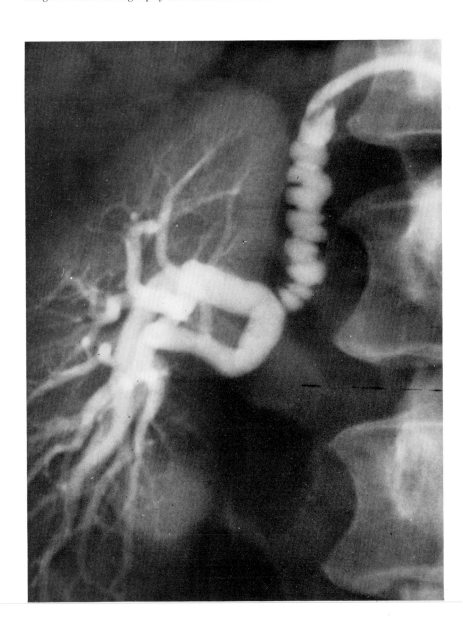

Fig. III.2 Fibromuscular dysplasia. Typical 'string of beads' appearance of medial fibroplasia subtype due to alternating regions of stenosis and aneurysmal dilatation. Note extension of process to renal artery bifurcation.

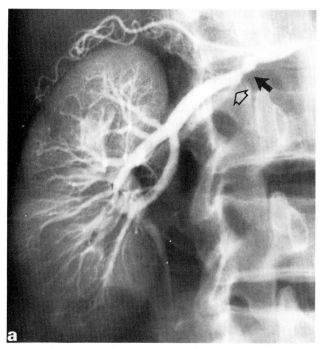 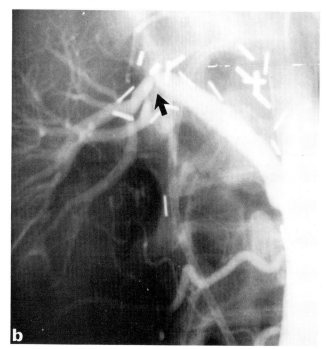

In patients with bilateral stenosis due to FMD or atherosclerosis the pertinent question is which kidney is responsible for hypertension? Again, renal vein sampling often shows the way to the renin-producing kidney.

Until very recently the arteriographer was asked only to demonstrate the anatomy of arterial lesion(s). Attempts to judge arteriographically whether a given stenosis was haemodynamically important were largely empirical and unreliable. Post-stenotic dilatation, originally thought to be important, is now known to indicate no more than turbulent flow and reveals nothing about the pressure gradient or likelihood of beneficial response to surgery. On the other hand, two arteriographic findings have emerged as true indicators of a haemodynamically significant lesion, i.e. a lesion which is causing enough flow or pressure aberration to cause renin release and hypertension: (1) diameter of stenosis less than 1·5 mm; and (2) presence of collateral arteries. It now appears that demonstration of collateral arteries circumventing a stenosis is about as good an indicator of surgical curability as lateralizing renins.

Bookstein's novel approach of pharmacoangiography allows one to make a positive statement about the presence or absence of collaterals in about 95% of patients (Bookstein *et al*, 1976). His review is well worth reading for the nuances of technique, but its rationale can be summarized: (1) If collaterals are shown directly on the aortogram, no pharmacoangiography need be done. (2) If on the selective renal arteriogram, 'wash in' defects are detected, this is prima facie

Fig. III.3 Progression of fibromuscular dysplasia: 20-year-old woman.
a Arteriogram shows multifocal stenosis of main renal artery (solid arrow) extending to the bifurcation. Major branch is narrowed proximally (open arrow). Superior capsular artery is enlarged and serves as bypass collateral. Renins lateralize to right kidney.
b Two months after saphenous vein bypass graft, hypertension recurred. Aortogram shows narrowing near the anastomosis (arrow) and persistent stenosis of major branch. Hypertension cured by nephrectomy. Specimen showed widely patent anastomosis but severe stenosis due to progression of intimal and subadventitial fibroplasia.

evidence of collaterals bringing non-opaque blood to the kidneys, and again no pharmacoangiography is needed (Fig. III.4). (3) If neither of the above is shown, renal artery injection of either angiotensin or epinephrine to raise renal vascular resistance, or acetylcholine to lower it, can be done just prior to selective arteriography. The aim here is to see if changes in direction of blood flow (renopetal or renofugal) can be induced in the non-parenchymal branches of the renal artery—the pelvic, ureteric, and capsular arteries. Reversing flow in one or more of these branches indicates that the artery is serving as a collateral, and the haemodynamic significance of the stenosis is established. The technique is somewhat time-consuming, requires magnification arteriography and has not been practised widely, but its favourable comparison with renin measurements as a forecaster of beneficial response to surgery makes it an alternative worth considering. We have found it useful.

With magnification arteriography, segmental or more peripheral stenoses of the renal artery are being recognized more frequently (Fig. III.5). Moreover, a network of intrarenal, bridging collaterals has now been demonstrated, contradicting the previously held notion that intrarenal branches of the renal artery

Fig. III.4 Dilution defect as sign of collaterals.

a Selective arteriogram shows focal renal artery stenosis, post-stenotic dilatation, and aneurysm (black arrow). White arrow points to localized dilution defect caused by inflow of non-opaque blood.

b Late phase of aortogram shows lumbar-pelvic collateral (arrows) accounting for dilution defect in **a**. Collaterals always indicate haemodynamic significance.

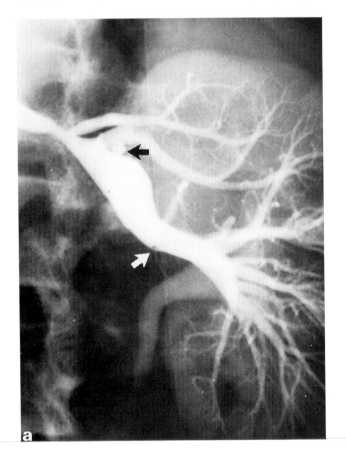

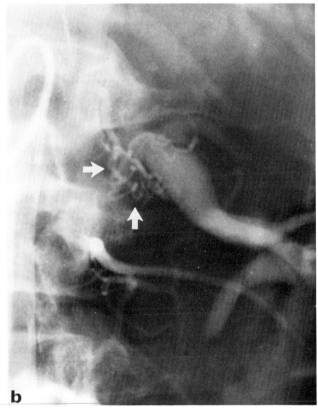

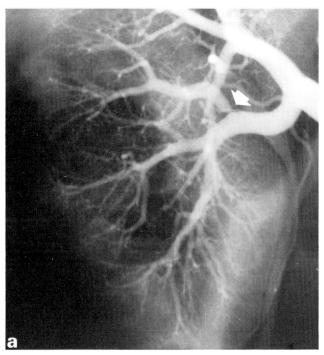

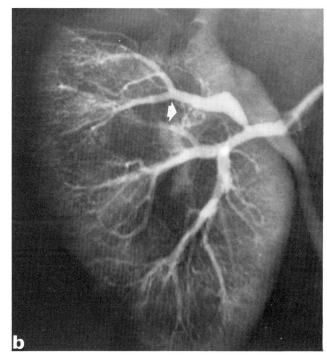

are end arteries with no possibility of collateralization. If a lobar artery is occluded, its distribution may be fed via pelvic or pericaliceal arteries from an adjacent lobar artery (Meng *et al,* 1973; Kirks *et al,* 1977) (Figs III.5 and III.6). Communications also exist between the extrarenal capsular arteries and peripheral intrarenal arteries. The direction of flow in intrarenal collaterals depends upon the site of renal ischaemia.

Renal vein sampling

Angiographers find themselves called upon to play the unfamiliar role of renal physiologist. A stenosis is found, the report goes out, and the referring physician asks to have 'some renins drawn'. Or probably more likely, the physician prior to angiography says, 'Draw some renal vein renins if you find something'. If the angiographer truly wishes to contribute something rather than add confusing data, he or she must become aware of the many renin-related pitfalls. These practical hints should help: (1) Venous blood must be drawn into iced syringes and immediately transferred to iced tubes containing the proper anticoagulant and transported promptly to the assay laboratory. (2) Samples must be labelled and recorded fastidiously, indicating both time and site of sampling. (3) Catheter position should be verified by a small test injection of contrast material after the sample is obtained, and this should preferably be documented

Fig. III.5 Interlobar artery stenosis—importance of magnification arteriography: 5-year-old hypertensive boy. Aortogram and non-magnified selective arteriogram were interpreted as normal.
a Magnification arteriogram of right lower pole shows focal narrowing at origin of interlobar artery (arrow).
b Subselective magnification study demonstrates stenosis better, and shows intrarenal collaterals (arrow) from neighbouring interlobar artery. Renins localized to right kidney 3:1, and hypertension was cured by nephrectomy after unsuccessful attempt at selective embolization.

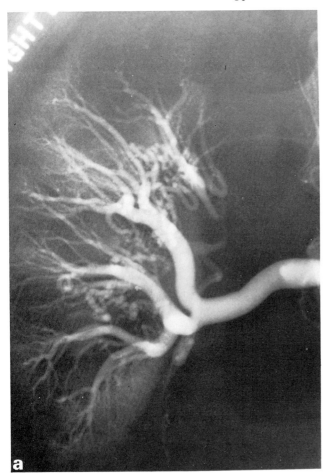

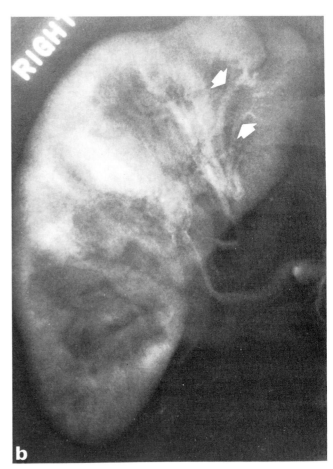

Fig. III.6 Intrarenal collaterals. Accidental surgical ligation of right upper pole artery during resection of juxtarenal phaeochromocytoma.
a Selective arteriogram shows absence of arterial branches to upper pole and extensive network of pericaliceal and peripelvic collaterals coursing cephalad.
b Capillary phase. Delayed opacification of upper pole arteries (arrow) reconstituted by collaterals. Note ischaemic shrinkage of upper pole.

by a spot film. Double renal veins are more common on the right (10–15%) than on the left. Watch for the circumaortic left renal vein. (4) Simultaneous, two-catheter sampling appears to improve reliability somewhat, but sequential sampling with a single catheter is still done in most hospitals. (5) Renal vein blood for renins should not be obtained directly after arteriography. Intra-arterial contrast material affects renin release unpredictably and may make data interpretation confusing. It is therefore better to do renin studies at a separate sitting after suitable preparation of the patient. (6) In the presence of segmental artery stenosis, intrarenal venous sampling should be attempted from involved and normal portions of the kidney. (7) Patients should be taken off all medications known to affect renin release or activity. Ideally this should be for 2–3 weeks. Drugs particularly to be avoided are propranolol, reserpine, alpha methyl dopa, and spironolactone (Youngberg *et al*, 1977). (8) Patients should be prepared in a standard fashion to maximize renin output from the kidney distal to a stenosis, and to increase chances of lateralization. When patients are not suitably stimulated, renin laterization occurs in only 60–70% of those subsequently cured or improved. With stimulation, renins should be about 90% sensitive, using a renal vein renin ratio (RVRR) of 1·5:1, relating the involved kidney to its mate.

Various preparations have been recommended, including low-salt diet plus diuretics for 3 days to achieve sodium depletion, upright posture during sampling, vasodilators on the table with the patient supine, and a host of others. We prefer 3 days of 2 gram sodium diet plus an oral diuretic. Intravenous furosemide at the time of venous sampling has been tried with poor results. Lateralization of renins can be obscured with this approach.

Even with meticulous attention to detail, renins fail to lateralize in approximately 10% of patients cured or improved by surgery for renal artery stenosis. This probably reflects sampling errors, poor handling technique, and assay variability.

Renal vein renin ratios have other problems. Ratios above 1·5:1 have been found in 20% of patients with essential hypertension, but they are rarely greater than 2:1 (Maxwell et al, 1975). In patients with renal artery stenosis, the higher the RVRR the more likely it is to be significant. Absolute values of renin activity less than 1 nanogram per millilitre per hour make for an inaccurate and misleading RVRR.

Laragh et al (1975) have published a series of papers stating that RVRR is not accurate enough, and that renin suppression must be demonstrated in the opposite kidney. This approach is controversial and beyond the scope of this section.

RVR studies in hypertensive patients with unilateral renal parenchymal disease have been disappointing, i.e. over half the patients cured of their hypertension by nephrectomy have not had lateralizing renins. Whether the mechanism of hypertension is related to something other than renin, or whether faulty technique can be blamed is not known (Bailey et al, 1978).

What is quite clear is that the RVRR is not perfect by any stretch of the imagination, but it is the best we have at present. We must hope that this area will become clarified and simplified as our understanding of the pathophysiology of hypertension continues to improve.

REFERENCES

ABRAMS H.L., MARSHAL W.H. & KUPIC E.A. (1967) The renal vascular bed in hypertension. *Seminars in Roentgenology* **2**, 157–197.

BAILEY R.R., McRAE C.U., MALING T.M.J. *et al* (1978) Renal vein renin concentration in the hypertension of unilateral reflux nephropathy. *Journal of Urology* **120**, 21–23.

BOOKSTEIN J.J., ABRAMS H.L., BUENGER R.E. *et al* (1972) Radiologic aspects of renovascular hypertension. Part II. The role of urography in unilateral renovascular disease. *Journal of the American Medical Association* **220**, 1225–1230.

BOOKSTEIN J.J., WALTER J.F., STANLEY J.C. *et al* (1976) Pharmacoangiographic manipulation of renal collateral blood flow. *Circulation* **53**, 328–334.

KIRKS D.R., FITZ C.R. & KOROBKIN M. (1977) Intrarenal collateral circulation in the pediatric patient. *Pediatric Radiology* **5,** 154–159.

KOROBKIN M., PERLOFF D.L. & PALUBINSKAS A.J. (1976) Renal arteriography in the evaluation of unexplained hypertension in children and adolescents. *Journal of Pediatrics* **88,** 388–393.

LARAGH J.H., SEALEY J.E., BÜHLER F.R. *et al* (1975) The renin axis and vasoconstriction volume analysis for understanding and treating renovascular and renal hypertension. *American Journal of Medicine* **58,** 4–12.

MAXWELL M.H., MARKS L.S., VARADY P.D. *et al* (1975) Renal vein renin in essential hypertension. *Journal of Laboratory and Clinical Medicine* **86,** 901–909.

MCAFEE J.G., THOMAS F.D., GROSSMAN Z. *et al* (1977) Diagnosis of angiotensinogenic hypertension: the complementary roles of renal scintigraphy and the saralasin infusion test. *Journal of Nuclear Medicine* **18,** 669–675.

MENG C.H., ELKIN M. & SMITH T.R. (1973) Intrarenal arterial collaterals. *Radiology* **109,** 59–64.

STEWART B.H., DUSTAN H.P., KISER W.S. *et al* (1970) Correlation of angiography and natural history in evaluation of patients with renovascular hypertension. *Journal of Urology* **104,** 231–238.

TALNER L.B. (1976) Renal complications of angiography. In *Complications in Diagnostic Radiology,* Ch. 4, Ed. G. Ansell, Blackwell Scientific Publications, Oxford.

TALNER L.B., STONE R.A., COEL M.N. *et al* (1978) Furosemide-augmented intravenous urography: results in essential hypertension. *American Journal of Roentgenology* **120,** 257–260.

YOUNGBERG S.P., SCHEPS S.G. & STRONG C.G. (1977) Fibromuscular disease of the renal arteries. *Medical Clinics of North America* **61,** 623–641.

DIVISION 1.
THE KIDNEYS

Renal size

This is one of the most useful IVU assessments. From the armchair there are obvious drawbacks to using renal length as an indicator of renal size. Kidneys have differing shapes in single two-dimensional projection: may not a short, squat kidney be as substantial as a long thin one? What about the falsely long but really normal duplex kidney? Or the small kidney of normal length where parenchymal shrinkage has occurred from within, i.e. where the renal sinus is now too large and filled with fat (Fig. IV.1.A1)?

In practice these are sensible provisos, but they do not detract from the important fact that measuring renal length is the single best guide to renal mass on the IVU (Griffiths *et al*, 1974). The measurement is usually straightforward, particularly when it is recalled that accuracy to less than half a centimetre is inappropriate: the kidney may undergo length changes of this order during the osmotic diuresis of the IVU. A number of methods and charts for normal renal length have been constructed: a good rough-and-ready rule is that the normal adult kidney is three and a half mid-lumbar vertebrae long, including disk spaces. In the child under 10 years a length of four vertebrae/disk spaces is sought. Absolute measurements like these have a wide normal range, and comparative measurements on serial examinations are therefore of particular value. In the child with a suspect kidney, plotting individual renal growth is especially rewarding (Lebowitz *et al*, 1975). In general, the growing kidney can be regarded as a healthy organ. At the other extreme of life, the elderly kidney tends to lose size, probably more influenced by vascular changes than the mere passage of years (Griffiths *et al*, 1976).

Note that the antero-posterior tilt of the kidney as between its lower and upper poles can lead to an underestimate of renal length, most pronounced in inspiration (Farrant & Meire, 1978).

A. UNILATERAL KIDNEY FAILURE

It is not uncommon to see one non-excreting kidney on the IVU (or non-functioning kidney on the radioisotope renogram). The clinical background to this finding is usually very helpful in diagnosis. Are there symptoms which prompted the examination, such as haematuria or unilateral pain? Or is this a chance finding, discovered at an IVU done for some quite different reason?

When unilateral renal failure is such a *silent finding,* the first question is whether there is a kidney at all on this side. It is closely linked with the possibility of a misplaced kidney, e.g. a pelvic kidney. However, an acquired lesion may present in this silent way, e.g. a kidney compressed by a perirenal haematoma dating from an old injury.

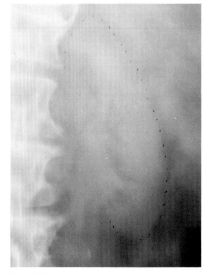

Fig. IV.1.A1 Chronic renal failure—renal length is deceptively normal, though there has been considerable volume lost, particularly in the renal sinus where there is fat replacement.

87

If a sudden dramatic symptom, such as *loin pain,* accompanies the non-excreting kidney, acute obstruction, infection or infarction need to be considered first. *Haematuria* as presenting symptom generally points to the presence of a well-established and perhaps far-advanced lesion; for instance a bladder tumour completely obstructing one ureteric orifice, or a kidney infiltrated by an extensive carcinoma.

Renal size

Probably the most immediately helpful distinction to try to reach about the non-excreting kidney is whether it is small, normal size, or large. This is because the tempo of clinico-radiological management will be dictated by this finding. The small kidney which has failed is of course likely to represent old disease. It is very unlikely to pose a threat to the patient's life chances, assuming there is a normal contralateral kidney. Depending on clinical circumstances, especially the patient's age, it will usually be right to find out why unilateral renal failure should have occurred. A timetable for such investigation is clearly much less pressing than for dealing with a recent, perhaps reversible lesion. The small kidney is further discussed in section B, Renal Failure (p. 112).

The normal size or large non-excreting kidney needs rapid, accurate diagnosis. In the acutely obstructed kidney each day that passes lessens the chance of complete functional recovery. There is obviously still greater urgency with fulminating renal infection, and arterial or venous occlusion.

1. ABSENT OR ECTOPIC KIDNEY

Ectopia and odd renal shapes

When the early contrast films of an IVU show no excretion from a normally sited kidney, the sensible next step is to take immediate careful films of the pelvis, particularly the presacral area. Tomograms may be needed here to reveal a suspected pelvic kidney.

The *pelvic kidney* can be a unilateral or rarely bilateral phenomenon (Fig. IV.1.A2). If unilateral, a normal contralateral kidney in the loin is the rule, but occasionally a patient may have a single pelvic kidney. This is a worrying finding because renal function in a pelvic kidney is generally poor. All may be well in childhood, but a single pelvic kidney may lead on to renal failure in adult life. This question of adequate function is the most important topic for a patient with a pelvic kidney. The possible obstetric complication of obstructed labour is an overrated hazard of this condition: most women with a pelvic kidney do not run into trouble on this account during delivery.

This is a convenient place for mentioning other anomalies of kidney shape and position. *Horseshoe kidney* produces a well-known deformity: the lower poles of the kidney are pulled in toward the midline and joined by a bridge of

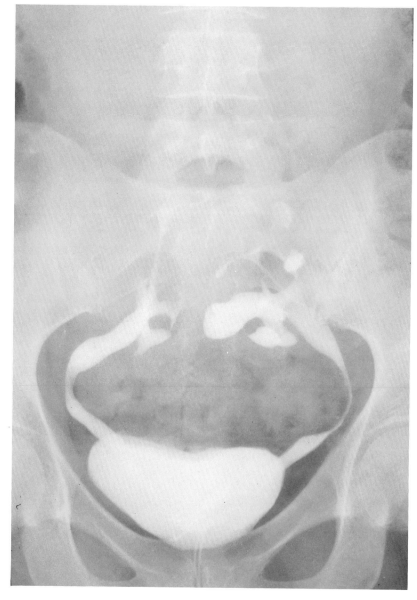

Fig. IV.1.A2   Bilateral pelvic kidneys.

either functioning renal parenchyma or fibrous tissue. The long axis of the
kidney is therefore parallel to the spine, instead of the normal slope with the
lower poles further away from the midline than the upper poles. An important
additional deformity concerns the pelvi-caliceal system and upper ureter: the
pelvi-ureteric junction in horseshoe kidney faces forward (anteriorly) instead of
inwards (medially). The upper ureter has to run anteriorly in order to cross the

joining bridge between the kidneys. These mechanical derangements are apt to impair urinary drainage from the horseshoe kidney, so that stasis and stone formation are frequent complications. It is often possible to diagnose the condition on the plain film because of the abnormal alignment of the kidneys there. This can be still easier when stones mark out the abnormally positioned lower pole calices (Fig. IV.1.A3).

There is a whole range of deformities between the classical horseshoe kidney (symmetrical about the midline) and *crossed renal ectopia* (asymmetrical). These variants go under names like 'sigmoid kidney', describing how one renal element is stuck on to the other. In crossed renal ectopia both renal elements are on

Fig. IV.1.A3 Stones in this horseshoe kidney outline the calices as a cast.

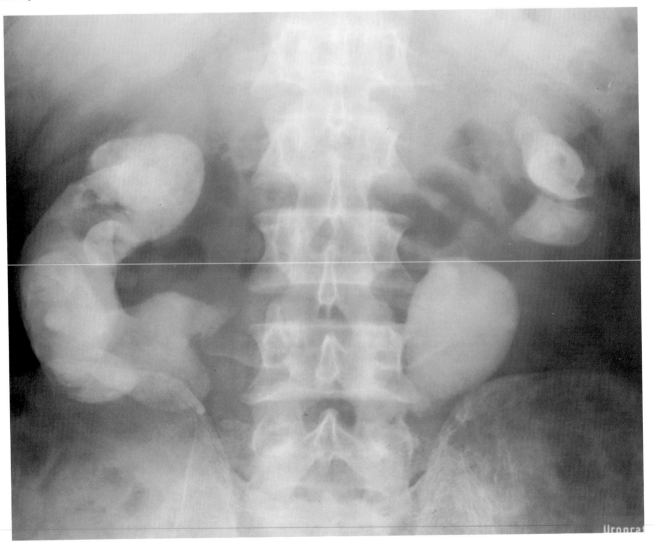

the same side of the body: a monster double kidney with its lower half representing the kidney meant for the opposite loin (Fig. IV.1.A4). The ureter of this lower renal half will always cross the midline to enter the bladder at the expected proper site on the trigone. This appears a firm embryological rule, however odd

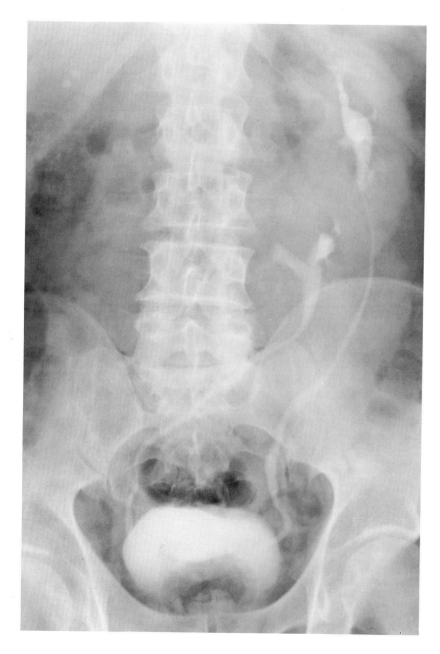

Fig. IV.1.A4 Crossed renal ectopia.

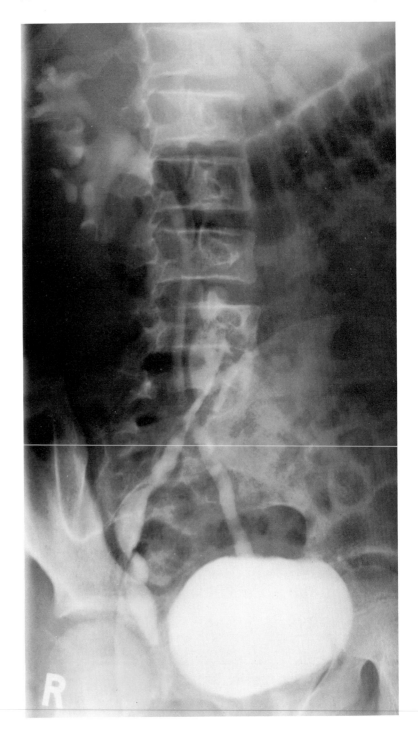

Fig. IV.1.A5 Oblique view of a patient
with crossed renal ectopia in whom the
two ureters wind round each other.
However, the lower right ureter belongs
to the normal right kidney, and the small
crossed kidney has a ureter entering the
bladder on the left.

the detailed plumbing in crossed renal ectopia (Fig. IV.1.A5). Even so, things are not always what they seem (Fig. IV.1.A6).

A further general rule applying to all the anomalies of renal shape and position is that the blood supply is likely to come via odd renal arteries. These are commonly multiple, arising from the lower aorta as well as iliac vessels. This fact is of special importance in the surgery of horseshoe kidney, where a whole string of anomalous renal arteries may be met.

Malrotation about the long axis of a kidney may be seen as a chance finding (Fig. IV.1.A7). The ureter will then follow an unusual course—the anomaly is of no clinical concern.

Absence

If no ectopic kidney can be found to account for unilateral failure of excretion, the possibility of an absent kidney on that side arises. It always needs more definitive proof than can be obtained from an IVU. Serious treatable disorders can masquerade as an absent kidney, for instance silent ureteric obstruction by tumour. A deformed asymmetric trigone, with no ureteric orifice, is a pathognomonic finding on cystoscopy. This is a better court of appeal than renal arteriography, for an absent renal artery is a negative piece of evidence. It can be

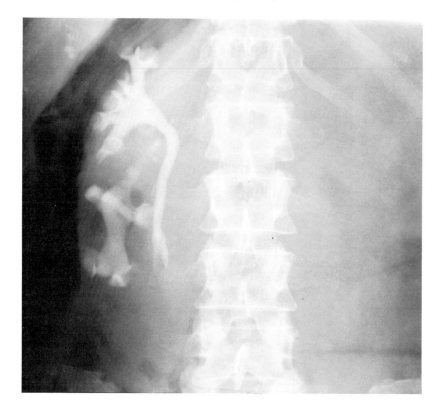

Fig. IV.1.A6 This may look like crossed renal ectopia, but the left kidney is in fact displaced by a large mass in the left loin (liposarcoma). Note the displaced stomach as additional clue.

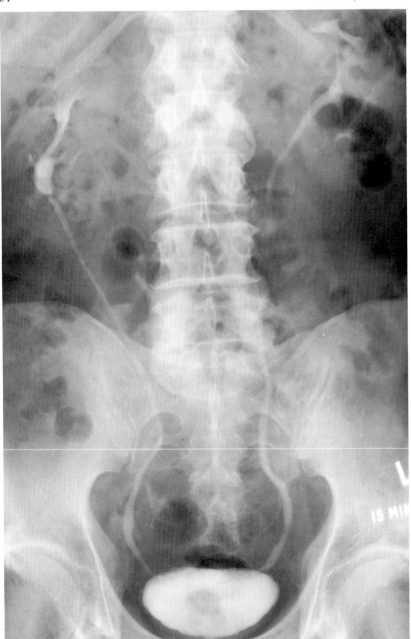

Fig. IV.1.A7 Malrotation of the right kidney about its long axis, with consequent lateral displacement of the right upper ureter.

closely mimicked by a renal artery shrunk away to nothing because of acquired renal disease (Fig. IV.1.A8). This illustration makes the point that ultrasound is the useful next diagnostic step in the investigation of a kidney thought to be absent on the IVU.

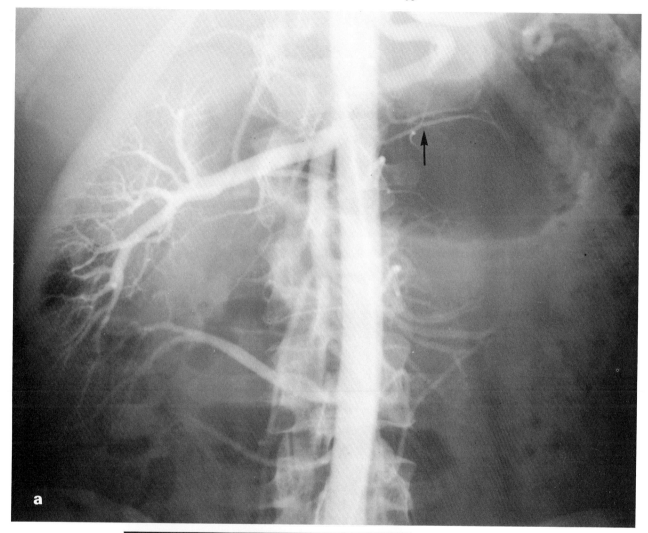

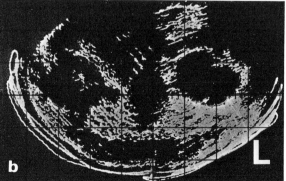

Fig. IV.1.A8a This patient was thought to have an absent left kidney, and the aortogram seemed to confirm this. In retrospect there is in fact a tiny left renal artery (arrow).

Fig. IV.1.A8b The ultrasound scan shows a large cystic mass in the left loin, later confirmed as a hydronephrosis (scan displayed supine).

Acute suppurative pyelonephritis can be a cause of unilateral renal failure in the adult. It is rare. On the IVU the functional deficit may be reflected in the absent pyelogram, but a nephrogram will usually occur in this condition. The nephrogram may grow increasingly dense during the day of the IVU, rather like the pattern of acute extrarenal obstruction. Indeed, intrarenal tubular obstruction by inflammatory debris may be an important mechanism of oliguria in this state. A characteristic streaky vascular nephrogram has been described during arteriography in severe adult pyelonephritis (Davidson & Talner, 1973a).

If fulminating infection occurs as a complication of diabetes, abnormal gas shadows may be seen in or about the kidney. This evidence of rampaging gas-forming organisms can present on the IVU as subcapsular or perirenal collections as well as intrarenal gas.

It is worth mention that severe renal infection short of this disaster picture can give rise to marked local deformity of the kidney. An apparent renal mass deforming the IVU in this state need not spell a large abscess requiring drainage: it may be oedema which will resolve with conservative management (Fig. IV.1.A9).

Fig. IV.1.A9a & b This young man suffered a severe acute infection of the left kidney, successfully treated with antibiotics. At the height of his illness there is considerable distortion of the left pelvi-caliceal system, which then returns to normal.

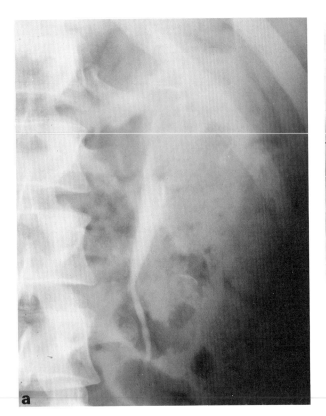
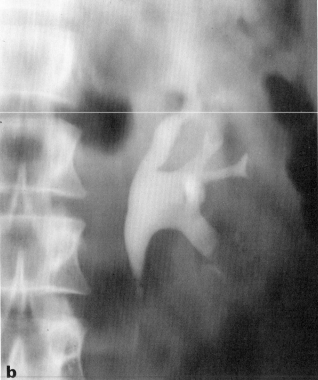

3. ARTERIAL STENOSIS OR OCCLUSION

Acute and chronic events need to be distinguished here. *Acute occlusion* of a
renal artery will commonly be related either to emboli (e.g. following myocar-
dial infarction) or to surgery (e.g. abdominal aortic aneurysm operation). A
dissecting aneurysm of the aorta may extend down to shear off the mouth of one
or both renal arteries. A dissecting aneurysm of the renal artery alone is a
specialized instance of renal infarction by arterial disease (Hare & Kincaid-
Smith, 1970). Unhappily, such dissection must be included as a radiological
hazard when listing the possible complications of selective renal artery catheter
procedures.

The immediate appearance of the grossly ischaemic kidney may be misleading on the IVU because a *large* non-excreting organ is seen. This represents the
oedematous stage of an infarct, familiar from many other territories. A *rim
nephrogram* may occur since the superficial renal cortex can be fed by blood,
reaching the capsular perirenal network via extrarenal arteries. The nephrogram proper is of course absent, and the gross perfusion defect will also be
obvious on radioisotope studies. Arteriography demonstrates the nature and
extent of the offending lesion (Fig. IV.1.A10). Whether it is necessary to have

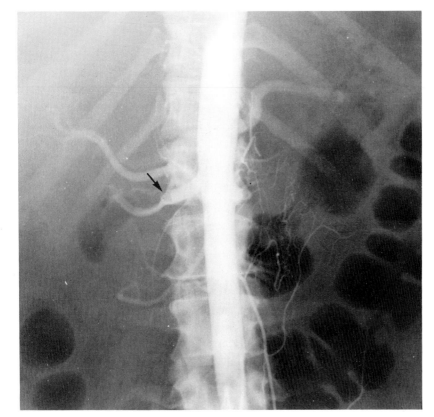

Fig. IV.1.A10 Acute renal failure
because of bilateral renal artery emboli.
The left renal artery is completely
occluded, and an arrow points to an
embolus in the right renal artery.

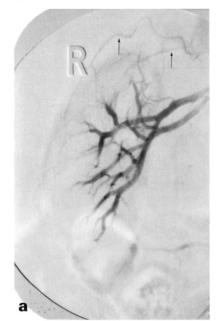
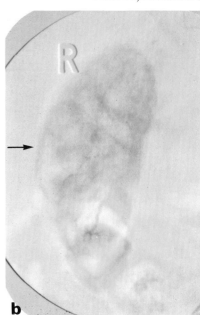

Fig. IV.1.A11a   Subtraction renal arteriogram 2 weeks after renal artery emboli. The cortex is grossly ischaemic, with hardly any flow into it. Note normal capsular arteries (arrows).

Fig. IV.1.A11b   A later frame shows a sliver of cortex (arrow) perfused by the capsular arteries. See also Fig. IV.1.F12 (cortical necrosis).

this information for any particular patient will naturally be dictated by the clinical background. The natural history of renal artery emboli is similar to that in other vascular beds: they break up into fragments which pass distally where there is a large vascular surface area, so that considerable recovery of function may occur. Arteriography can then help in judging prognosis by showing whether cortical ischaemia is diffuse or patchy (Fig. IV.1.A11).

The characteristic picture of the kidney with *chronic* severe ischaemia is of a small non-excreting kidney with no caliceal deformity. Renal atrophy is uniform so a small, smooth kidney results. It may show a long-lasting nephrogram (Fry & Cattell, 1972) because of feeble perfusion via collaterals. On arteriography late filling of the distal renal arterial tree may be seen, brought about by a similar pathway.

4. VENOUS OBSTRUCTION

Renal vein thrombosis is a very different entity in the adult as compared with the childhood problem. Infants presenting with an acute illness involving dehydration, predominantly gastroenteritis, may develop renal vein thrombosis as a complication. This will usually be bilateral, with resultant renal failure. Following recovery the kidneys show papillary deformities looking deceptively like papillary necrosis on the IVU (Chrispin, 1972). In the adult, renal vein occlusion is commonly a complication of some other renal disease, not a primary event. Usually this will either be a renal carcinoma with tumour extension into the vein, or a nephritis (glomerulonephritis) with reduced renal blood flow.

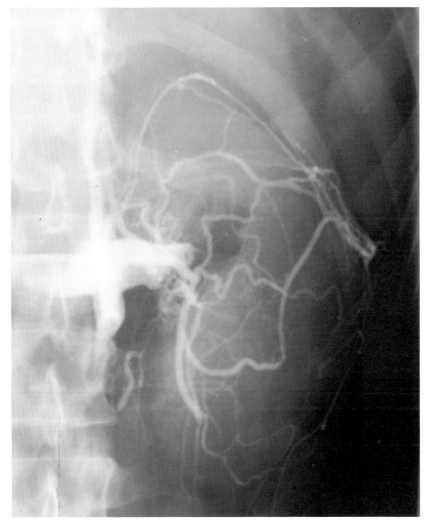

Fig. IV.1.A12 Amyloid renal disease
with renal vein block—note clot lying in
the main renal vein on this selective left
renal venogram.

Renal vein thrombosis is a particular hazard in the clinical setting of the
nephrotic syndrome. Its link with amyloid is well known (Fig. IV.1.A12).

In occlusion of the main renal vein the kidney is large (swollen), and the IVU
will probably show only a distinct long-lasting nephrogram, which may grow
denser with time. No pyelogram will be seen. These classical signs are sometimes taken as embracing the whole subject, but in fact apply only to complete
main renal vein occlusion. Many patients with multiple thrombi in the peripheral renal venous tree will show a perfectly good pyelogram, though the
kidney will still tend to be large. Clinico-radiological suspicion that there may
be renal vein thrombi should not be put off by a normal-looking IVU. Providing
that patient management will be influenced by the answer, renal venography is
a rewarding and decisive investigation here.

5. OBSTRUCTION

This is the most common reason for unilateral renal failure. In *acute obstruction* presenting with pain, there is generally little difficulty with the diagnosis. The IVU shows a large kidney with a characteristic, increasingly dense nephrogram (see Division 2 section B). Diagnosis can be harder in *chronic obstruction*. The early 'soap-bubble' nephrogram outlining dilated non-opacified calices is certainly characteristic, but may not be seen on every occasion. Upright films can be helpful here (Fig. IV.1.A13).

An *ultrasound scan* is of obvious help for clinching the diagnosis. Because of the importance of obstruction in the differential diagnosis of unilateral renal failure, ultrasound is almost always the sensible next diagnostic step following the discovery of a large non-excreting kidney on the IVU.

Obstruction is also the commonest cause of unilateral renal failure in childhood. The differential diagnosis of the finding in this age group includes a Wilms' tumour and the multicystic kidney (see section H p. 170). Wilms' tumour is unlikely to be mistaken since there is usually evidence of a mass severely distorting the kidney, i.e. an indented rather than an absent nephrogram/pyelogram. The non-excreting multicystic kidney is a congenital anomaly, probably also based on obstruction as primary disorder. There is an atretic ureter, accompanied by cystic deformity of the kidney. The 'cysts' may in fact represent the 12–20 obstructed calices. Calcification can occur in the kidney, and a renal

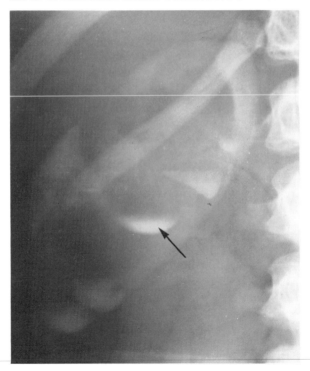

Fig. IV.1.A13 Upright IVU in chronic right renal obstruction. Calices are grossly distended by non-opacified urine. The arrow points to one of several contrast medium/urine fluid levels in this static system.

artery is not identifiable on arteriography. The differentiation of this disorder
from obstruction owing to other causes, e.g. pelvi-ureteric junction obstruction,
can be difficult in the infant. It is an important decision because the multicystic
kidney is harmless. It does not need surgical attention whilst the obstructed
kidney will perish without it. The ultrasound scan of a hydronephrosis is of
course characteristic, with more or less symmetrical communicating fluid-filled
spaces. The cluster of small cysts in a multicystic kidney will not be obviously
communicating, or symmetrical. Renal puncture may well be helpful in the
difficult patient in order to arrive at a certain diagnosis.

6. TUMOUR

A kidney diffusely infiltrated by a renal carcinoma can become largely destroyed without giving rise to alarming symptoms. As in Wilms' tumour, it is
likely that with care something of the distorted renal anatomy will be seen, e.g.
a displaced calix (Fig. IV.1.A14).

Fig. IV.1.A14 The left kidney is almost
entirely replaced by tumour—this is
infiltration rather than a local mass.

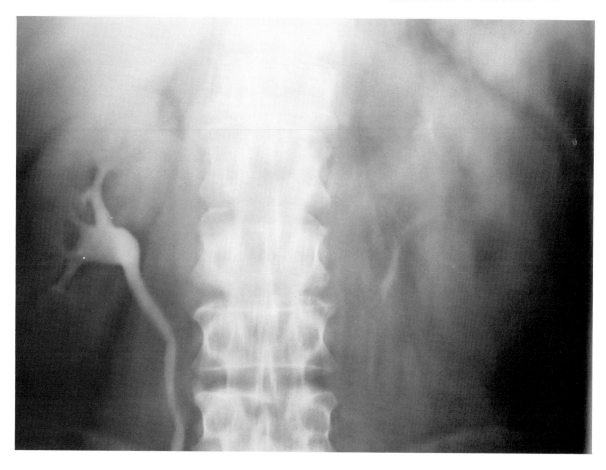

7. COMPRESSION

A kidney compressed by an extrarenal collection may be lit up as a non-excreting problem long after the original event. The past history may then reveal an episode of trauma to explain a lesion such as a subcapsular haematoma. This group of causes can be a common explanation of the non-excreting, unobstructed kidney (Koehler *et al*, 1973).

SUMMARY COMMENT

If there is a non-excreting kidney, look first for an ectopic site, and remember the value of ultrasound scanning.

B. RENAL FAILURE

When a patient first presents with renal failure, the immediate diagnostic problem is whether this could be prerenal (i.e. circulatory) failure. The classical divisions of renal failure are:

a. Prerenal, e.g. salt and water depletion;

b. Renal, e.g. glomerulonephritis;

c. Postrenal, e.g. bilateral ureteric obstruction.

Radiology plays no specific diagnostic part in the first group. Radiologists should recognize this and steer such patients away from the IVU in particular. Hypotension, hypovolaemia or heart failure are conditions to be diagnosed in the initial clinical assessment of the renal failure patient. They are also the very conditions where the IVU may do harm, and make up *contraindications* to the examination. It is a sound general rule that reversible factors in renal failure should be corrected before any patient comes for special radiological examinations.

By contrast the diagnosis of postrenal disorders is a wholly radiological challenge and responsibility. Since urinary tract obstruction is a reversible cause of renal failure, the radiologist cannot sleep quietly till he has diagnosed or excluded this condition in every patient.

The renal parenchymal disorders in the second group (b) of intrinsic renal failure states often do not have distinctive radiological features. This does not mean that radiological studies have no place here: they are vital to proper management of these patients.

Initial radiographs on admission of the renal failure patient

Plain films of the *chest, abdomen* and *hands* are necessary at this stage (not an IVU).

Chest: An important baseline observation in the renal failure patient, often fluid overloaded—pulmonary oedema may mimic almost any chest X-ray abnormality. Lung bleeding in *Goodpasture's syndrome* shows characteristic sequences (Fig. IV.1.B1).

Abdomen: There may be decisive clues here, e.g. bilateral renal stone disease, calcareous papillary necrosis (Fig. IV.1.B2), or bilharzial bladder calcification. Such complete diagnoses are rewarding but uncommon outcomes of the plain film. It is also worthwhile for the renal outlines that can be seen in many patients. An informed guess can then be made whether the kidneys are of normal size.

Hands: Hyperparathyroid (osteitis fibrosa) changes are a reliable but insensitive index of long-standing renal failure, i.e. of chronic rather than acute mischief (Fig. IV.1.B3) (Doyle *et al,* 1972). The importance of this distinction makes a hand X-ray worthwhile at this stage, even if little can be concluded from the normal appearances usually seen in most renal failure patients.

INTRAVENOUS UROGRAPHY

The IVU was thought to be useless and dangerous in renal failure until the early 1960s. Certainly a good pyelogram will not usually be seen. This is irrelevant to the important radiological questions to be answered in renal failure:

1. How large and where are the kidneys?

2. Could they be obstructed?

3. What is the cause of renal failure?

The nephrogram occurring in the great majority of patients having an IVU, however severe their renal failure, is the key to these questions.

Contraindications

Prerenal, correctable uraemic factors, e.g. salt and water depletion, hypotension, hypovolaemia. These are much more important than multiple myeloma, widely feared on the hypothesis that contrast media react with the abnormal urinary protein to form precipitates in the nephron. There is no good evidence to support this mechanism (Saxton, 1969), and inappropriate dehydration before the IVU is the likely culprit accounting for the disasters reported with the investigation. Certainly the indications for the IVU in myeloma should be subjected to particularly searching inquiry, and the examination then carried out under conditions of a known fast diuresis. Performing an IVU in oliguric renal failure in myeloma still appears unwise.

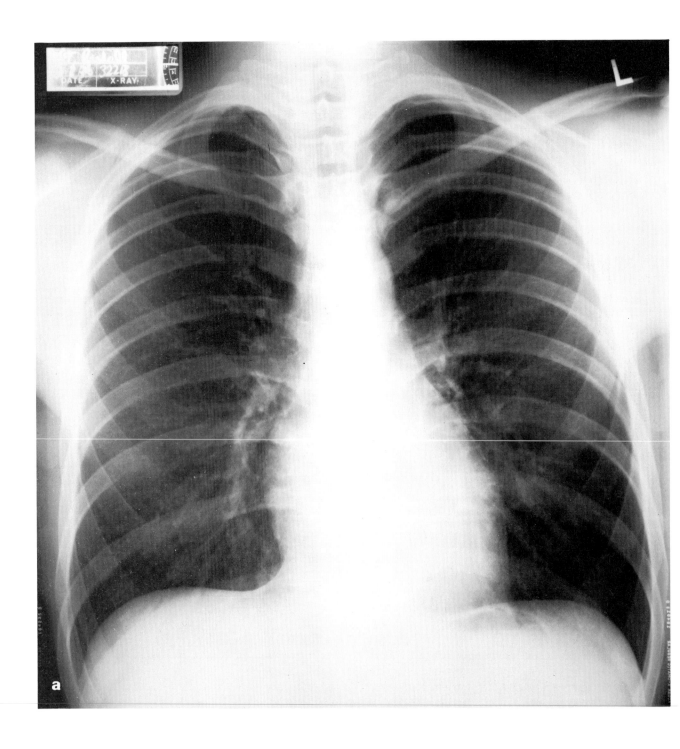

Safety

The possibility of contrast medium reactions exists, as with patients having normal renal function, and needs no further discussion. The confidence that the properly performed IVU offered no additional hazard to the renal failure patient

Fig. IV.1.B1a & b Goodpasture's syndrome—the patient is already bleeding into his lungs on the first film, as determined by labelled carbon monoxide studies, but the picture of florid alveolar shadowing is only seen 24 h later.

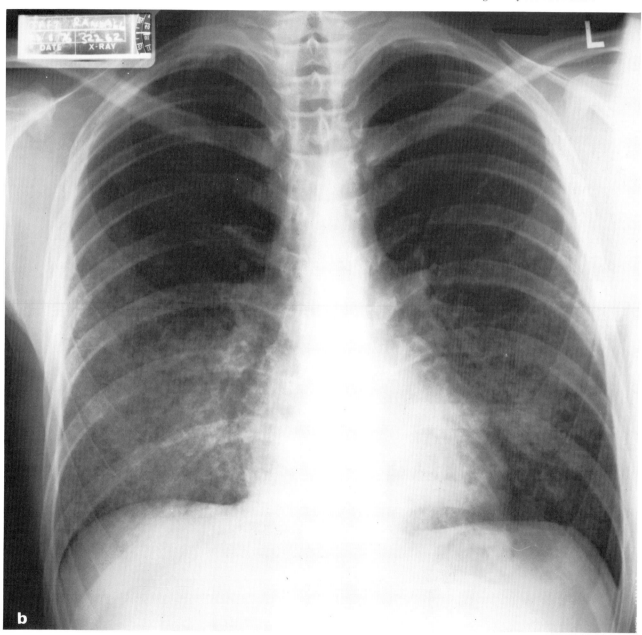

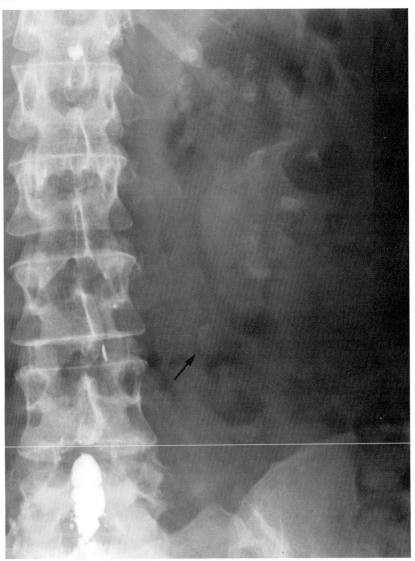

Fig. IV.1.B2 Multiple calcified papillae are seen in this kidney, and one of them has dropped down (arrow), obstructing the ureter. Note the tell-tale myelogram (analgesic abuse).

has been dented a little recently. Studies across the IVU in severe renal impairment had at first suggested that there were no ill effects on the kidney (Davidson *et al*, 1970). This is still broadly true, but certain high risk groups whose kidneys may be further hurt by the IVU have been recognized. The young infant and the adult diabetic patient in renal failure are the outstanding examples. If the clinical value of the radiological information to be gained is considerable, it may outweigh the further risk of the IVU in these patients. These questions always demand joint clinico-radiological discussion over the individual patient.

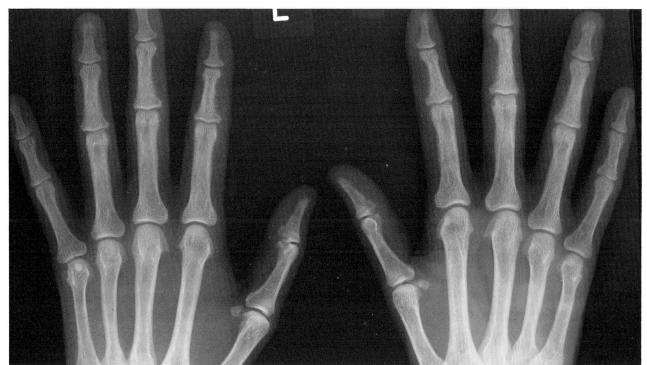

Inappropriate dehydration before the IVU is again the villain to avoid at all cost in these high risk groups.

Fig. IV.1.B3 Chronic renal failure—note erosions on the radial side of the phalanges.

Contrast medium and dose

There are theoretical advantages in keeping the sodium load low by choosing meglumine as the main cation in renal failure, but these are not important in practice. 600 mg iodine per kg body weight of a standard IVU preparation is a common dosage, adopted by a number of centres, doubling the usual dose given to patients with normal renal function (about 300 mg iodine per kg). There is an obvious advantage in keeping to a few standard contrast medium preparations within any one department, so that there is less room for confusion or error.

For a time the way the contrast medium was given was thought rather important, with particular enthusiasts for drip infusion methods. Our understanding now is that it is the contrast medium dose that matters most for producing good IVUs, not the method of administration. Whatever is most convenient and cheap will be best, and this will usually mean simple injection by syringe. There are two reservations to this:

1. If radiographic staff are not familiar with renal failure work, then instilling the contrast medium by drip infusion can provide a certain useful error margin for obtaining the early nephrotomograms. Should these not be perfect at first attempt, they can be repeated whilst the infusion is still running and keeping plasma contrast levels high for the best nephrogram.

2. There is preliminary evidence (Stadalnik *et al,* 1977) that patients with cardiac disease, particularly ischaemia, are at risk from dysrhythmias induced by the large load of contrast medium given in renal failure. It is probably best to give the medium slowly to such patients.

Dehydration

It cannot be too strongly emphasized that fluid deprivation is useless and dangerous in preparing a patient with renal failure for an IVU. There is still sometimes a block about this message at one of the links in the chain organizing IVUs. This chain may involve radiographers, nurses and clerks, and everyone should be clear on this single most important safeguard in renal failure IVU work. In practice anyone with a raised blood urea is best considered in renal failure for this purpose.

Radiographic technique

Tomography and a low kV are essential points for seeing the best possible nephrogram. The skill and interest of radiographers who understand what is at stake are even more important.

The important radiological questions in renal failure

1. How large (and where) are the kidneys?

For the patient admitted in oliguric acute renal failure, the demonstration of normal size or large kidneys spells a potentially reversible disease state. Finding such kidneys is the proper cue for a major diagnostic and therapeutic endeavour to save the patient's nephrons. The nephrogram occurring in the great majority of patients, however severe their renal failure, will therefore be a sign of great importance for correct clinical management.

However, not all patients with long-standing renal disease have small kidneys. Finding kidneys of normal size is therefore no guarantee that renal failure is of recent onset. The two chronic renal failure states particularly likely to mislead, because both kidneys may still be of normal size, are accelerated (malignant) hypertension and chronic glomerulonephritis.

Large kidneys in renal failure are found in polycystic disease, urinary tract obstruction, renal vein occlusion, and renal infiltration, for instance by amyloid. Amyloid kidneys are not always large, however. In the later stages of the disease they shrink (Ekelund, 1977). *Renal vein occlusion* occurring in amyloid kidneys is a good example of the pathway to acute-on-chronic renal failure: an already compromised kidney tipped over the edge into sudden failure by a new insult. It is worth noting again that renal vein occlusion in the adult is almost always secondary to pre-existing renal disease, e.g. amyloid or glomerulonephritis. The argument that renal vein thrombosis might act as the primary insult, bringing about a glomerulonephritis, is unconvincing (Trew *et al,* 1978). This contrasts with renal vein occlusion in the infant which commonly occurs in normal kidneys, precipitated by a systemic insult such as gastroenteritis with dehydration.

The question of *acute arterial occlusion* is considered in section A p. 97—see also Part II section A (p. 45).

Ultrasound is clearly an excellent alternative to the IVU for estimating renal size.

2. Are the kidneys obstructed? (diagram 1)

IVU sequences

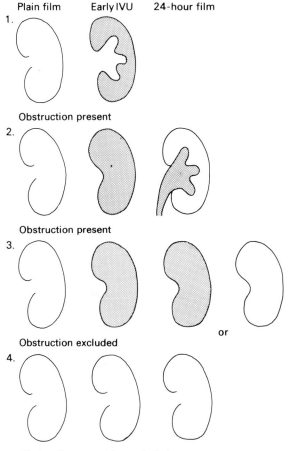

1

The confident exclusion of obstruction is a vital matter in all patients with renal failure. To this end retrograde pyelography used to be the standard approach, and is still practised with advantage by some centres (Kingston *et al*, 1977). The IVU provides so much more useful information that it is at present the investigation of choice. Ultrasound also shows promise in being able to detect the patient with early obstruction—its usefulness in the gross pelvicaliceal distension seen in the later stages of obstruction is not in doubt.

a. The early nephrogram may at once point to the diagnosis of obstruction by outlining large regular radiolucent spaces within the kidney: the dilated, non-opacified calices (Fig. IV.1.B4).

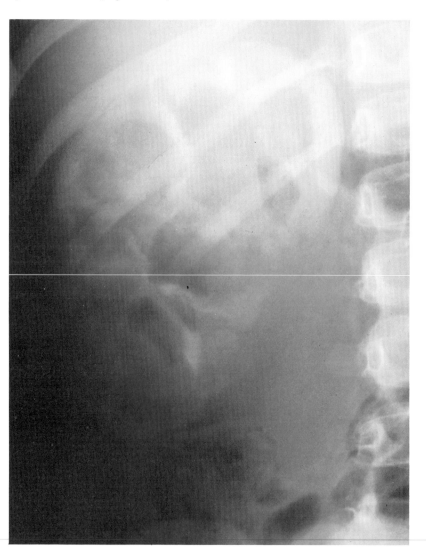

Fig. IV.1.B4   The 'soap bubble' nephrogram of obstruction, outlining non-opacified calices.

b. The early nephrogram may however be homogeneous. Obstruction may still be present, and careful follow-up films up to at least 24 h are needed for its diagnosis or exclusion. Providing enough contrast medium has entered the nephron to produce a nephrogram, then the late films will reveal an obstructive state by outlining opacified dilated renal calices, pelvis or ureter (Fig. IV.1.B5). This is because there is always some onward movement of glomerular filtrate even in severe obstruction, e.g. by lymphatic reabsorption. It is important to note that this reasoning only holds when an early nephrogram has been seen, i.e. the nephron has been sufficiently primed with contrast medium to allow later opacification of collecting structures.

c. If an early nephrogram occurs, and either persists or fades at 24 h with no sign of dilated opacified collecting structures, obstruction can be taken as excluded.

d. If no nephrogram occurs on the early films, there is no chance of having enough contrast medium in the right place to see possibly obstructed urinary collecting structures. This small minority of renal failure patients with no nephrogram is the group which still needs a routine retrograde examination for excluding obstruction.

Fig. IV.1.B5a This chronically obstructed kidney only has a thin rim of parenchyma left, producing a shell nephrogram early on during the IVU (arrows).
Fig. IV.1.B5b Twenty-four hour film—even following such a poor nephrogram, enough contrast medium has now entered the calices to opacify them.

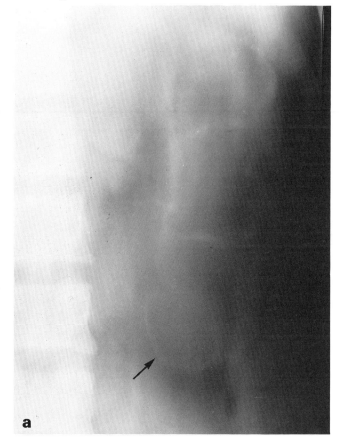

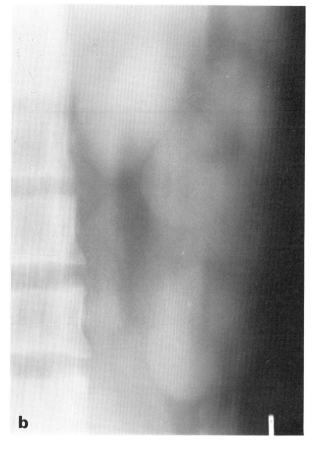

The diagnosis of obstruction as a correctable cause of renal failure is of such great moment to the uraemic patient that it is worth being obsessional about it. This means going on to further studies, i.e. a retrograde or antegrade pyelogram at the slightest suspicion of a questionable IVU. The kidney which becomes obstructed on a background of existing renal disease is a particular worry in this respect, e.g. the patient with renal impairment because of analgesic abuse who obstructs her ureter with a necrotic papilla. An overzealous normal retrograde/antegrade pyelogram carries no dishonour, but to miss the diagnosis of obstruction is a tragedy.

3. Can the nephrogram be used for specific diagnoses?

It is clearly attractive if the nephrogram pattern occurring during the renal failure IVU can be used for arriving at a final diagnosis. An obvious example is the chaotic, patchy nephrogram of polycystic disease (Fig. IV.1.B6). Sudden decrease in the size of one kidney known to be normal previously will point to a main renal artery lesion. Particular attention has been paid to the density/time pattern of the nephrogram, and three common patterns (Fry & Cattell, 1972) are:

a. Immediate faint persistent nephrogram, characteristic of impaired perfusion/-filtration states, e.g. glomerulonephritis.

b. Increasingly dense nephrogram, familiar in acute obstruction (e.g. by a ureteric stone), also seen in acute hypotension and many other states.

c. Immediate distinct persistent nephrogram, characteristically seen in acute renal failure linked with the diagnosis of acute tubular necrosis.

Such divisions make a useful framework for considering nephrograms, but they are far from hard-and-fast rules. Acute tubular necrosis, for instance, most commonly presents an immediate distinct persistent nephrogram, but at least one third of patients show an increasingly dense nephrogram (Fig. IV.1.B7) (Sherwood *et al,* 1974). The nephrogram must therefore be looked at in the clinical setting of any individual patient, not in isolation, if unhappy mistakes are to be avoided.

Small kidneys in renal failure

Rule-of-thumb: In chronic pyelonephritis, IVU changes (scars etc.) are always well in advance of functional renal impairment. In chronic glomerulonephritis such functional impairment is well ahead of any IVU changes (renal shrinkage).

Small kidneys generally point to an end stage in renal failure. This is naturally a depressing finding. With the fight for the patient's nephrons lost, there may be little point in accurate diagnosis of the remaining renal ruins. This is in sharp contrast to the vital drive toward accurate diagnosis demanded by a recoverable renal failure state.

However, correctable factors are worth seeking even in advanced renal failure. The exclusion of obstruction is a particular radiological responsibility.

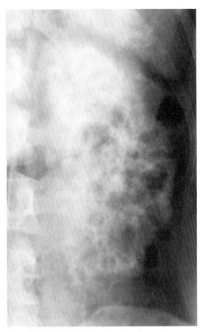

Fig. IV.1.B6 Characteristic nephrogram of polycystic disease.

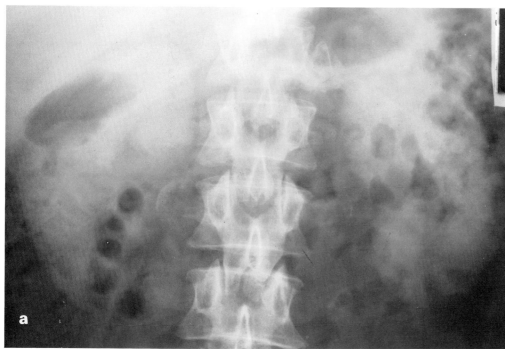

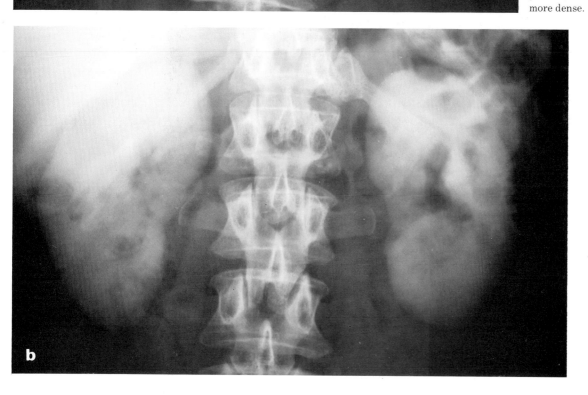

Fig. IV.1.B7a Acute renal failure/acute tubular necrosis—immediate nephrogram on the IVU.
Fig. IV.1.B7b Eighteen hours later, the nephrogram persists, and is notably more dense.

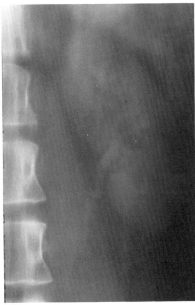
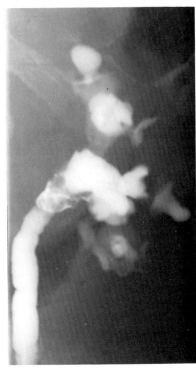

Fig. IV.1.B8 *(left)* Chronic renal failure with glomerular filtration rate below 10 ml/min—enough is seen of the pelvicaliceal system and upper ureter to exclude obstruction.

Fig. IV.1.B9 *(right)* Gross papillary necrosis, with necrotic debris obstructing the ureter (retrograde examination).

This is often quite straightforward on chronic renal failure IVUs, since a pyelogram or uretogram is seen with good radiographic technique (Fig. IV.1.B8). Papillary necrosis is an important example of the chronically impaired kidney thrown into sudden severe failure. Obstructing papillae may lie in both ureters (Fig. IV.1.B9). In such patients there is usually multiple ureteric debris rather than one obstructive papilla. Removal may then return the patient to several years' independent existence.

Hodson (1977) has put forward extremely useful schemes for analysing small kidneys on the IVU, and these have also been advanced independently by Davidson (1977). These authors should be read at source. Three common varieties of the small kidney are:

1. Small kidney with normal IVU architecture, e.g.
   vascular lesion
   chronic glomerulonephritis
   atypical post-obstructive atrophy (rare).

2. Small kidney with uniform papillary deformities and even parenchymal thinning, e.g.
   post-obstructive atrophy
   renal papillary necrosis (late).

3. Small kidney with irregular papillary deformities and uneven parenchymal thinning, e.g.

chronic pyelonephritis
renal papillary necrosis
tuberculosis etc.

Distinctive arteriographic changes are claimed for the common causes of the
endstage kidney (Mena *et al*, 1973). They are of interest, debatable (Davidson &
Talner 1973b), and do not generally contribute to the management of the patient
with chronic renal failure. Polyarteritis nodosa is a spectacular exception (Fig.
IV.1.B10) (see also section K p. 202).

Renal fascia sign

The small kidney shrinks away from the perirenal fascia. This structure may
therefore be seen as a separate sliver surrounding the nephrogram (Fig.
IV.1.B11). This sign can also be helpful on arteriography, since the misnamed

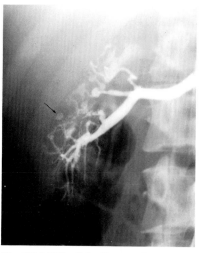

Fig. IV.1.B10 Selective renal
arteriogram with multiple aneurysms in
polyarteritis nodosa (arrow).

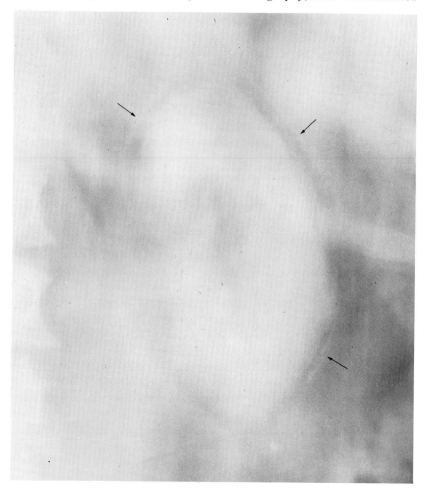

Fig. IV.1.B11 IVU in
glomerulonephritis: the shrinking kidney
has left the perirenal fascia in its normal
site, now discernible as a separate shadow
(arrows). (Courtesy of Dr R. Eban).

capsular arteries are really the perirenal fascia vessels, separating away from the renal parenchymal outline as the kidney shrinks (Meyers *et al*, 1967).

C. HYDRONEPHROSIS

This is a useful if rather vague term. It indicates a dilated pelvi-caliceal system, and is often used to imply a narrow pelvi-ureteric junction as the cause.

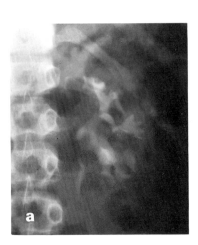 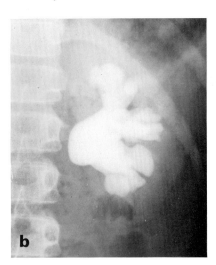

Fig. IV.1.C1a & b This child's left kidney looks normal enough during one examination (a), but on another occasion 3 months later (b), she clearly has a pelvi-ureteric junction obstruction.

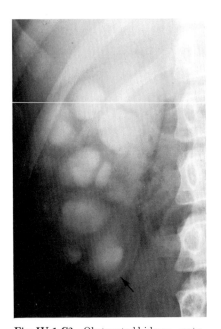

Fig. IV.1.C2 Obstructed kidney—note the caliceal crescent sign (arrow), pointing to stasis in the distorted collecting ducts at the periphery of the calix.

Pelvi-ureteric junction obstruction is a common condition. It may present as a non-excreting kidney in infancy—it is the most frequent cause of such an event. An adult patient may suffer a dramatic onset of loin pain, or may have a long history of intermittent attacks, perhaps precipitated by a large fluid intake (Fig. IV.1.C1). If the IVU is performed during the attack of pain, there is no difficulty with the diagnosis (Fig. IV.1.C2). Indeed, pelvi-ureteric junction obstruction can be most usefully excluded from the differential diagnosis in this way: a normal IVU performed in a patient writhing with loin pain exonerates the urinary tract from blame. The Casualty Officer's IVU (see Division 2 section B) can be very helpful here, for instance in the patient addicted to opiates who has found the simulation of ureteric colic a ready door to his desires.

However, most commonly in suspected pelvi-ureteric junction obstruction the IVU is carried out 'cold', i.e. by appointment and prompted by a history of intermittent loin pain. Occasionally the upper urinary tract can look entirely normal at these times (Fig. IV.1.C3). Such patients are a very particular worry. If clinical suspicion is strong, a diuresis IVU (see Division 2 section D) can be helpful in lighting up a doubtful pelvi-ureteric junction obstruction (Fig. IV.1.C4). Whitfield *et al* (1977) have shown that monitoring the area increase of the renal pelvis during such an IVU is a good way of nailing an obstructive state. Pressure/flow studies at antegrade pyelography may have to be done in

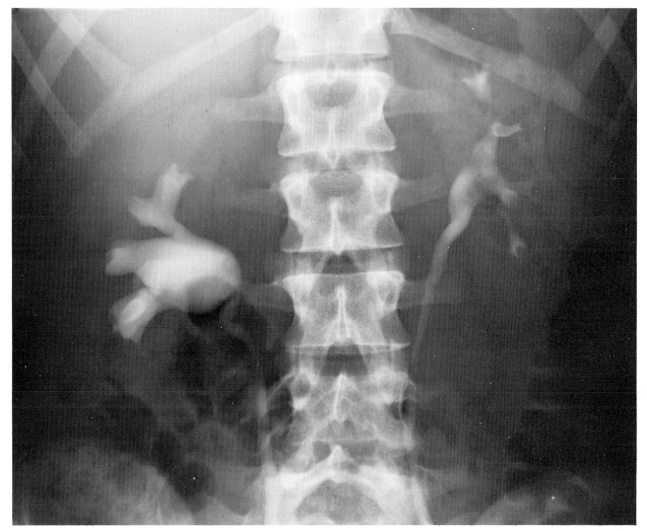

the difficult patient with a doubtful pelvi-ureteric junction whose symptoms suggest an obstruction (Whitaker, 1973). Radioisotope studies show some promise of helping to unravel these difficult problems. The standard renogram is not well suited to this task, and deconvolution techniques are required (Whitfield *et al*, 1977).

The difficulty lies in the distinction between stasis and obstruction (see Division 2 section D). The perfect renal pelvis, with ideal urinary drainage from the kidney to the ureter, is a funnel-shaped muscular organ which merges into the upper ureter. The two behave as one structural and functional unit, with no way of telling where one ends and the other begins (diagram 2A). Not all renal

Fig. IV.1.C3 The right renal pelvis may look a little full during this IVU, but the ureter fills readily enough, and there is no pain.

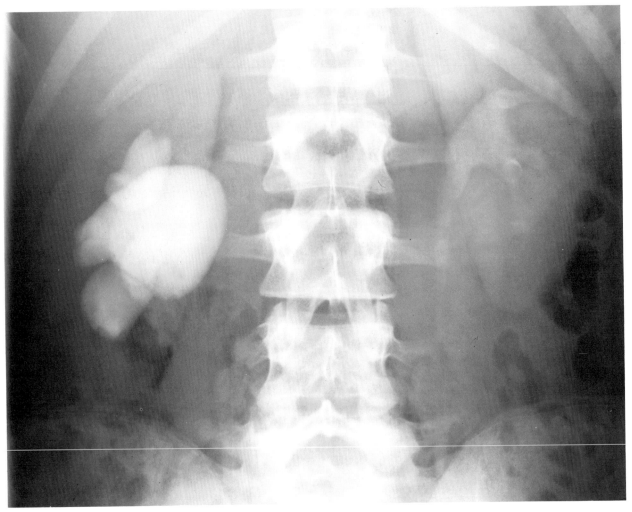

Fig. IV.1.C4 Same patient as in Fig. IV.1.C3, but after the injection of an intravenous diuretic—the left kidney has washed out its contrast medium very satisfactorily, but an obvious pelvi-ureteric junction obstruction has been precipitated on the right.

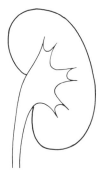

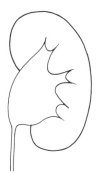

2A   **2B**

pelves are like this. Many have a distinct take-off for the ureter, and clearly do not behave as a single structural/functional unit (diagram 2B). Such renal pelves are part of the normal spectrum, given to less than perfect emptying and to mild urinary stasis, of no importance to the nephron population or the patient's comfort. The pelvi-ureteric junction obstruction problem begins when this variant crosses the boundary into the pathological, and the diagnostic difficulty is to define this line (see Division 2 section D).

D. UROTHELIAL TUMOURS

Filling defects in the upper urinary tract may be urothelial tumours (Fig. IV.1.D1). Haematuria may have been the presenting symptom to raise particular suspicion on this score. Or the IVU may be following up a patient with a bladder tumour, at special risk from new upper tract tumours.

Radiolucent filling defects in the pelvi-caliceal system or upper ureter may be:

    extrinsic impressions
    urothelial tumours

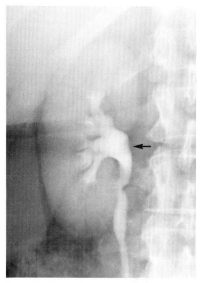

Fig. IV.1.D1 A small urothelial tumour is present in the right renal pelvis (arrow). This patient's antegrade pyelogram is illustrated in Part I Fig. I.5.

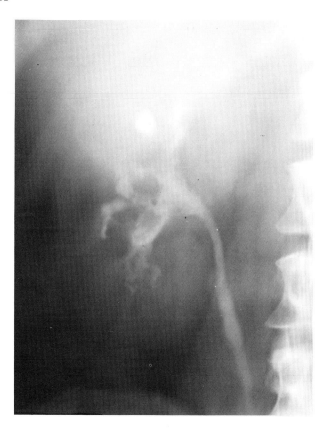

Fig. IV.1.D2 Malacoplakia—note multiple filling defects in the pelvicaliceal system.

radiolucent stones
blood clot
necrotic papillae
pelvi-ureteritis cystica
infective material, e.g. fungus
infiltrations, e.g. leucoplakia, malacoplakia, amyloid.

How to tell them apart? Uncommon lesions like *malacoplakia* (Fig. IV.1.D2) or *amyloid* hardly deserve further consideration. They will only be diagnosed with confidence by the pathologist, implying an exploratory operation and at least partial resection. Amyloid in the renal pelvis may calcify.

Fungus balls or other infective material is to be expected only in diabetics.

Pelvi-ureteritis cystica is a more frequent problem. The usual explanation of this interesting condition of multiple small fluid-filled blebs in the upper urinary tract is past inflammation. Gross infection may indeed accompany these lesions. But pelvi-ureteritis cystica is now commonly discovered as a chance finding

Fig. IV.1.D3 Pelvi-ureteritis cystica—note multiple filling defects in both upper urinary tracts (arrow). This patient has never had a urinary infection—she has a uterine carcinoma.

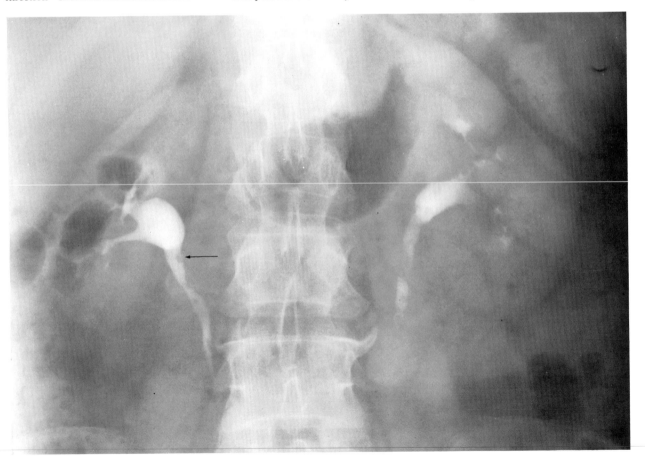

(Fig. IV.1.D3). Regular radiolucent spheres, half projecting into the ureteric lumen (the other half in the wall) are the characteristic signs (Fig. IV.1.D4). Diagnosis from multiple urothelial tumours can be difficult on occasion.

Necrotic papillae will be accompanied by tell-tale caliceal changes; the condition is further discussed in section G p. 146.

Blood clot presents very real difficulty in differential diagnosis. It may simulate urothelial tumour very closely, and is an obvious diagnostic problem in the patient presenting with haematuria (Fig. IV.1.D5). A changing picture because of clot moving about is the most helpful sign, but difficult to obtain during any single examination. A retrograde ureterogram is often arranged to try to unscramble the filling defect, but a follow-up IVU 1–2 weeks after the initial examination can also be very helpful. If the defect continues absolutely unchanged, the suspicion of tumour will naturally harden. Cytology of the urine, looking for the abnormal cells commonly shed by urothelial tumours, is very helpful here. Brushing such lesions with a steerable ureteric catheter for obtaining material for cytology has been described (Gill *et al*, 1973), but is not practised widely.

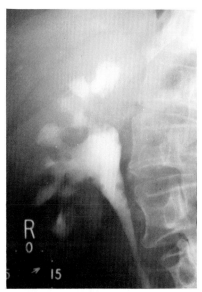

Fig. IV.1.D4 Multiple cysts in the renal pelvis—chance finding in a man complaining of bladder outflow obstruction.

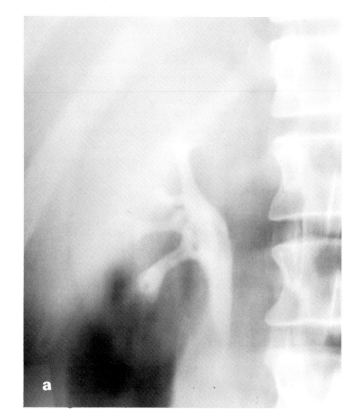

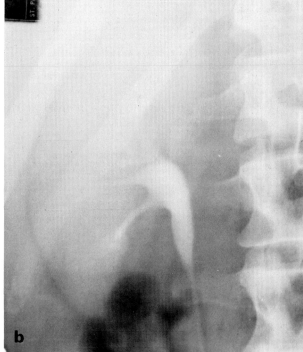

Fig. IV.1.D5a A number of filling defects are present in the right renal pelvis of this man suffering from haematuria. They are clots.

Fig. IV.1.D5b Several weeks later the pyelogram is back to normal.

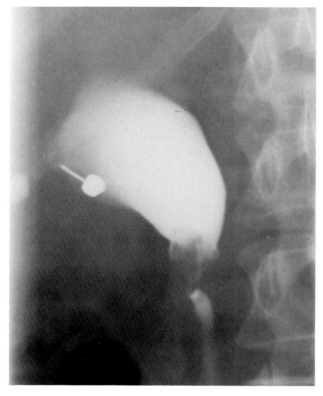

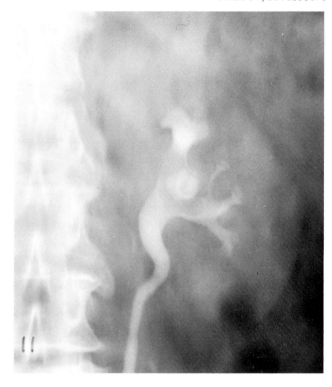

Fig. IV.1.D6 *(above left)* A large lesion is clearly obstructing the pelvi-ureteric junction, demonstrated by an antegrade pyelogram. Although this man has already had a bladder tumour, and is therefore at risk from new urothelial growths, his story is now of pain and urinary infection. This was a non-opaque stone.

Radiolucent stones do not generally cause difficulty in diagnosis from tumours. A large uric acid or matrix stone linked with pain or urinary infection makes up a different clinico-radiological picture to the urothelial tumour problem (Fig. IV.1.D6). However, misdiagnoses can certainly occur here (Fig. IV.1.D7).

Fig. IV.1.D7 *(above right)* The large non-opaque filling defect in this symptom-free woman was thought to be a probable tumour, but it was a stone.

Fig. IV.1.D8 *(right)* Non-excreting left kidney presenting with 1 week's haematuria—a large renal pelvis tumour is present (arrow). This infiltrated the kidney extensively, and must have been growing for a long time. Note contrast medium backflow into the tumour at this retrograde examination (pyelo-tumour backflow).

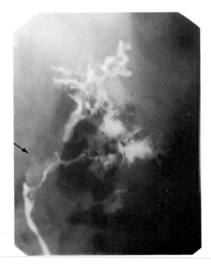

Fig. IV.1.D9 *(facing page—top)* Prone film during an antegrade pyelogram, to show the urothelial tumour invading the upper calices.

Fig. IV.1.D10a & b *(facing page—bottom)* Serial IVUs done because of a bladder tumour. The kidney appears normal enough at first, but the arrow points to a caliceal deformity which was the first sign of the tumour obvious on the later film.

Urothelial tumours

Whilst haematuria is the expected presentation of these lesions, they can be quite silent until they reach large size (Fig. IV.1.D8). Most characteristically they produce irregular filling defects in the renal calices, pelvis or ureter. If the significance of a suspicious defect is unclear on the IVU, a retrograde pyelo-ureterogram can be helpful, and will also offer a chance of collecting urine from that side for cytological studies. The difficult filling defect can often benefit from careful examination by multiple projections, e.g. prone films (Fig. IV.1.D9).

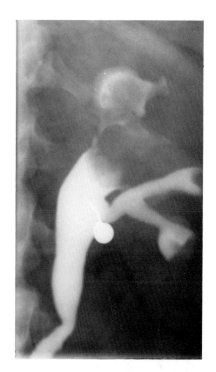

Recurrent urothelial tumours

Bladder carcinoma can be regarded as overt neoplastic disease in just one part of a potentially unstable urothelium. Such patients are more likely to develop new primary urothelial tumours in the upper urinary tract than the population at large, even after successful treatment of the bladder lesion. New pelvicaliceal tumours can be hard to diagnose, even on careful follow-up of these patients (Fig. IV.1.D10). The desirable frequency of follow-up examinations is under debate at present, since only a small minority of patients with bladder cancer run into upper urinary tract tumour problems. There is the hope that cytological and tumour immunological studies will be able to pinpoint patients at special risk, so that this minority can be selected for repeated IVU follow-up.

Extrinsic impressions (see section G)

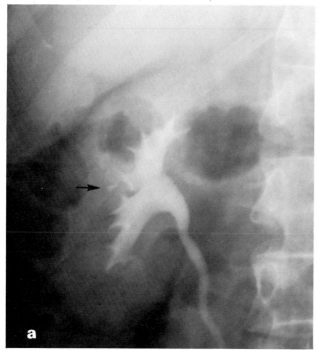

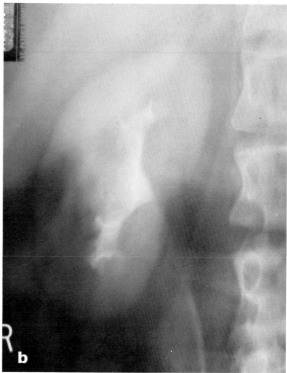

E. STONES

Concretions within the pelvi-caliceal system are classically renal stones; 'nephrocalcinosis' is best reserved for calculi, however big or small, lying within the renal substance (medulla or cortex).

Most renal stones are radio-opaque, and therefore the plain film is all-important in making or excluding this diagnosis. Additional plain views will often be needed to sort out whether an opacity seen on the first film is intrarenal or not. It is essential that this decision is made by adequate plain films before contrast medium is given: the problem will not be resolved by contrast films. Plain tomograms can help with the difficult case.

Type of stone

1. Radiodense

Much ingenuity and effort sometimes goes into guessing what the renal stone is made of. The accuracy of such guessing is poor. The vast majority of stones are dense because of their calcium content; this goes for the common infected mixed stone as well as for a pure calculus like calcium oxalate. The more jagged shape of the latter ('mulberry stone') is occasionally a useful distinguishing mark.

2. Poorly radiodense

Cystine stones, visible on radiographs owing to their sulphur content, are the example usually cited here. Cystinuria, however, is a very rare metabolic disorder. Of greater everyday importance is the problem of the poorly calcified infective stone largely made up of *matrix* material. Matrix stones have a protein base, and may be wholly radiolucent. They are always associated with urinary infection, often involving proteus (see Fig. IV.2.B4).

3. Radiolucent

Uric acid and *matrix* stones are the most common in this group. Uric acid stones can be treated with remarkable success by alkalinizing the urine (Fig. IV.1.E1). Other causes of apparent radiolucent stones need to be remembered, particularly necrotic papillae (see section D p. 119).

Causes

Passing too much calcium in the urine ('idiopathic hypercalciuria') and infection are the common background to patients forming stones in this country. Dehydration is an important cause in hotter countries. Metabolic causes are always worth excluding in anyone presenting with a renal stone, but a detailed consideration of such causes is outside the useful scope of the radiologist.

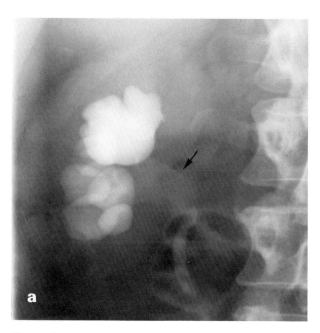

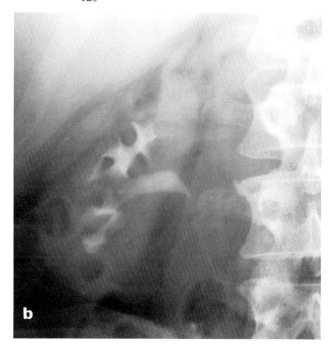

Clinical presentation

Most stones probably come to light as the result of pain, but this presentation is now closely followed by urinary infection. They may be chance findings on IVUs performed for other reasons, and may even produce painless haematuria as their first clinical sign. Infection and haematuria are particularly important in children with renal stones.

Clinical significance of size and site

Renal stones might be divided arbitrarily into three major groups:

1. The small caliceal stone

This finding may be a useful explanation of a patient's haematuria (having excluded a bladder carcinoma), or a sequel to having already passed a stone from that kidney. Biochemical screening will have to be done to exclude a treatable metabolic disorder. Beyond this, there is usually little cause for clinical alarm. Patients with small caliceal stones are unlikely to come to harm. They need to be followed up with plain films at long intervals to make sure a stone is not growing. They will of course have to be advised about the painful possibility of passing the stone down the ureter. Surgical removal of small caliceal stones is difficult, and not indicated in the absence of pressing symptoms. This thinking does not necessarily apply to children, where the growing kidney is at risk from infection.

Fig. IV.1.E1a A large non-opaque stone is present in the right renal pelvis (arrow). This was a uric acid stone treated conservatively with sodium bicarbonate alone.

Fig. IV.1.E1b Three months later the stone has disappeared.

2. The obstructive renal stone

Quite small stones may become impacted in the pelvi-ureteric junction, or indeed anywhere along the ureter. Management of the small stone which has already passed through most of the length of the ureter before it becomes obstructive may well be conservative on a cautious wait-and-see basis. By contrast the stone impacting in the renal pelvis/upper ureter will usually demand early surgery.

Impaction in caliceal necks is not a common clinical problem, probably because it is painless. Caliceal neck strictures are a theoretical hazard of caliceal stones. Calices harbouring stones are often distorted (ballooned), but the stones remain freely mobile within them. Localized renal atrophy is the likely explanation.

3. Large or growing renal stones

The staghorn calculus (Fig. IV.1.E2) is the best example of the large harmful

Fig. IV.1.E2 Large staghorn calculus in the left kidney.

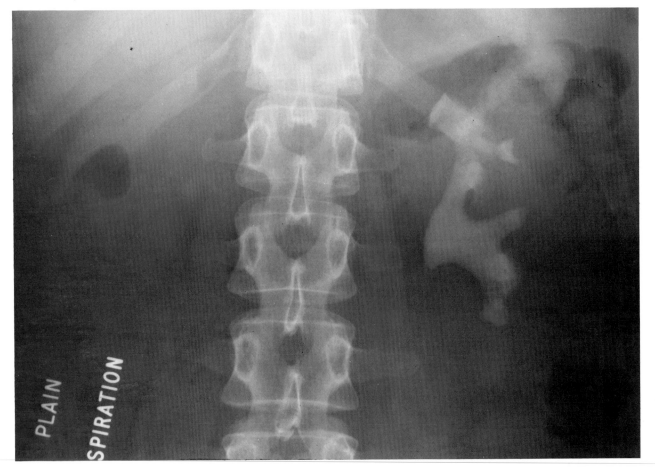

renal stone. Its name derives from the branching shape of these stones as they become casts of the whole pelvi-calciceal system. Such giant growths may be quite silent clinically, but there is no doubt that they are a bad thing. They threaten not only the survival of this kidney, but of the patient (Singh *et al*, 1973). The individual with a staghorn calculus carries a renal time bomb which may blow up into a pyonephrosis. He needs skilled surgical advice. Careful plain film follow-up of smaller stones is done in order to catch the growing calculus which will require surgical interference, well before it has become too large.

Summary comment

Renal stones are common and potentially very serious afflictions. The radiologist can play a vital part in their proper management, and contribute enormously to patients' well being. Failing over a rare, small-print diagnosis may do no more than bruise the radiologist's ego, but missing a large renal stone because of inattention to the plain film means a human and professional disaster (Fig. IV.1.E3).

Fig. IV.1.E3 This is the IVU of the patient illustrated in Fig. IV.1.E2. If a look at the plain film had been omitted, the large stone would have been missed—it is now obscured by contrast medium.

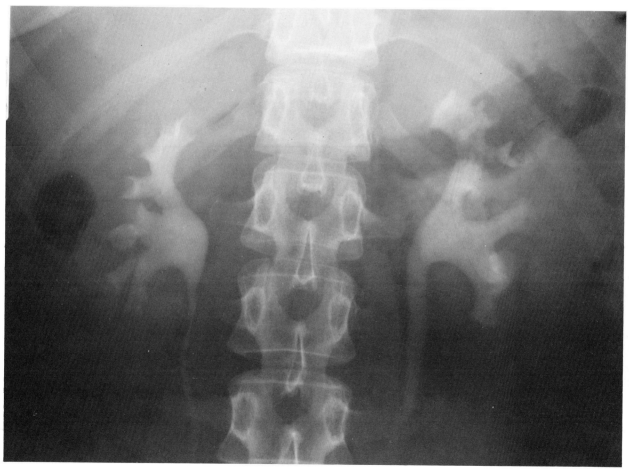

F. NEPHROCALCINOSIS

This term sensibly means calcification within solid renal territory (cortex or medulla). When looking through the microscope there may be some point in semantic quibbles whether parenchymal nephrocalcinosis (as in hyperparathyroidism) is something different from concretions in abnormal collecting ducts (medullary sponge kidney). For the practical radiologist there is no value whatever in such nitpicking: the radiological eye sees a patient with nephrocalcinosis on the plain film, and the problem is to sort out what is the underlying disorder. The attraction of the radiological diagnosis of nephrocalcinosis is that good detective work will make sense of the great majority of these patients, as between well-defined disease groups. This is in contrast to finding calcium in the pelvi-caliceal system (renal stones) where the final answer is all too often 'we don't know' (or 'idiopathic hypercalciuria' in Latin/Greek).

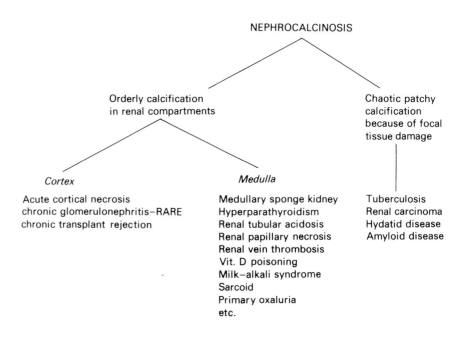

A suggested scheme for thinking about nephrocalcinosis is given. The essential initial distinction is between orderly calcification in anatomical renal compartments, usually in the medulla, and the chaotic calcium found on a focal damage basis, e.g. in tuberculosis. Orderly medullary nephrocalcinosis is much the most common form seen. The list of causes even here is intimidating, but in fact the top three diseases account for about 70% of all patients, and are the only ones worth considering in detail here. For a fuller discussion, see Wrong & Feest (1976).

Medullary sponge kidney

This is a structural disorder of the terminal nephron: the collecting ducts are dilated. Because of this, concretions tend to form within them, presumably because of urinary pooling, though a third of patients with this condition are also said to have hypercalciuria, i.e. a metabolic abnormality. It is clearly possible to have an early sponge kidney with no nephrocalcinosis.

The condition is most commonly bilateral, but can be unilateral (Fig. IV.1.F1). Indeed, only part of one kidney may be involved, with the remainder perfectly healthy (Fig. IV.1.F2).

Nephrocalcinosis in this disease is naturally on a medullary pattern, i.e. the site of the collecting duct. Some authorities imply that because of this, a diagnosis can be reached on the plain film alone, but this notion does not stand up to critical examination—the plain film of other medullary calcification patterns, e.g. in renal tubular acidosis, can be identical.

Fig. IV.1.F1a & b Plain film (a—*below*) and IVU (b—*overpage*) in right medullary sponge kidney. See also Fig. IV.1.F3. Note post-obstructive folds in right renal pelvis—this patient had suffered ureteric obstruction in the past.

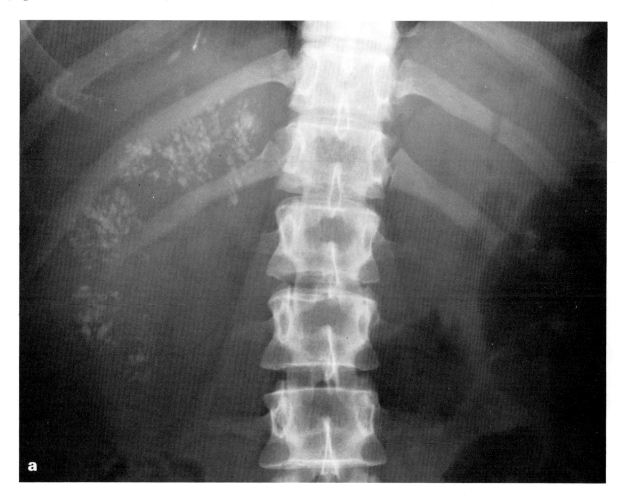

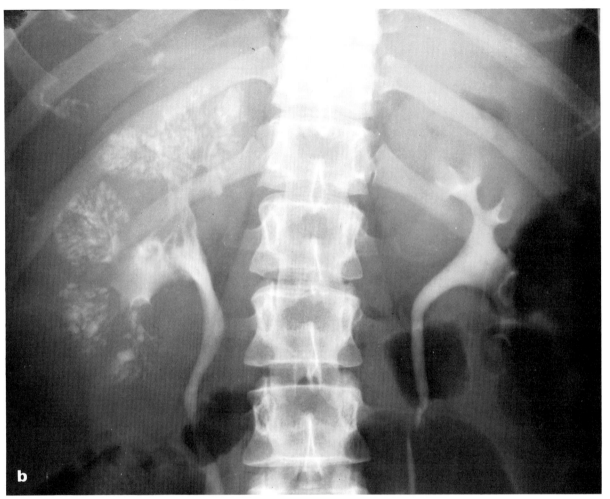

The key sign in making the diagnosis is the demonstration of the dilated collecting duct. The contrast film will therefore show additional medullary abnormalities to those of the nephrocalcinosis on the plain film: contrast medium spills around the concretions (Fig. IV.1.F3). In short, there are more medullary blobs on the contrast film than on the plain film.

With this guide, the diagnosis is usually straightforward. Care is needed to distinguish the coarse, discrete streaks of the abnormal collecting ducts from the phenomenon of 'papillary blushing'. In current large dose urography practice, it is not uncommon to see diffuse, homogeneous opacification of normal papillae—this is after all the area of final urinary concentration (Fig. IV.1.F4). The uniformity of the picture is quite different from the streaky sponge kidney.

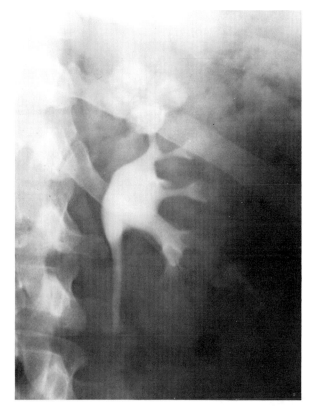

Fig. IV.1.F2 Localized medullary sponge kidney at the left upper renal pole only.

Clinical significance

Medullary sponge kidney disease is now quite often a chance IVU finding. Many patients do not come to harm with their sponge kidneys. Some will have repeated painful episodes of ureteric colic. A very few will have severe disability because of pain and perhaps renal parenchymal destruction by mammoth nephrocalcinosis—I have seen a patient die as a result of severe disease. The diagnosis is of value as an explanation of symptoms, and as a guide to management—a large fluid intake is to be encouraged as a lifelong measure.

Associations

Skeletal hemi-hypertrophy is a rare accompaniment (Fig. IV.1.F5). It need not imply unilateral sponge kidney, and indeed can occur on the opposite side to a unilateral renal disorder.

Infantile polycystic disease can give rise to a sponge kidney picture on the IVU. The usual clinical background is a child with only mild cystic disease who has been able to survive well into the first or even second decade of life because of this fact. The effects of hepatic changes (fibrosis) then begin to dominate the clinical picture. The renal changes are mild in the sense that only a fraction of nephrons are affected—these dilated structures are responsible for the coarse, sponge-kidney-like features on the IVU (see Fig. IV.1.H13).

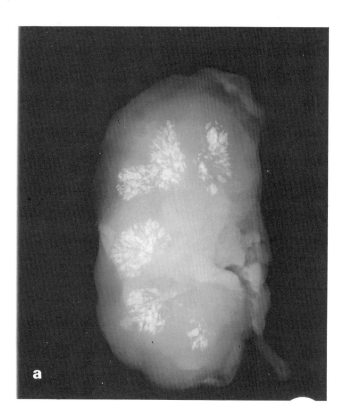
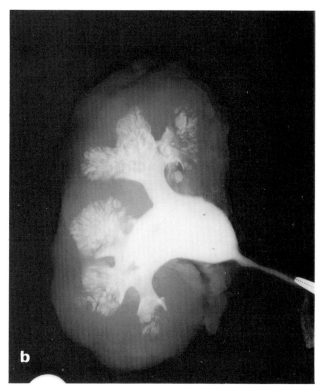

Fig. IV.1.F3a & b Plain film (a) and retrograde contrast injection (b) after removal of the kidney shown in Fig. IV.1.F1. Note that contrast flows around the concretions in the dilated collecting ducts.

The rare *EMG syndrome* (exomphalos, macroglossia, gigantism) also shows a sponge kidney appearance on the IVU. Variants of this syndrome exist where the odd facies are accompanied by a sponge kidney picture which does not ring quite true, some contrast spaces looking like multiple caliceal diverticula.

These variations are all rare, and should not be allowed to detract from the

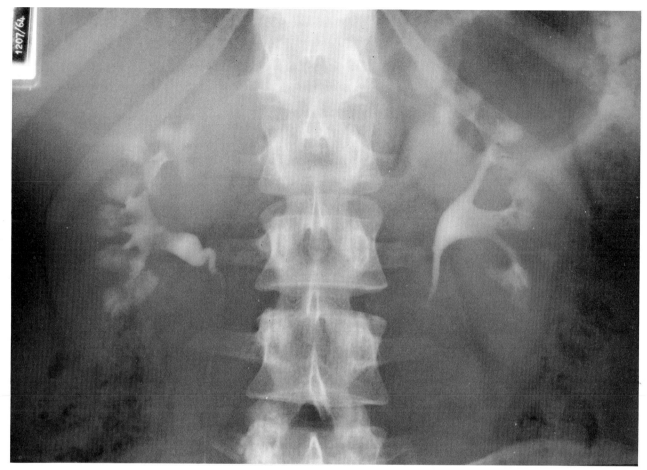

generally straightforward diagnosis and management of simple medullary sponge kidneys.

Fig. IV.1.F4 Homogeneous blushing of papillae during the IVU—a normal finding.

Primary hyperparathyroidism

This is usually held to be the commonest cause of nephrocalcinosis. It is of medullary pattern (Fig. IV.1.F6). It is worth noting that primary hyperparathyroidism may itself give rise to renal failure in time, and so renal shrinkage may be observed in this condition.

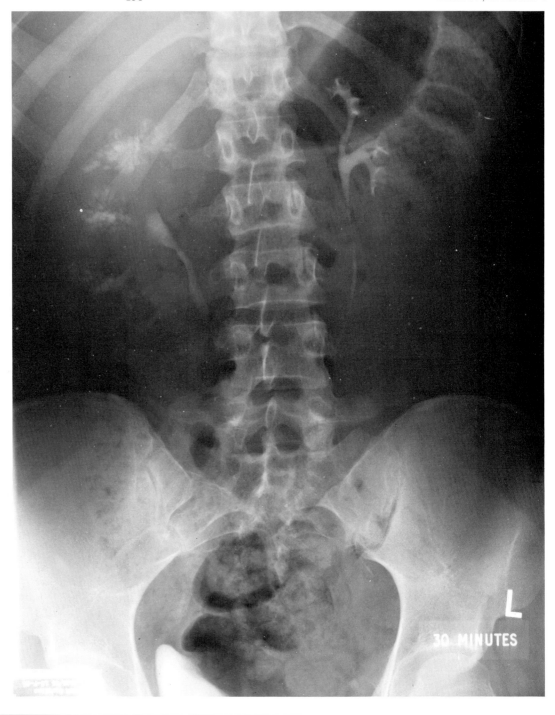

Fig. IV.1.F5 *(facing page)* Right
medullary sponge kidney—there is also
hemihypertrophy of the whole right side.

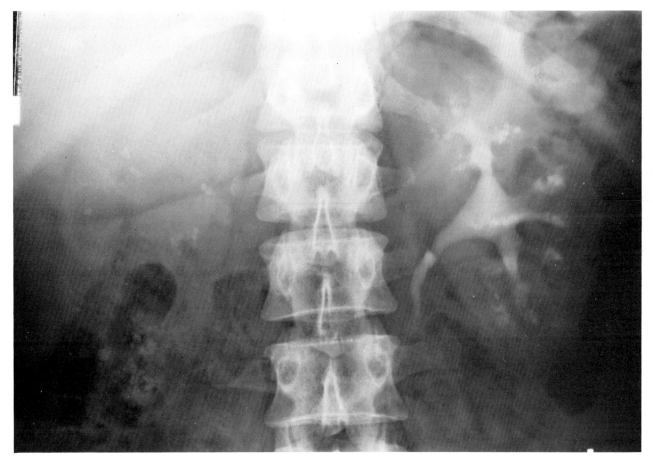

Fig. IV.1.F6 Hyperparathyroidism with
extensive medullary calcification. On this
IVU the right kidney is severely
obstructed by stones in the lower right
ureter.

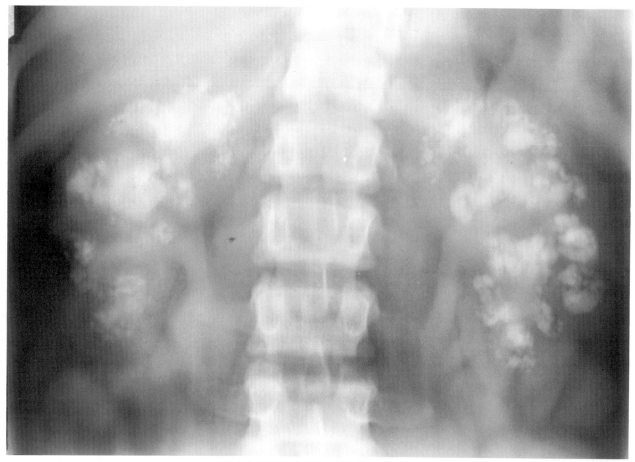

Fig. IV.1.F7 Renal tubular acidosis—IVU showing widespread medullary calcification.

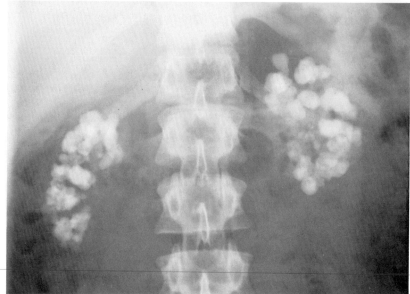

Fig. IV.1.F8 Plain film in oxaluria.

Renal tubular acidosis

The congenital, not the acquired, form of this disorder is accompanied by nephrocalcinosis (Fig. IV.1.F7). There is nothing distinctive about this medullary pattern, but it is sometimes found together with rather large calculi, also seen in oxaluria (Fig. IV.1.F8).

Renal papillary necrosis

Calcification of necrotic papillae presents as nephrocalcinosis because they

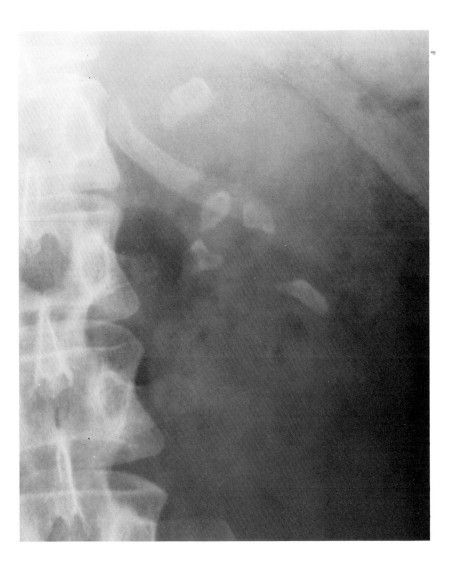

Fig. IV.1.F9 Multiple calcified, necrotic papillae—note odd shapes and radiolucent centres.

may remain in place, i.e. are not shed. The triangular shape and dense rim of calcareous papillae are distinctive (Fig. IV.1.F9).

Renal cortical necrosis

Classically this is a sequel to an obstetric disaster—ante-partum haemorrhage

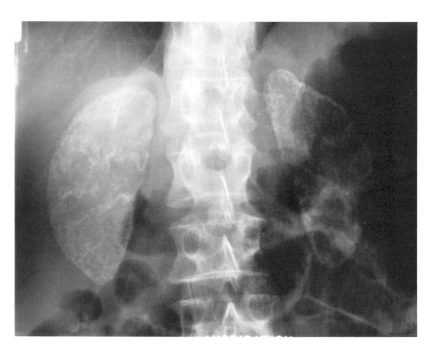

Fig. IV.1.F10   Bilateral cortical necrosis—plain film.

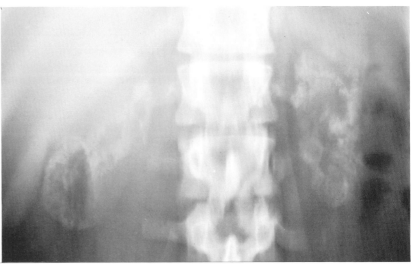

Fig. IV.1.F11   Late stage of cortical necrosis, with severely shrunken kidneys, 1 year ago this patient suffered a severe accident with hypotension, followed by acute renal failure.

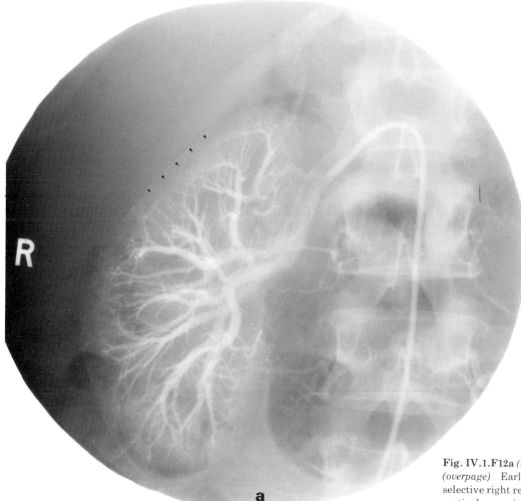

a

Fig. IV.1.F12a *(left)* **& b**
(overpage) Early and late frames from a
selective right renal arteriogram in acute
cortical necrosis (ante-partum
haemorrhage). Note the ischaemic renal
cortex (arrowheads) (see also Fig.
IV.1.A11).

(Fig. IV.1.F10). Because the calcification involves the whole renal cortex, it will
be projected on the two-dimensional radiograph as a kidney which is dense
throughout. Where the cortex is seen in profile as the renal rim, calcification
will appear still more dense. A 'tramline' effect of two parallel calcareous lines
projected along this cortical rim may rarely be seen.

   This classical presentation is not the only path to cortical necrosis. It is
probable that this state can also come about as the severe, irrecoverable end of
the spectrum of acute renal failure, then dubbed acute tubular necrosis (Fig.
IV.1.F11). Angiography can be particularly helpful when this diagnosis is
suspected. The ischaemic cortex is seen as a zone of diminished perfusion in
irrecoverable cortical necrosis (Fig. IV.1.F12).

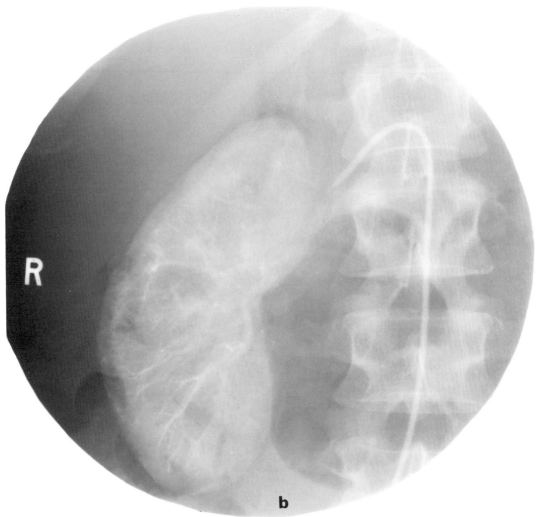

G. HURT CALICES/PAPILLAE

The emphasis on study of the pelvi-caliceal system during the IVU is reflected by
the former term 'pyelogram'. It has given way to understanding the additional
importance of the nephrogram as a vivid, direct demonstration of renal parenchyma. Similarly, the calix can be regarded as a window through which to look
in on another vital renal structure—the renal papilla. Calices are inverse
images of papillae, and it is helpful to be dominated by the idea of a cup-and-egg
calix/papilla relationship when judging calices on the IVU.

The deformed calix is a frequent radiological problem on the IVU. 'Clubbed calix' for a balloon-like deformity is a favourite term, and there is sometimes a temptation to equate this expression with the diagnosis of chronic pyelonephritis. This section attempts to put the hurt calix seen on the IVU into a practical diagnostic framework (Table IV.1.1).

Table IV.1.1

Deformed/destroyed calix/papilla
    Chronic pyelonephritis
    Renal papillary necrosis $\begin{cases} \text{total} \\ \text{partial} \\ \textit{in situ} \end{cases}$
    Tuberculosis

Ballooned calix with narrow neck
    Stricture $\begin{cases} \text{tuberculosis} \\ \text{calculus} \end{cases}$
    Extrinsic impression by artery
    Hydrocalicosis

Ballooned calix with wide neck
    Post-obstructive atrophy
    Megacalices
    Polycalicosis

DEFORMED/DESTROYED CALICES

Chronic pyelonephritis (see also Division 2 section C)

The work of John Hodson looms large over this topic, as indeed over so much of renal radiology. Thanks to him there is now general agreement that the diagnosis of chronic pyelonephritis is to be made on quite specific radiological signs, and offers a meeting ground between clinician, microbiologist, pathologist and radiologist. We are concerned with a *patchy renal disease of predictable distribution*. The hallmark of chronic pyelonephritis is the linear scar developing across the renal medulla and cortex. It will pull at the calix to deform it into a clubbed shape, and may also indent the renal outline. We can sometimes follow the development of the pyelonephritic scar in the growing kidney (Fig. IV.1.G1). Scarring occurs at the upper renal poles first and foremost. When the condition is seen in the adult, we are looking at the scars of battles waged long ago in childhood: in the absence of gross derangements of ureteric drainage, pyelonephritic scarring does not occur beyond childhood. Compensatory hypertrophy of surviving normal islands of parenchyma in the badly scarred kidney may give rise to marked deformities (Fig. IV.1.G2).

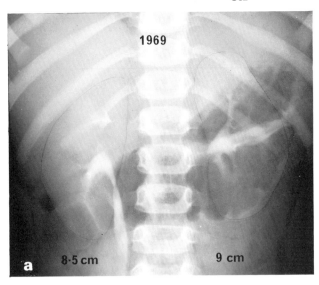

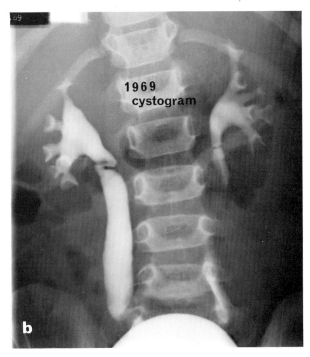

Fig. IV.1.G1a   Normal IVU in a young
child with urinary infections.
Fig. IV.1.G1b   The cystogram shows
bilateral reflux, worse on the right.
Fig. IV.1.G1c   Two years later there is a
characteristic scar deforming the
uppermost calix in the right upper renal
pole. Note that this kidney has not grown
in the interval.

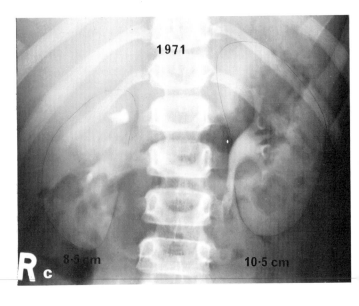

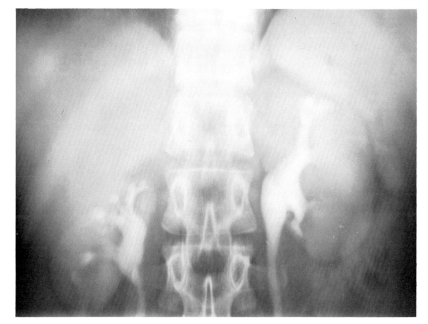

Fig. IV.1.G2 Small scarred right kidney, and also scarring at the left upper renal pole. Overgrowth of the remaining normal parts of the left kidney, with apparent deformity.

Rules of thumb

1. In adults the onset of renal infection ('pyelonephritis') is a florid clinical presentation, but there is no subsequent scarring.

2. In infants and small children urinary infection is either silent, or presents as unexplained fever, vomiting, or failure to thrive. Renal scarring may occur. It is usually already established by the time the child comes to have an X-ray, and does not progress further.

3. A proven urinary infection in a child is a good indication for radiological studies, but this is not so in adults.

Vesico-ureteric reflux will be considered in Division 2 section C. That there is a connection between reflux and pyelonephritic scarring has been accepted for some time, but many questions about the precise relationship between the two remained unanswered. Particular puzzles have been:

1. Why are the scars predominantly at the upper renal poles?

2. Why do only some children with reflux develop scars?

3. What is the importance of infection in the reflux/scarring story?

The work of Hodson *et al* (1975) and of Ransley and Risdon (1978) has illuminated these problems in a remarkable way. They have shown that intrarenal reflux is a key event, i.e. reflux not only from the bladder into the pelvi-caliceal system, but onward into the nephron via the collecting ducts opening on the renal papilla (see Fig. I.13). Papillary shape is all important in determining intrarenal reflux. Complex fused papillae are those that allow this reflux to occur, whilst simple conical papillae do not. Scars are seen predominantly at the upper renal poles because that is where we have fused papillae. About a third of children have no refluxing papillae at all, and in them vesico-ureteric reflux, however severe, will not be followed by scarring. It does not look as if sterile intrarenal reflux on its own causes scarring—it is infection, introduced into the renal lobe by reflux, which sets up a renal lobar pneumonia leading on to scarring.

In the adult, characteristic 'childhood' pyelonephritic scarring generally arises only with gross disorders of ureteric drainage, e.g. in ureteric diversion, particularly in uretero-colic anastomosis, and in the neuropathic bladder (Fig. IV.1.G3).

Whilst the characteristic scar dominates the picture of kidney damage, two other forms of renal insult need to be considered in chronic pyelonephritis. Uniform caliceal distension and renal atrophy is sometimes seen, very reminiscent of the obstructive atrophy kidney (Hodson *et al*, 1975). Whether repeated high pressure reflux waves alone could cause this is questionable—transformation of non-refluxing into refluxing papillae, with consequent widespread scarring (Ransley & Risdon, 1975), is a possible explanation. There is also a strong clinical impression, supported by scarce individual cases (Fig. IV.1.G4), that the kidney affected by severe reflux may not grow normally, even when infection is

Fig. IV.1.G3a Normal right kidney in a young adult with ureteric diversion.
Fig. IV.1.G3b Eight years later severe renal scarring has developed.

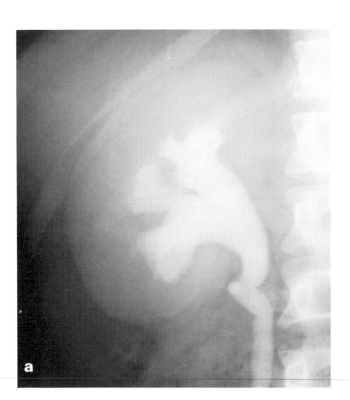

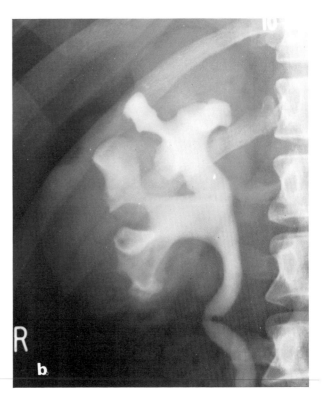

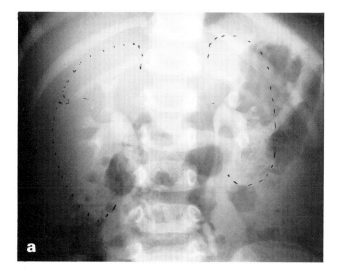

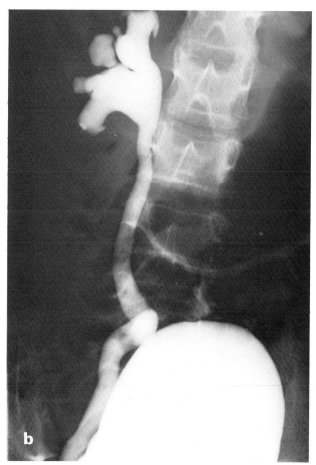

controlled. However, such isolated instances do not appear to be of much importance when the subject is reviewed in large series (Edwards *et al*, 1977, Asscher *et al*, 1978).

The continental European writing on this subject includes a curious 'segmental aglomerular hypoplasia' or Ask-Upmark kidney. This is said to be a renal deformity of congenital origin, with distinctive clinico-pathological features. It looks exactly like the acquired chronic pyelonephritic disease to the radiological eye, and indeed there is now good evidence from a key case report that this is the correct interpretation of this non-entity (Johnston & Mix, 1976).

Fig. IV.1.G4a Normal IVU in a 3-year-old girl with urinary infection.
Fig. IV.1.G4b The cystogram shows rightsided reflux. Infections were controlled medically.

Summary comment

It seems that pyelonephritic scarring happens extremely early in childhood, often in the first year and only rarely after the fifth year of life. When the child then presents with a urinary infection, radiological studies simply document

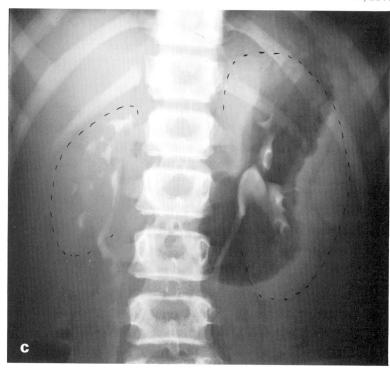

Fig. IV.1.G4c Seven years later the right kidney is shrunken.

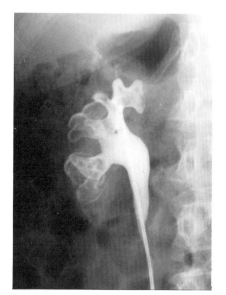

Fig. IV.1.G5 Retrograde study with multiple necrotic papillae lying in calices.

the established damage. Whatever is done as a result probably does not influence the natural history as much as was once thought. The battle to save nephrons from chronic pyelonephritis may have to be directed toward much earlier diagnosis in high risk groups. The near relatives of patients with known scars, for instance, have a high prevalence of reflux threatening their kidneys, put at about 10% (de Vargas *et al,* 1978).

Renal papillary necrosis

This is now a common disease, and a radiologist in a district hospital will probably encounter several patients with the condition each year. Such patients often see many doctors before the right diagnosis is made, and the radiologist has a particular opportunity and responsibility to be on the look-out for cutting short the usual diagnostic labyrinth. Papillary necrosis is an important cause of renal failure, and early recognition offers the chance of saving the patient from the 'end stage kidney' by arresting further renal impairment. This will usually mean dissuading the patient from further abuse of analgesics.

The disease is much more common among women (5:1). Patients often hide their analgesic addiction, and more persistence and indeed clinical detective work is needed than accepting a simple answer: 'No, I don't take any drugs'.

Causes

Analgesic abuse
Diabetes
Sickle cell haemoglobin
Obstruction with infection
Acute suppurative pyelonephritis (adults)
Hypoxaemia and dehydration (infants)
Chronic transplant rejection
Cryoglobulinaemia ⎤
Polyarteritis nodosa ⎬ Rare
Chronic alcoholism ⎦

Main forms of renal papillary necrosis

1. Total. A whole renal papilla sloughs off, presenting as a filling defect in the pelvi-caliceal system (Fig. IV.1.G5), and leaving a rounded hole in the medulla. These rounded spaces can be mistaken for 'clubbed calices' (Fig. IV.1.G6).

2. Partial. Dissection occurs around the base of the papilla into the caliceal fornix, or centrally into the apex of the papilla. Abnormal clefts or cavities therefore appear around or inside the papilla (Fig. IV.1.G7). Those tunnelling around the base will form 'ring shadows' when projected on to the two-dimen-

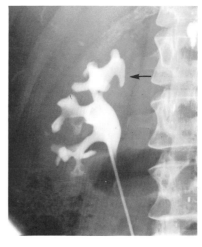

Fig. IV.1.G6 *(above)* Excavated calices in papillary necrosis. Note particularly a characteristic medial hook from the uppermost calix (arrow).

Fig. IV.1.G7 *(below left)* The arrows point to contrast medium in dissection spaces in renal papillae.

Fig. IV.1.G8 *(below right)* Multiple necrotic, calcified papillae are seen in place in the left kidney. By contrast, there are none on the right because surgical debridement was carried out on this side.

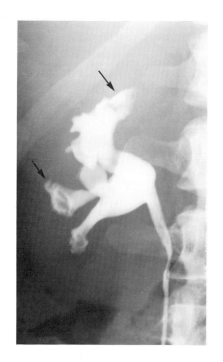

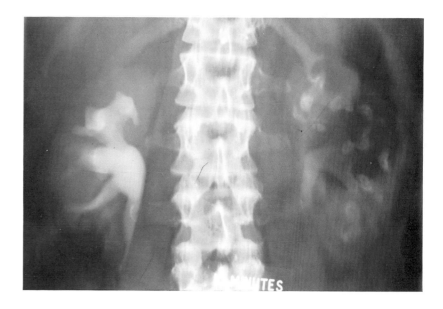

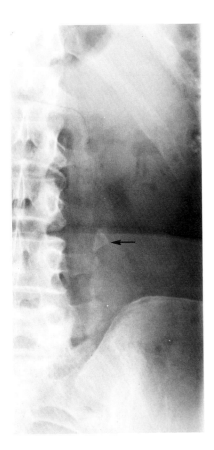

sional X-ray film. This particular term has acquired too much weight. Ring shadows are not all that frequent, and not needed to make the diagnosis; indeed many cases of papillary necrosis will be missed if we are to wait on the appearance of these circles.

3. In situ. Poynter and Hare (1974) have shown that the necrotic papilla may simply stay in place, without developing clefts or cavities. Calcification is then a helpful sign toward diagnosis, and indeed part of the differential diagnosis of medullary nephrocalcinosis (Fig. IV.1.G8).

4. Ureteric obstruction. The shed papillae may cause acute ureteric hold-up, with acute renal failure if this is bilateral (Fig. IV.1.G9). Infection and dehydration are often part of this disaster story.

5. Chronic renal failure. A diagnosis is particularly difficult when renal function has deteriorated so much that a good pyelogram can no longer be seen. Help may then be obtained from the 'lumpy-bumpy' pattern of renal atrophy seen on the nephrogram: there is relative sparing of the septa of Bertin, with centrilobar atrophy in between (Hodson, 1972a) (Fig. IV.1.G10).

Summary comment

Renal papillary necrosis is not a difficult diagnosis—the real problem is to be on the look-out for it, particularly in unexplained adult renal infection or failure.

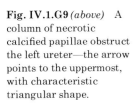

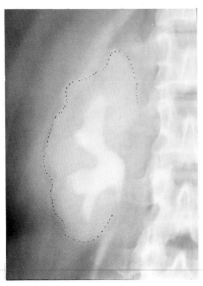

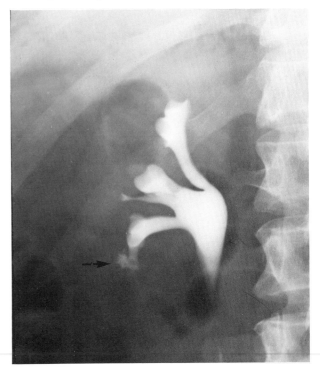

Fig. IV.1.G9 *(above)* A column of necrotic calcified papillae obstruct the left ureter—the arrow points to the uppermost, with characteristic triangular shape.

Fig. IV.1.G10 *(left)* Papillary necrosis with 'lumpy-bumpy' atrophy.

Fig. IV.1.G11 *(right)* Early erosion in renal tuberculosis (arrow).

Diabetes and sickle cell disorders are important additional causes to analgesic abuse.

Tuberculosis

A similar comment applies to tuberculosis. Just because this is less common now, it is particularly important to be hot on the heels of this treatable disease. Most large district hospitals will see several new patients with renal tuberculosis each year.

The earliest radiological sign is an erosion of the papilla (Fig. IV.1.G11). This may look like the characteristic central cavity of renal papillary necrosis. Soon additional signs appear.

1. Cavitation. Any cavity within the kidney could be a tuberculous one, and it is as well to keep this possibility in mind. There is often advanced destruction when the patient is first seen (Fig. IV.1.G12).

Fig. IV.1.G12 Extensive tuberculosis of the left kidney, with calcification at its lower pole. Note also tuberculous involvement of two adjacent lumbar vertebrae, and a calcified psoas abscess (arrow).

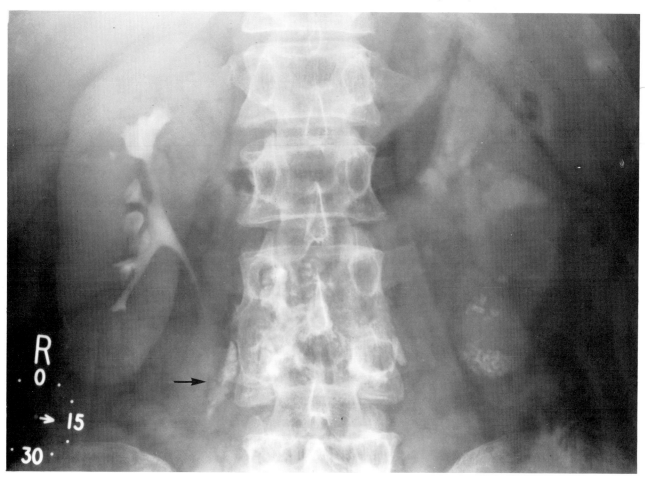

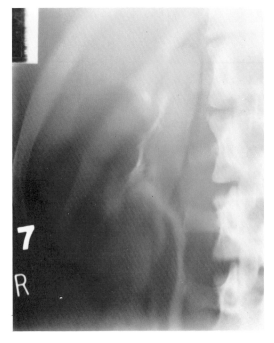

Fig. IV.1.G13 Right renal tuberculosis—a number of caliceal necks have become stenosed, so that the obstructed calices have blown up, giving a soap bubble effect on the nephrogram.

2. Fibrosis. Stenoses appear particularly in caliceal necks (Fig. IV.1.G13) and in the ureter (Fig. IV.1.G14). Fibrosis may rampage ahead even once the disease is being treated; indeed, there is an impression that the early treatment phase is especially dangerous for allowing this attempt at healing and repair to progress (see Management below).

3. Multiple involvement. That the urinary tract is abnormal at several sites is a particular characteristic of the disease. Combined renal, ureteric and bladder lesions should always raise high suspicion of tuberculosis. A small contracted bladder is a well known part of the story (Fig. IV.1.G15).

4. End stage renal destruction. If renal tuberculosis advances unchecked, the whole kidney may die, transformed into a calcareous mess (so called auto-nephrectomy) (Fig. IV.1.G16).

Management

Once the diagnosis is made and the patient begins treatment, a close watch must be kept on the possibility of fibrosis with obstruction. A brief (one or two film) follow-up IVU should be done 6 weeks later. If all is well, the next examination may be delayed for 2–3 months, and again repeated at 1 year. Beyond this, in a healthy patient with a sterile urine, the value of further follow-up is doubtful.

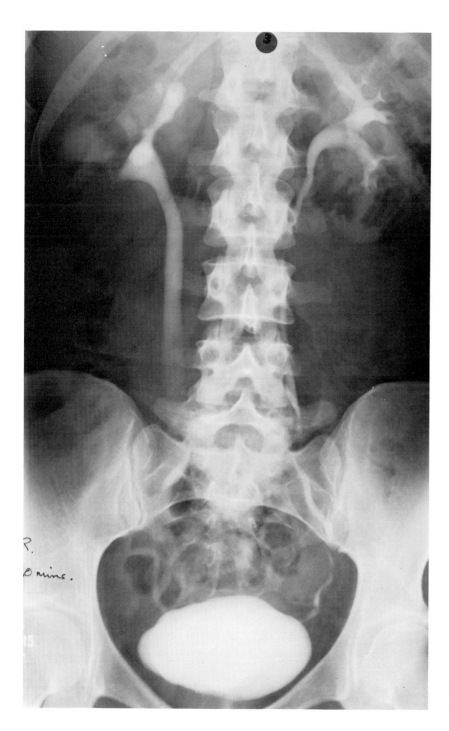

Fig. IV.1.G14 Same patient as in Fig. IV.1.G13—1 month after beginning antituberculous treatment, the right ureter is now obstructed as it crosses the sacrum.

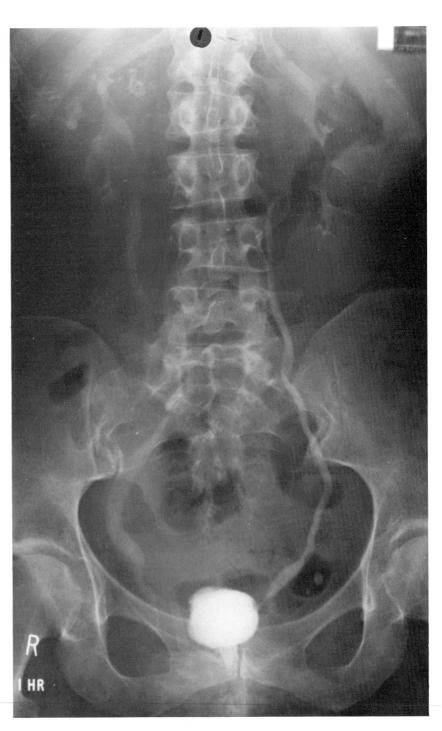

Fig. IV.1.G15   Note the small
contracted bladder, with contrast
staining below because the patient
cannot hold her water. There is
widespread calcification and
destruction in the right kidney, and
the right ureter is wide. Involvement
of the whole urinary tract is
characteristic of tuberculosis.

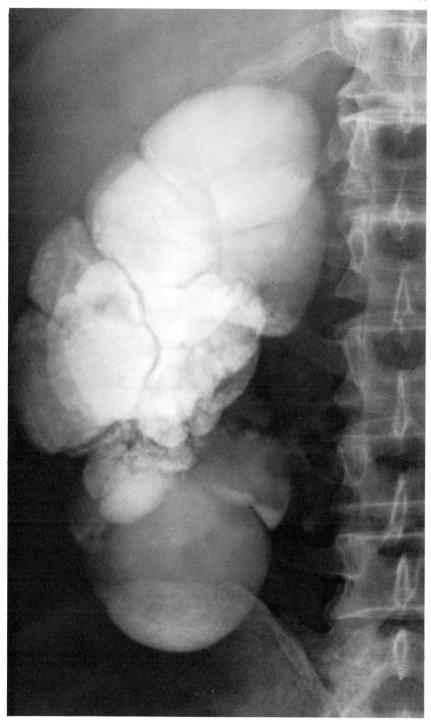

Fig. IV.1.G16 The right kidney is a calcified bag of tuberculous pus—auto-nephrectomy.

Established renal distortion and cavitation will remain as lifelong scars of the disease, and there is little point in looking at them year by year. However, any flare-up of symptoms (e.g. frequency) needs renewed investigation: it is possible to see fresh activity even years later in supposedly burnt out disease.

Summary comment

It is a tragedy to miss this treatable disorder.

NARROW CALICEAL NECKS

Stricture

Tuberculosis straddles the subjects of the destroyed and the strictured calix (see previous section). Calices may go on dilating because of advancing fibrosis of their necks, even when the urine has become sterile (Fig. IV.1.G17).

There are not many other common causes of caliceal stricture. Caliceal stones are a theoretical possibility, but not very important in practice. Renal tumours may occasionally grow so as to obstruct a single caliceal system (Fig. IV.1.G18).

Fig. IV.1.G17a & b Left upper renal pole tuberculosis—although this patient is on effective anti-tuberculous treatment, calices have become obstructed over 8 months.

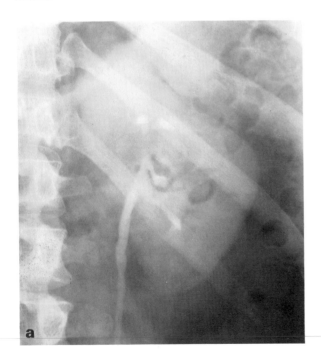
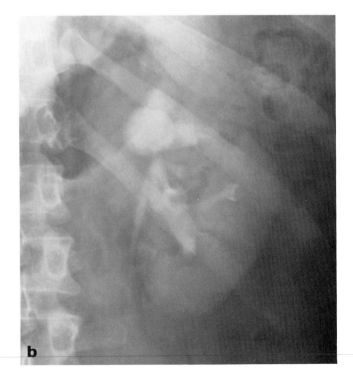

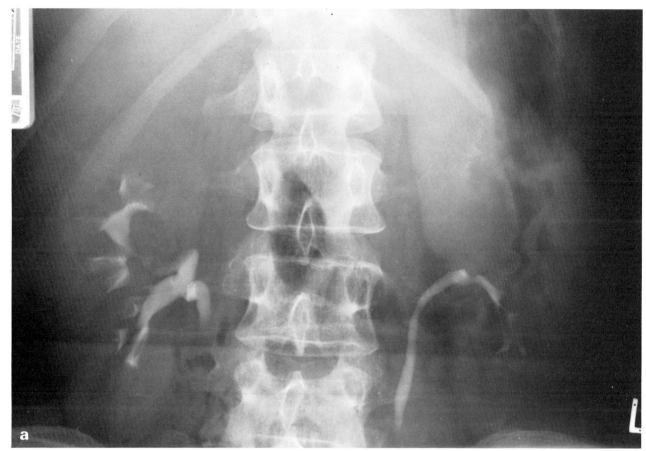

a

Fig. IV.1.G18a The left upper pole calices are not seen on this early film from an IVU (haematuria).

Fig. IV.1.G18b *(overpage)* The 24-hour film shows the obstructed calices now filled. There is a large carcinoma in the middle of this kidney.

Extrinsic impression

It is not uncommon to see the renal calices or pelvis indented by vessels, usually arteries. They are generally distinguished by their linear shape, and only rarely give rise to diagnostic difficulty (Fig. IV.1.G19). However, calices may distend where such impressions cross their necks. This happens most often in the upper caliceal group of the right kidney, where a posterior division of the renal artery is closely applied to the draining neck. This relationship can be shown on arteriography (Fig. IV.1.G20), but the clinical relevance of the finding is highly doubtful. In most patients this anomaly is a chance finding, not related to any symptoms (Rusiewicz & Reilly, 1968). Against this background, there should be very considerable hesitation in ascribing even suggestive symptoms such as right flank ache to what is simply a quite common normal variant. The IVU picture is not usually improved by operation.

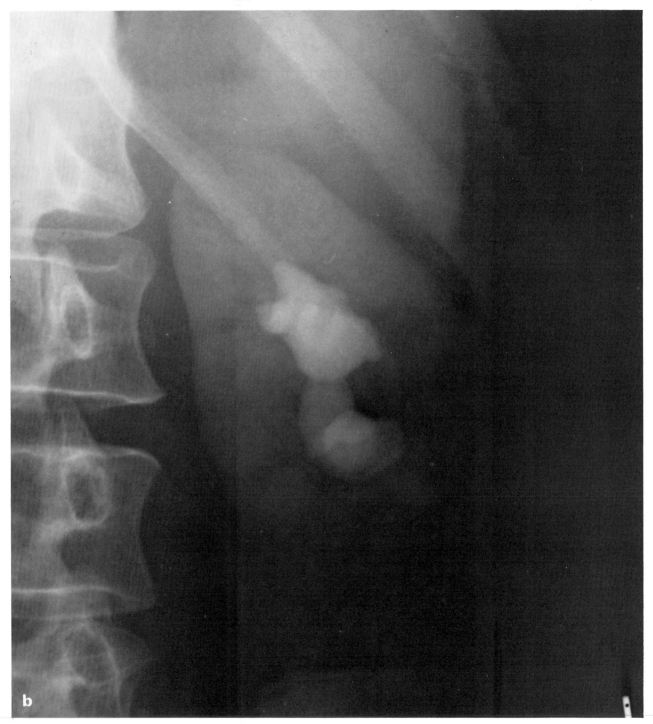

b

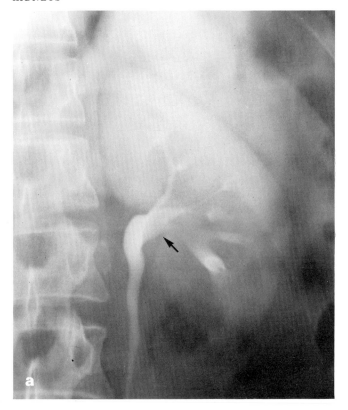

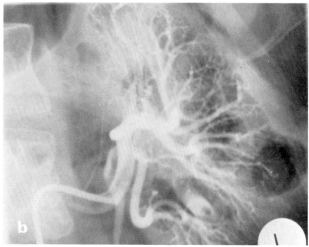

Fig. IV.1.G19a & b There is a prominent shoulder impressing the lateral border of the renal pelvis (arrow). The selective arteriogram shows that this is caused by the main renal artery.

Hydrocalicosis

Narrow caliceal necks may occasionally be a congenital abnormality (Fig. IV.1.G21). This condition can only be safely diagnosed in children, where renal tuberculosis is extremely uncommon. It is not a diagnosis to be made every day of the year.

WIDE CALICEAL NECKS

Post-obstructive atrophy

It is again particularly to Hodson (1972b) that we owe our understanding about the distinctive changes to be recognized in the kidney which has been hurt by obstruction. When obstruction has been relieved, generalized dilatation of varying severity of all calices may remain, together with uniform renal parenchymal thinning (Fig. IV.1.G22). If this picture is met for the first time in a patient having an IVU for some other reason, careful inquiry will often elicit a past history of urinary stones. What is not known is what critical threshold there is to the severity or length of obstruction for firing off renal atrophy. Certainly patients with ureteric stones may have severe obstruction of one

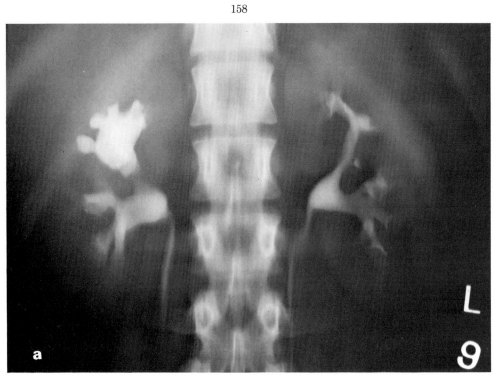

Fig. IV.1.G20a & b   Considerable
dilatation of right upper renal pole
calices, bounded by a transverse
impression at the base of the calices. The
selective arteriogram shows the
responsible renal arteries.

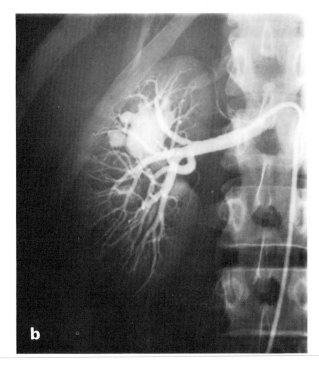

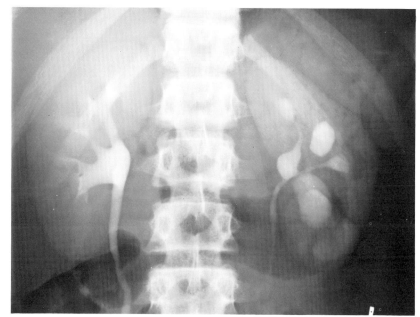

Fig. IV.1.G21 Hydrocalicosis—note distended calices and narrow caliceal necks in this child's left kidney. Exploration confirmed that these were congenital lesions (normal urothelium).

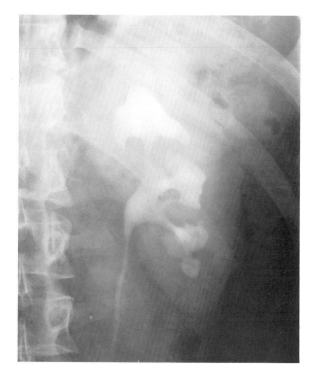

Fig. IV.1.G22 Post-obstructive atrophy in a patient with a history of passing left-sided stones. One stone remains in the lowermost calix. Note uniform caliceal deformity.

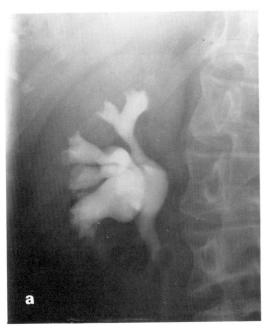

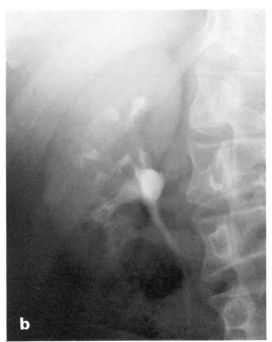

Fig. IV.1.G23a IVU during obstruction of the lower right ureter by a stone.
Fig. IV.1.G23b One month later—the stone has just been passed, with a characteristic 'floppy', post-obstructive appearance of the caliceal system.

kidney, and yet in most there are no residual long-term changes once the stone is passed. In the immediate post-stone period subtle changes can sometimes be recognized (Fig. IV.1.G23). The whole process of post-obstructive atrophy may be seen at work in the vulnerable kidney of the child (Fig. IV.1.G24).

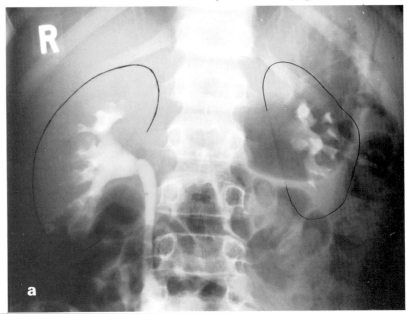

Fig. IV.1.G24a This young boy suffers from urinary infections and left ureteric reflux. Note that the right kidney is normal.

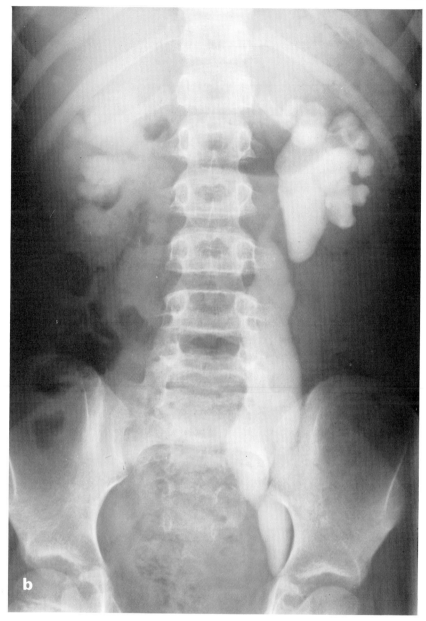

b

Fig. IV.1.G24b   IVU 6 months after bilateral ureteric reimplantation—both ureters have been obstructed by surgery.

It is worth noting one other post-obstructive sign. This is the formation of longitudinal folds in the upper urinary tract, indicating a pelvis or ureter which has once been distended, and will not return to complete normality (Fig. IV.1.G25). It is a most characteristic sign in the collapsed ureter seen on the IVU of a child who then has severe reflux on cystography. The alternative explanation that it represents a ureteritis appears unnecessarily complex.

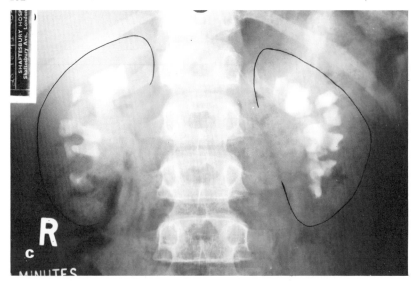

Fig. IV.1.G24c Following correction of ureteric obstruction by a second operation, the right kidney now shows post-obstructive atrophy. Note uniform caliceal deformity.

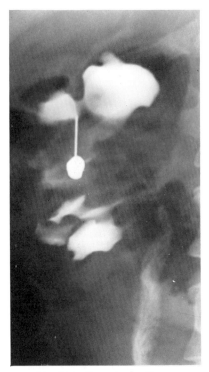

Fig. IV.1.G25 Post-obstructive longitudinal ureteric folds shown during an antegrade pyelogram. The same picture can be seen in the right kidney of the patient illustrated in Fig. IV.1.F1.

Megacalices

Puigvert, followed by Talner and Gittes (1974), has pointed to a picture of generalized caliceal distension which is to be distinguished from post-obstructive atrophy. This is most commonly seen in children and adults as a chance finding on the IVU (Fig. IV.1.G26). They have no history of obstruction, the functioning renal cell mass is normal on isotope studies, and there is no renal cortical atrophy on angiography. Indeed angiography defines a normal cortex but malformed medulla. The suggestion is that this is an anomaly of medullary shape, so that calices simply mirror this structural oddity.

One practical difficulty is that these baggy calices may collect stones in them as a secondary event, consequent on urinary stasis. It may therefore be permissible to make the diagnosis of megacalices rather than post-obstructive atrophy, even in the presence of renal stones. This should only be done with much caution.

The more fundamental difficulty is to explain the deranged embryology of this supposed congenital disorder. How can the medulla possibly grow in this way? The alternative explanation is that megacalices is really a burnt out obstruction, perhaps dating from intrauterine life (Johnston, 1973).

Whatever the aetiology, for practical management it is as well to recognize that some children and adults may have this functionally unimportant renal state. It does not require surgical or medical treatment. The diagnosis can be made on characteristic IVU findings, and does not need arteriography to substantiate it.

Polycalicosis

Whilst there are cross-relations with megacalices, it is probably helpful to

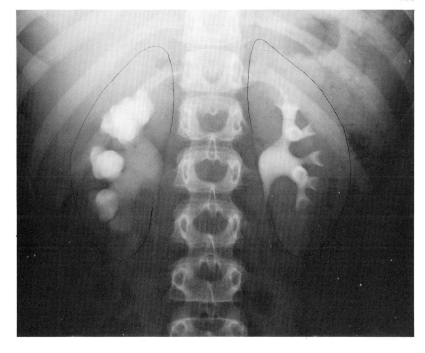

Fig. IV.1.G26 Megacalices on the right side. All the calices are deformed, but there is no obstruction, and a normal cortical width is the expected finding on angiography.

regard the grossly dysplastic kidney with obviously too many papillae/calices under a separate heading (Fig. IV.1.G27). Such children may have associated renal impairment or ureteric abnormalities. This is a rare diagnosis.

OTHER PAPILLARY/CALICEAL ODDITIES

Dysplastic kidneys

The badly made kidney is primarily a histopathological diagnosis. Abnormal renal elements are seen under the microscope. For the radiological eye such kidneys present obvious deformities (Fig. IV.1.G28). They may be associated with drainage abnormalities (e.g. ectopic ureterocele). The depth of renal substance as seen on the nephrogram may be misleading here: these may be poor nephrons even when renal bulk appears adequate. 'Oligomeganephronia', i.e. too few too large nephrons, is a telling example.

Caliceal diverticula

Small diverticula of calices are common unimportant chance findings (Fig. IV.1.G29). The fact that they have a neck usually serves to distinguish them from acquired cavities, e.g. tuberculosis. The neck may occasionally be so narrow that the diverticulum blows up, and is then a potential source of

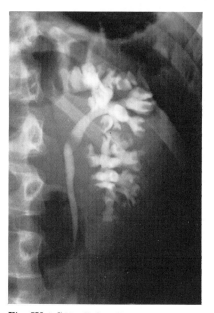

Fig. IV.1.G27 Polycalicosis.

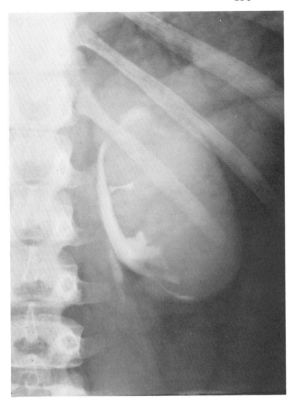 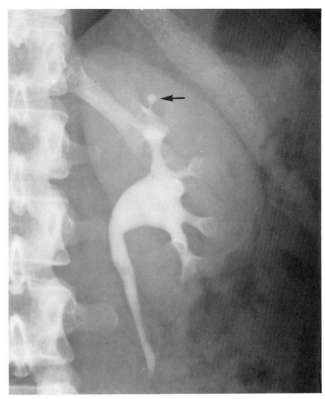

Fig. IV.1.G28 *(left)* Dysplastic kidney, with characteristic caliceal deformities. In such a badly made kidney, the volume of renal parenchyma is not a good guide to functional reserve.

Fig. IV.1.G29 *(right)* Small caliceal diverticulum arising from the uppermost calix (arrow).

infection and therefore pain. Such obstructed diverticula tend to collect stones (Fig. IV.1.G30).

Multiple caliceal diverticula are a rare congenital anomaly, for instance in the Bardet-Biedl syndrome (Alton & McDonald, 1973). There are cross-relations in this IVU picture with other rare disorders, e.g. EMG syndrome (see Medullary Sponge Kidney, p. 132).

Renal infarct

A small renal infarct classically does not lead to caliceal deformity, since there is simply loss of renal parenchyma by atrophy, not fibrosis. In practice, infarcts are sometimes seen where renal thinning is so severe that the calix does become deformed, taking up atrophy space (Fig. IV.1.G31). This is an uncommon diagnostic problem.

Chyluria/renal lymphatic obstruction

Filariasis is the common background to this syndrome. Lymphograms show spectacular disarrays of the abdominal lymph node chains, with reflux into the

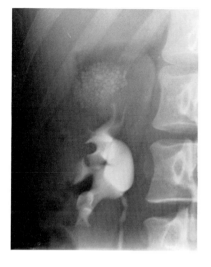

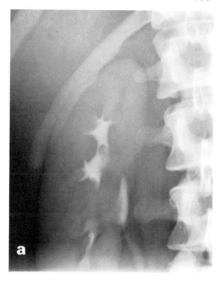

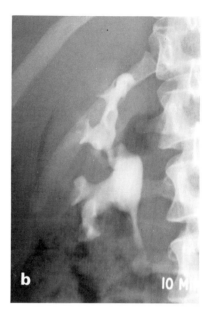

Fig. IV.1.G30 *(above left)* A collection of small stones is present in a large caliceal diverticulum at the right upper renal pole.

Fig. IV.1.G31a *(above centre)* Normal right upper renal pole—this patient's kidney is about to be explored because of a small stone.
Fig. IV.1.G31b *(above right)* At operation a small accessory artery to the right upper renal pole was severed. On follow-up the resulting infarct has produced caliceal deformity very like a pyelonephritic scar (arteriogram proof).

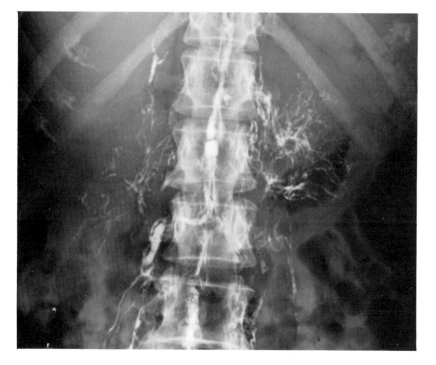

Fig. IV.1.G32 Filariasis—destruction of para-aortic nodes, with contrast refluxing into renal lymphatics.

renal lymphatics (Fig. IV.1.G32). The contrast medium, travelling up from the feet, may outline calices via lymphatico-caliceal communications, thus demonstrating the mechanism of chyluria (Fig. IV.1.G33).

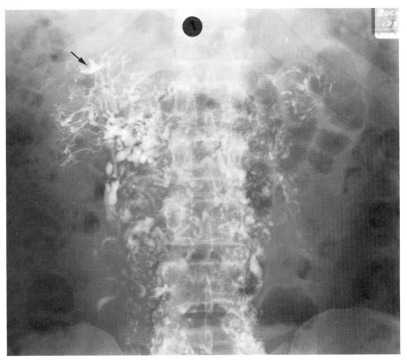

Fig. IV.1.G33 Another patient with chyluria, reflux into renal lymphatics, and thence into a calix (arrow).

H. RENAL MASSES

Clinical presentation and likely diagnoses are generally so different between adults' and children's renal masses that the two are best considered separately. A few diagnoses are of course shared between both groups, notably renal abscess, described in the adult section.

Normal variants: the renal island

Recognizing unusual variants is a problem with children's as well as adults' kidneys (Fig. IV.1.H1). The normal kidney is made up of 12–14 lobes, and it is remarkable that the congenital and acquired disarrays arising from this arrangement have only been understood fairly recently (Hodson 1972a). Elements of renal lobes may become displaced or just exaggerated during lobar fusion. Lobes are of course normally separated from each other by layers of cortex dipping down to the renal sinus—the septa of Bertin. A septum may grow unusually large, forming in effect a deeply placed renal cortical island. It will then present as a mass on the IVU. The resulting picture is characteristic: the renal pelvis is often bifid, and at the junction of the upper third and lower two-thirds of this potential duplex kidney a mass is seen (Fig. IV.1.H2). It may blush during the early films of the IVU, just like the peripheral renal cortex. If investigation is driven as far as angiography because of doubt over the true diagnosis, no abnormal vessels are seen, simply a highly vascular cortical lump

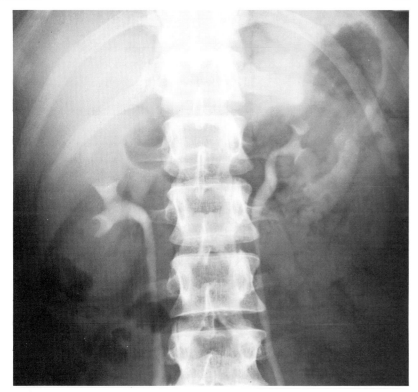

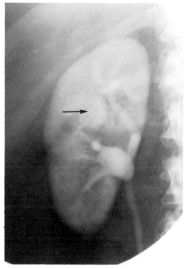

Fig. IV.1.H1 *(left)* Two-lobed kidneys—note that there are just two papillae in each kidney. Chance finding.

Fig. IV.1.H2 *(above)* Characteristic renal island (arrow) in a bifid kidney.

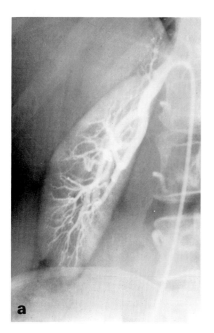

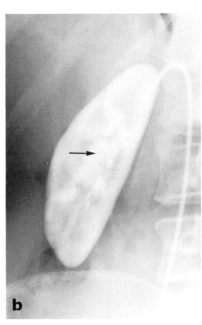

Fig. IV.1.H3a & b Early and late frames from a selective renal arteriogram showing a renal island (arrow).

(Fig. IV.1.H3). Nuclear medicine studies have an important place here—see Part II section A.

With this characteristic picture, the diagnosis should in fact be obvious from the IVU, and need not be taken further. Occasionally, difficulty arises because a whole miniature renal lobe may be displaced deeply in the kidney. It will then have a relatively avascular centre (medulla) and a miniature calix draining it. Rarely, the displaced renal island is stuck onto the periphery of the kidney (Fig. IV.1.H4). There is a well-known, left-sided 'dromedary hump' variant (Fig. IV.1.H5).

This subject has been bedevilled by the awful term *pseudo-tumour*, which is perhaps best forgotten. It may possibly have some point for the odd lumps and bumps sometimes seen in the badly scarred kidney, where surviving normal renal islands stand out sharply against the wasteland of destroyed renal parenchyma.

The ageing kidney with renal sinus fat

Fat is a normal constituent of the renal sinus, and increasing amounts are often laid down with advancing years. This can take on the appearance of a renal

Fig. IV.1.H4 *(left)* Small additional lobe on the renal surface—the arrow points to the projecting shoulder.

Fig. IV.1.H5 *(right)* Selective renal arteriogram showing normal dromedary hump (arrow).

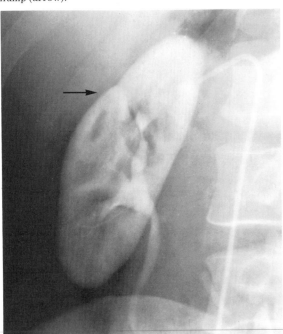

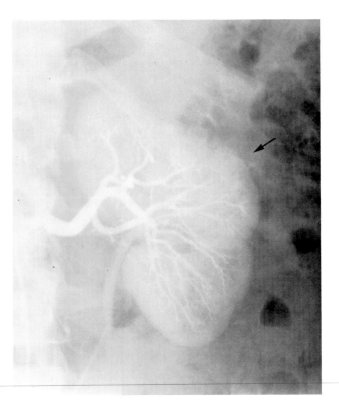

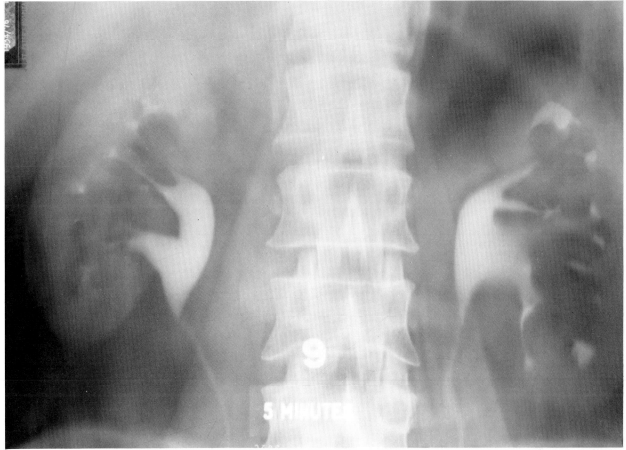

Fig. IV.1.H6 *(above)* Fat in both renal sinuses making for stretched caliceal necks.

Fig. IV.1.H7 *(right)* IVU nephrogram showing the renal sinus packed with fat.

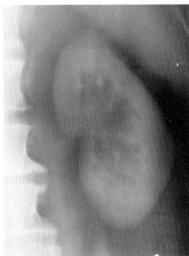

lump, particularly if it is sited peripherally (Fig. IV.1.H6). This picture of radiolucent masses obeying renal sinus boundaries is harmless and character-istic, needing no further investigation (Fig. IV.1.H7).

Technical pitfalls

A poor IVU may mimic renal masses because of underfilled calices. This can be a problem in the adult as well as the child (Fig. IV.1.H8). The obvious lesson is that the serious diagnosis of a renal mass should only be made on good IVU grounds. It is better to repeat a questionable IVU than to catapult a patient into a chain of unnecessary further investigations. Radioisotope scans of the kidney can be very useful in the worrying individual case: a normal scan is good evidence toward the diagnosis of a normal variant.

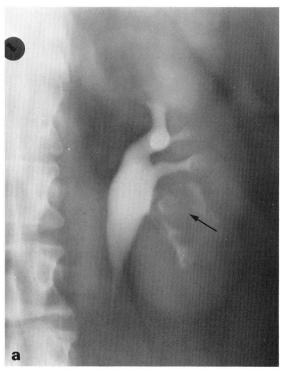

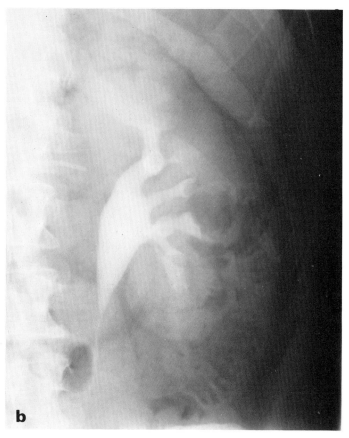

Fig. IV.1.H8a This man was thought to have a mass in his left kidney, displacing calices (arrow).

Fig. IV.1.H8b An unnecessary arteriogram was done—at this examination calices are properly filled out, showing that there is no mass at all.

CHILDHOOD RENAL MASSES

The renal lump itself is often the presenting symptom and sign in childhood, in contrast to the adult, where such a mass effect is quite uncommon. By further distinction, haematuria is a rare presenting sign in children.

A greatly enlarged non-excreting kidney may occasionally be found in children presenting with a flank mass. *Hydronephrosis* or *multicystic* disease must then be considered, with ultrasound as very helpful next diagnostic step toward these diagnoses. If a solid mass is shown, Wilms' tumour is high on the differential diagnostic list, even with a non-excreting kidney.

Wilms' tumour

Most children presenting with this tumour are less than 5 years of age. The IVU shows a mass distorting the kidney, arising from within, rather than an extrinsic deformity as in neuroblastoma.

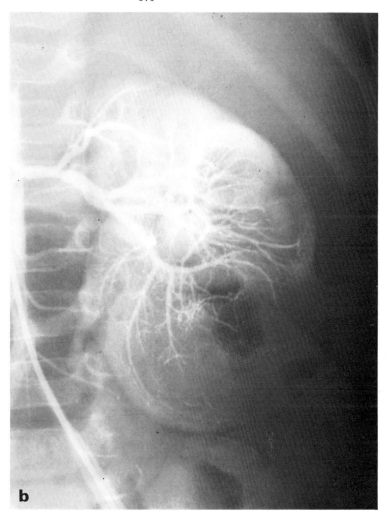

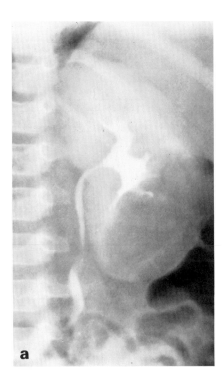

The question of further renal investigation in the presence of this highly characteristic picture is debatable (Fig. IV.1.H9). Arteriography produces splendid images of the abnormal circulation within the tumour, but its impact on management is rather doubtful. The arteriographic picture is not specific for either this tumour or indeed a malignant lesion—an inflammatory or cystic mass may also have abnormal vessels. Staging of the tumour is done at laparotomy in any event.

An obvious claim for arteriography is the ability to diagnose a tumour in the contralateral kidney. The incidence of bilateral tumours is about 10% (*British Medical Journal*, 1976). On the less satisfactory IVUs of two or three decades ago, missing a contralateral tumour certainly occurred more readily than with present day IVU techniques (Fig. IV.1.H10).

Fig. IV.1.H9a & b IVU and selective arteriogram showing a large Wilms' tumour at the lower renal pole. (Courtesy of Dr C. D. R. Flower).

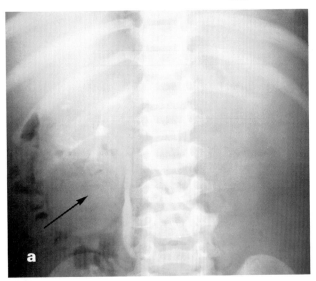

Fig. IV.1.H10a Non-excreting left
kidney in a young girl—Wilms' tumour.
There is also a mass at the right lower
renal pole (arrow), i.e. bilateral tumours.
A left nephrectomy was done, and the
right lower renal pole irradiated.
Fig. IV.1.H10b Nineteen years later,
the rightsided tumour is again growing
uncontrollably (selective arteriogram).

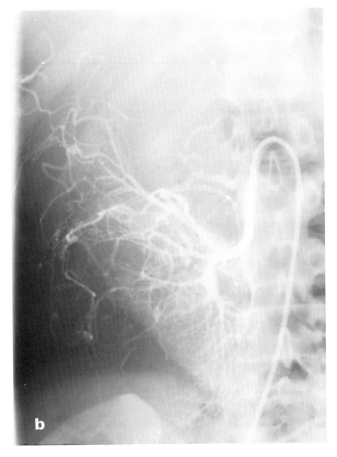

The case for arteriography is not proved at present, and in this country
children with obvious unilateral Wilms' tumours usually have urgent surgery
without the additional handling or even delay of such further investigation. A
chest X-ray is an essential part of the preoperative assessment. A useful investigation which can be done without further ado is an *inferior vena cavagram* to
demonstrate the medial extent of the tumour. It is readily obtained on the early
films of the IVU if foot veins are chosen for the injection in a child with a renal
mass.

Infantile nephroma (fetal hamartoma)

The renal tumour presenting at birth or during the first year of life formerly
classed as congenital Wilms' tumour appears to be a different entity (Bolande,
1974). It is generally benign, and cure can be expected following simple surgical
removal.

Neuroblastoma

Whilst tumour calcification may be seen on the plain film of a child suffering from a Wilms' tumour, this finding is rather more common with neuroblastoma. The fact that there is an extrinsic deformity distorting the kidney from without is generally the most helpful sign in differentiating a neuroblastoma from a Wilms' tumour. With large tumours this distinction can become very difficult. Because of the likelihood of bony deposits, a radioisotope bone scan or radiographic skeletal survey is important as part of the preoperative assessment.

Summary comment

Considerable strides have been made in the treatment of malignant renal and suprarenal tumours of childhood in recent years. They demand expert surgical and oncological attention, including accurate staging of the disease. At present these patients are best treated in a small number of specialist centres, and the radiologist should not hesitate to seek similar expert help on the diagnostic side.

The distended non-excreting moiety of a duplex kidney

It is as well to remember this entity as part of the childhood problem, though urinary infection will be the common presenting story. This diagnostic possibility is particularly important in an upper pole mass, because of the impaired urinary drainage which may occur with a duplex anomaly here (see Division 2 section A). Awareness of the diagnosis is usually enough, though such children can be driven as far as angiography without it (Fig. IV.1.H11).

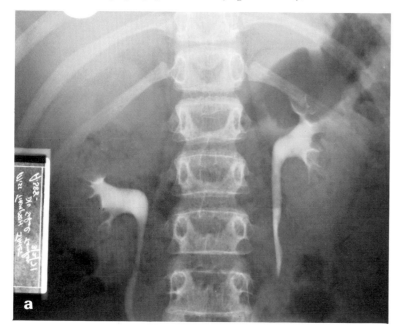

Fig. IV.1.H11a *(left)* & **b** *(overpage)* IVU and aortogram in a duplex right kidney with a non-excreting upper moiety. Note the distended calices, producing a cystic right upper renal pole mass.

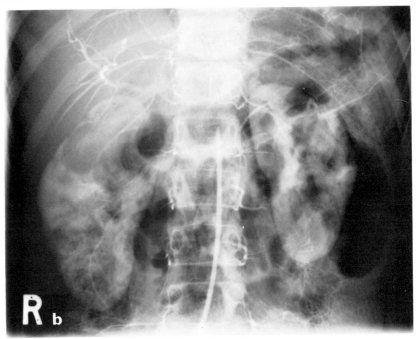

Other problems may of course occur in childhood, e.g. infiltration of the kidneys by leukaemia, or by an inflammatory process producing a renal abscess. However, the most important conditions straddling the subject of renal masses in the child and adult are the *renal cystic diseases* (diagram).

Multicystic kidney

This is a gross renal anomaly with a distinctive array of signs—the ureter is atretic, the kidney made up of a collection of cysts, the renal artery so small that it is thought absent, and renal calcification possible on the plain film. The atretic ureter is a constant finding, and indeed obstruction has been put forward as the starting point of the whole anomaly. The cysts might then be shut off calices, and are often about the right total number for this idea. In further support caliceal crescents of contrast medium have been described during the IVU (Felson & Cussen, 1975). However, the multicystic kidney is ordinarily a functionally useless, non-excreting organ.

Once diagnosed with the help of a retrograde examination to show the atretic ureter, there is little cause for alarm or even surgical interference. The multicystic kidney may present as a lump in infancy or as a chance finding later, perhaps picked up by its calcification on a plain abdominal X-ray done for another reason. As a strictly unilateral finding, it does no harm. However, it is not always unilateral. Survival is of course impossible with both kidneys involved by the full blown anomaly. But a number of patients with one multi-

Radiolucent masses on the nephrogram

OBSTRUCTION

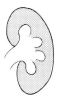

Orderly caliceal arrangement

ADULT POLYCYSTIC
DISEASE

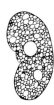

Chaotic, innumerable cysts

INFANTILE POLYCYSTIC
DISEASE

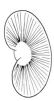

Streaky
nephrogram

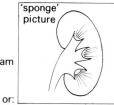

'sponge'
picture

or:

MULTICYSTIC KIDNEY

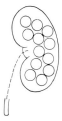

Atretic ureter, with small
number of cysts

MEDULLARY CYSTIC DISEASE

Small unremarkable kidneys
(renal failure)

MULTIPLE ACQUIRED
ADULT CYSTS

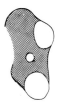

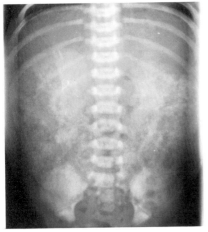

Fig. IV.1.H12 Characteristic streaky, long-lasting nephrogram in infantile polycystic disease. This 2-week-old infant did not survive. (Courtesy of Prof. T. M. Barratt).

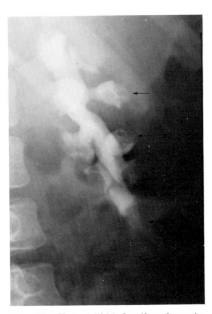

Fig. IV.1.H13 Mild infantile polycystic disease—the arrows point to dilated collecting ducts, rather like the medullary sponge picture. (Courtesy of Dr A. Warner).

cystic kidney are found to have a ureteric narrowing on the contralateral side, pointing to a forme fruste of the disease, not usually of clinical importance.

Medullary cystic disease

Juvenile nephronophthisis is a synonym stressing the common presentation of this odd familial disorder: young patients in the first and second decade of life develop chronic renal failure, often a salt-losing nephritis. Their kidneys are of normal or small size, and generally unremarkable on the IVU. The cysts found in the medulla are small, and difficult to make out, even on angiography (Junghagen & Lindqvist, 1973). Though the disease is rare, it may account for a sizeable proportion of chronic renal failure in the teens.

Infantile polycystic disease

This is a different condition to the well-known adult disease of the same name. It is better not to cavil about this muddle: there are fascinating cross-relations between the two diseases, hinted at below.

Infantile polycystic disease is of recessive inheritance. The essential renal deformity is a dilatation of the distal nephron. There is also accompanying hepatic disorder, marked by progressive periportal fibrosis. The fate of the child is determined by the number of nephrons involved (Blyth & Ockenden, 1971).

With near total nephron involvement, renal failure develops immediately after birth. The IVU is remarkable and distinctive: a dense streaky nephrogram is seen, with multiple radiating lucencies—the disordered distal tubules (Fig. IV.1.H12). The nephrogram is long lasting, and does not usually advance to a pyelogram. These babies do not survive.

At the other extreme only a small proportion of nephrons is involved. These children survive to be overtaken by hepatic failure in their second decade as periportal fibrosis advances. The few dilated nephrons present coarse striated papillary shadows on the IVU, very much like the medullary sponge kidney picture (Fig. IV.1.H13). A predictable muddle has arisen on the lines 'sponge kidneys are usually innocuous, but sometimes associated with liver disease', and needs no further comment.

Between these two ends there is a spectrum, some children with, say, 50% of nephrons involved presenting with renal failure during their first decade before hepatic symptoms or signs have got under way. However, there are odd individual instances and families where infantile polycystic disease moves on to classical adult polycystic disease (Ritter & Siafarikas, 1976). They are fascinating but ill understood.

ADULT RENAL MASSES

Adult polycystic disease

This disorder of dominant inheritance is an important cause of chronic renal

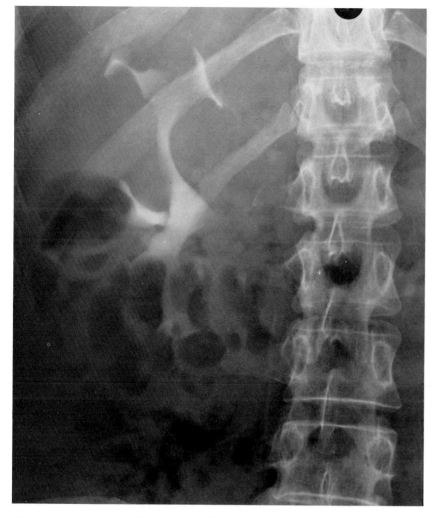

Fig. IV.1.H14 Polycystic disease with obvious caliceal deformities.

failure, hypertension and haematuria. It may rarely present in childhood, but is *not* then a variant of the infantile disease of the same name.

The IVU is the investigation of choice, though ultrasound can also be very helpful. The nephrogram shows innumerable cysts of all sizes (see Fig. IV.1.B6). It is more important for the diagnosis than the pyelogram, where obvious multiple deformities are a later sequel (Fig. IV.1.H14). An angiogram is the most sensitive test (Fig. IV.1.H15), possibly to be rivalled by very careful ultrasound (Fig. IV.1.H16).

Pitfalls

1. The kidneys may not be enlarged.
2. The pyelogram may be normal (Fig. IV.1.H17).

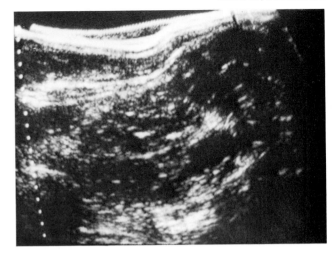

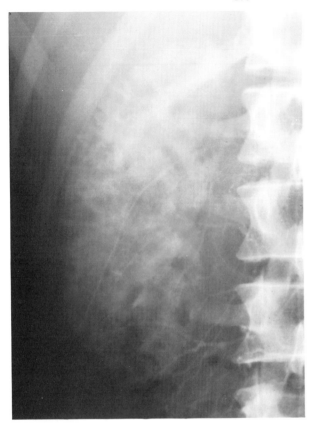

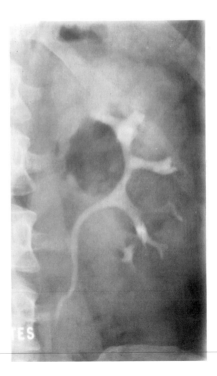

Fig. IV.1.H15 *(above left)* Late frame from an arteriogram showing innumerable small renal cysts.

Fig. IV.1.H16 *(above right)* Prone longitudinal ultrasound scan in polycystic disease—note the multiple echoes arising throughout this kidney as evidence of the disturbed architecture.

Fig. IV.1.H17 *(right)* This kidney is on the large side, but its pyelogram is remarkably normal. The nephrogram from this patient with polycystic disease is shown in Fig. IV.1.B6.

3. The disease may be markedly asymmetric between the two kidneys (Fig. IV.1.H18).

Cyst puncture

There are now no grounds for believing that renal function can be improved by this means, though the discomfort from very large cysts can certainly be lessened.

Fig. IV.1.H18 Asymmetric polycystic disease—both kidneys are involved, but the left has been largely destroyed by the disease.

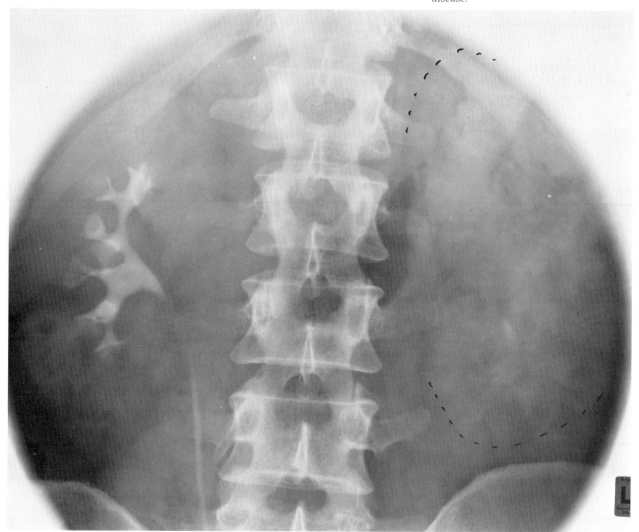

Malignant change

Curvilinear calcification may occur in cyst walls as a benign finding, but extensive diffuse calcification must raise the suspicion that a carcinoma has supervened. There is obvious difficulty with this diagnosis in a kidney riddled with masses, and angiography is usually needed (Tegtmeyer *et al*, 1978).

Acquired renal cyst

This is now a very common chance finding on IVUs carried out for some quite different reason, e.g. bladder outflow obstruction in elderly males. A sharply defined radiolucent mass is shown, perhaps with a beak of normal parenchyma lifted up over its edge if peripheral (Fig. IV.1.H19).

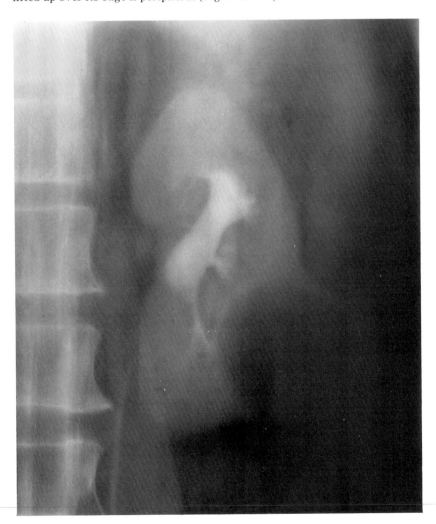

Fig. IV.1.H19 Characteristic simple cyst on the lower lateral renal border.

There has been a reorientation in the past two decades over this lesion. Renal cysts were not so common on earlier, less satisfactory IVUs. If seen, the mass was a dramatic finding, and had to be distinguished from a carcinoma. This led to the search for characteristic IVU signs. The paper-thin wall of the cyst on nephrotomography, the beak sign mentioned above etc. appeared helpful for a time. However, mistakes inevitably occurred, and surgical exploration of all renal masses was sensibly advocated in the 1950s.

Angiography then opened up a new era. The accuracy of the arteriogram in the diagnosis of renal cyst is certainly high when a wholly avascular lesion is shown, with a sharp demarcation between the lesion and normal parenchyma (Fig. IV.1.H20). But these signs too turned out to be fallible, since a small proportion of renal carcinomas are avascular, and may mimic these appearances (Fig. IV.1.H21).

At this point the much older technique of cyst puncture was rediscovered, and used to check on the angiographic diagnosis of benign renal cyst. In the 1970s ultrasound arrived, allowing radiologists to build a critical diagnostic pathway for the renal mass problem. This is discussed below. A few further

Fig. IV.1.H20 *(left)* Selective renal arteriogram—simple cyst at the lower renal pole.

Fig. IV.1.H21 *(right)* Avascular mass at the lower renal pole (selective arteriogram)—this was a carcinoma.

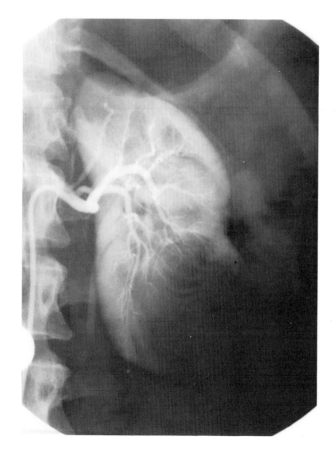

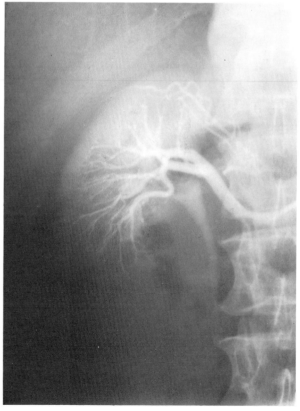

points on renal cysts are worth making now:

1. Autopsy series suggest that about half of all adults harbour at least one renal cyst at death—we are dealing with a common disorder.

2. Any policy of exploring all cysts at surgery is bound to carry morbidity and mortality in its trail, including needless nephrectomy. This risk is probably greater (Plain & Hinman, 1965) than missing the very rare association of cyst/carcinoma as a single lesion.

3. For multiple renal masses the teaching has grown up that the presence of one cyst makes it most likely that the others will also be cysts. Because cysts are so frequent, this is not a good guide. The commonest association between cyst and carcinoma is for a kidney to harbour an unrelated cyst and carcinoma at separate sites. Each renal mass should be diagnosed on its own merits.

Renal carcinoma

The classical triad of flank mass, pain and haematuria is a thing of the past. Few renal carcinomas now advance this far before presentation. Unexplained fever, malaise and weight loss have become particularly important as non-specific

Fig. IV.1.H22a A small mass at the left lower renal pole was missed on this IVU (arrow).

Fig. IV.1.H22b Seven years later the patient remains well apart from his prostatic troubles, but the left renal carcinoma is now very obvious, and has grown.

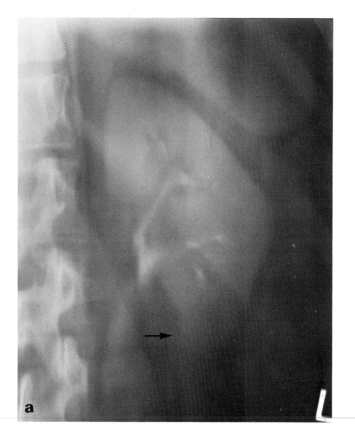
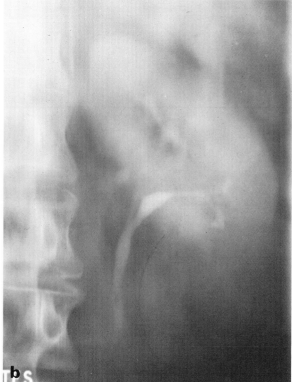

features present in perhaps 20% of patients. They may be accompanied by abnormal liver function tests without implying liver or any other metastases. Renal carcinomas may also be discovered by chance in the absence of any relevant symptoms or signs on IVUs done for other reasons. Certainly the natural history of these tumours is of slow growth, often extending over many years (Fig. IV.1.H22). When a carcinoma comes to light, there is a natural anxiety to deal with it urgently, but it has probably been there a very long time.

Diagnostic pathways for the renal mass (diagram)

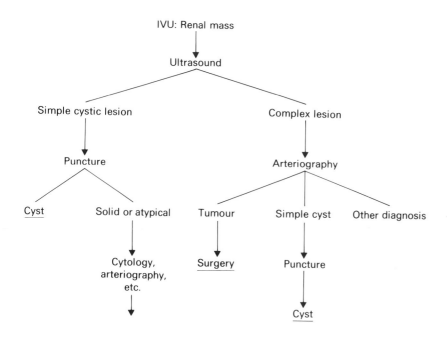

The IVU may provide clues on the central problem of differentiating a renal cyst from a carcinoma. The sharply demarcated, 'punched-out' picture of the radiolucent cyst is obviously different from the ill-defined, vascular, infiltrating cancer (Fig. IV.1.H23). The observation whether calices (normal in number) are simply displaced rather than invaded and amputated (fewer in number) can be very helpful.

Calcification is always a worrying sign in a renal mass, particularly if it is amorphous and central: most of these lesions are carcinomas (Fig. IV.1.H24). Curvilinear calcification in the periphery of the mass may be in the wall of a simple cyst (Fig. IV.1.H25)—only 20% of lesions with this sign are carcinomas (Daniel *et al,* 1972).

However, the IVU diagnosis is a guess with an inadequate accuracy, and ultrasound is the next sensible step. This comparatively cheap outpatient test

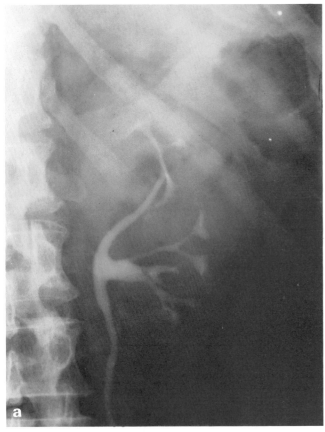

Fig. IV.1.H23a & b IVU and selective
arteriogram in an infiltrating renal
carcinoma. Note that the calices show
only minor deformities with this large
tumour.

will help to separate the patients with a likely cyst (the majority) from those
with a possible tumour requiring further inpatient investigation.

The ultrasound criteria of a simple cyst are:

1. A well defined echo-free space.

2. A sharp interface between cyst and normal parenchyma at the exit of the
ultrasound beam.

3. Enhanced transmission of the sound beam through the cystic space.

This contrasts with complex lesions as possible tumours, where:

1. Echoes are present within the mass.

2. There are no sharp interfaces.

3. The sound beam is attenuated by passage through the lesion.

As always, these differences are clear enough in the textbook examples (Fig.
IV.1.H26), but in practice some doubts, difficulties and misdiagnoses occur. For

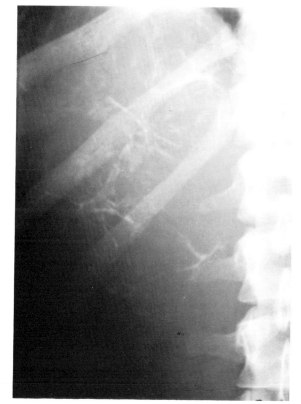

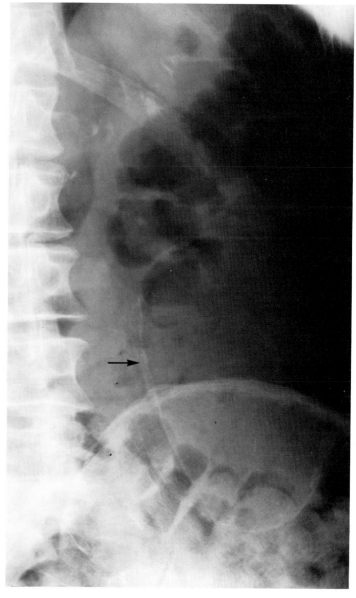

these reasons most ultrasound diagnoses of the one or other lesion must be taken further for confirmation, in order to avoid tragic mistakes. Clinical judgement is of course always essential. An example is the elderly unfit man with a poor life expectancy, presenting with prostatism. Here the chance finding of a renal cyst with characteristic IVU and ultrasound signs can very properly rest at this stage, since little good can be expected for the patient from the search for an unlikely tumour.

Fig. IV.1.H24 *(left)*   Extensive spidery calcification in a right renal carcinoma.

Fig. IV.1.H25 *(right)*   Curvilinear calcification (arrow) in the wall of a renal cyst (autopsy proof).

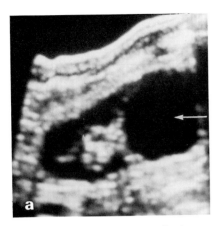

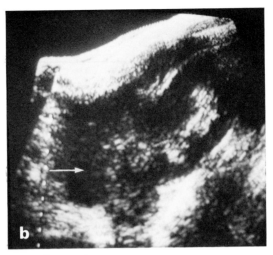

Fig. IV.1.H26a Prone longitudinal ultrasound scan, with a large cyst at the upper pole (arrow).

Fig. IV.1.H26b By contrast this prone ultrasound scan shows a mass deforming the lower renal pole containing multiple echoes (arrow). This is the patient illustrated in Fig. IV.1.H22.

Ultrasound diagnosis: cyst→puncture

Puncture of renal lesions thought to be cysts on ultrasound is generally straightforward and safe. Any needle of adequate length (15 cm) and calibre (about 20 gauge) is suitable. The procedure is done in the prone position under local anaesthesia. The target can be chosen on fluoroscopy after an intravenous injection of contrast medium. It is best to insert the needle vertically above the cyst, following a straight path down. With oblique paths there is difficulty about predicting where the needle tip will go next.

Cyst puncture during ultrasound scanning is an alternative method. This is most elegantly done through a special transducer with a central lumen for the needle. This method will allow very accurate monitoring of the needle path, but by comparison with fluoroscopy it is more difficult to fulfil requirement 2 below.

The prime aim of cyst puncture is accurate diagnosis. To this end there are two requirements:

1. Clear fluid is aspirated from the lesion.

2. The whole of the renal mass is accounted for by a cyst with smooth walls.

Contrast medium is instilled into the cyst in order to check on point 2 if the procedure is done under fluoroscopy. More elaborate techniques can be carried out to study the cyst wall, e.g. introducing air as well as urographic contrast medium into the cyst for a double contrast cystogram. This is of course done in the search for the rare cyst-wall carcinoma. However, irregularities are then frequently found in what are simple cysts by every other criterion (Fig. IV.1.H27). This is because normal renal parenchyma bulges into the cyst, particularly when it is no longer fully distended (Fig. IV.1.H28). There is therefore no persuasive clinical reason for such studies: the diagnosis of simple cyst, if established on every other count, will not be changed.

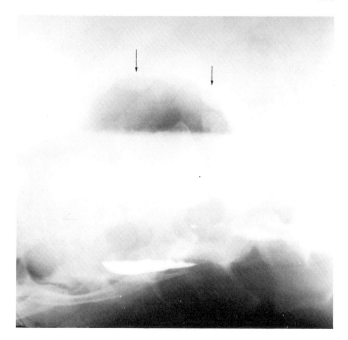

Fig. IV.1.H27 Horizontal beam film of a simple renal cyst which has been filled with air and oily contrast medium, seen lying as a small puddle in the most dependent part. Cyst fluid is seen between these two contrast media. The arrows point to bulges in the cyst wall—these are not tumours.

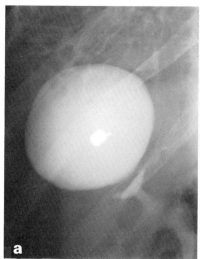
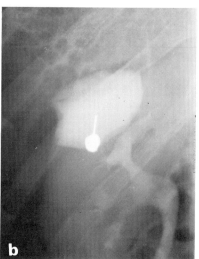

Fig. IV.1.H28a & b Simple renal cyst, seen completely filled and partially aspirated. Note that as the cyst becomes smaller, bulges appear in the wall.

The whole anxiety-ridden topic of cyst/carcinoma is further discussed below.

Therapeutic cyst puncture. The fact that the cyst is made to disappear at aspiration has obvious attractions, but these are superficial. Most cysts will recur after simple aspiration. Methods for preventing this have been advanced, for instance injecting 2–3 ml of iophendylate ('Myodil') (see Fig. IV.1.H27). Cysts will recur even after such manoeuvres, though with less frequency. These efforts have the drawback of introducing foreign materials with unknown long-term hazards. A further objection is that such efforts are misdirected: most renal cysts do no harm. The important thing is to know their nature, i.e. diagnosis. Renal cysts are potentially harmful in two circumstances:

1. If they are so large that they compromise normal renal parenchyma by pressure atrophy.

2. If they are parapelvic in position, obstructing calices (Fig. IV.1.H29).

A case can be made for treating cysts of this sort surgically in the fit patient with a good life expectancy.

Solid mass at puncture. If the needle is clearly in the lesion and there is no fluid aspirate, it may be in a carcinoma. This is unattractive because of the theoretical risk of spreading tumour cells, now substantiated by a case report (Bush *et al,* 1977). However, this risk is very small indeed against the background of the

Fig. IV.1.H29a   There is a para-pelvic mass in this kidney, distorting calices.
Fig. IV.1.H29b   Puncture shows a multi-locular cyst as the responsible lesion.

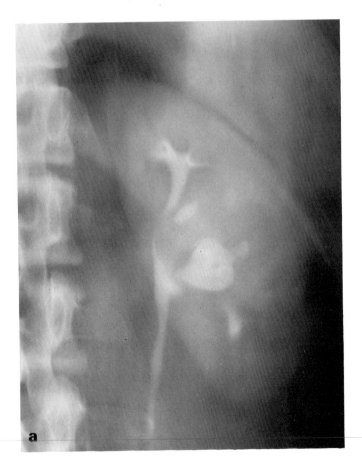
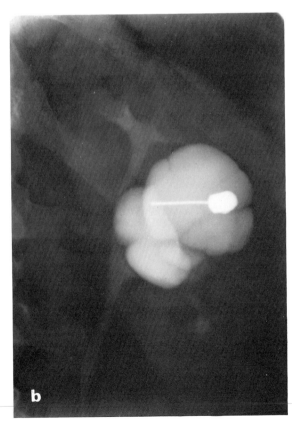

large number of cysts punctured every day—a comparative series was unable to show any difference in 5 year survival related to fine-needle puncture (von Schreeb *et al*, 1967). Indeed, fine needle puncture of a suspected renal carcinoma can be used with advantage for the definitive diagnosis; it is a direct and easy method in the elderly patient by comparison with angiography.

It is important to aspirate hard on the needle when it is in a solid lesion. Cytology comes into its own here. Cytological examination of ordinary clear cyst fluid is usually carried out, but is most unlikely to reveal a dramatic unsuspected diagnosis. However, careful washing of the needle after aspirating a solid mass will often produce vital cytological material for diagnosis. False negative results still occur, but false positive cytological answers are unlikely (Highman & Sherwood, 1978).

Individual clinical circumstances will dictate the next move after solid mass puncture with negative cytological findings. Arteriography can be useful for confirming a carcinoma. As a rule, surgical exploration will be the right final step. However, inspection of a kidney is generally agreed to be a poor diagnostic manoeuvre, and the radiologist must always aim to establish a likely preoperative diagnosis for guiding the surgeon toward correct management at operation.

Hazards of renal puncture. These are slight. Blood will often be aspirated because of hitting a vessel, and the intrepid can then obtain a needle angiogram of the kidney (Fig. IV.1.H30). Complications from this are so rare that renal

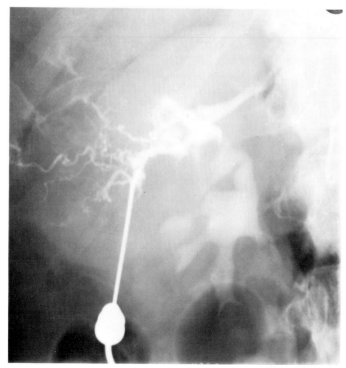

Fig. IV.1.H30 Mixed arteriogram and venogram obtained during renal puncture (carcinoma).

puncture is increasingly performed as an outpatient procedure. The patient should be warned that transient haematuria may occur, and provisions made that he can report back at once if untoward complications occur.

A *pneumothorax* may be induced with upper pole punctures. It is a rare complication, and not usually severe when it occurs. It is wise to avoid beginning the puncture at a higher level than absolutely necessary—it may therefore be better to angle the needle upwards under the twelfth or eleventh rib, ignoring the point about vertical needle paths made earlier.

There is an obvious worry about puncturing an unsuspected *hydatid cyst*— could the disease be spread disastrously? This does not seem to be so on the strength of one case report (Roylance *et al*, 1973). The condition may of course be suspected if there is renal calcification, or unusual ultrasound findings (multiple septa in the cyst). Plasma tests can then be done. The whole subject does not look like presenting an undue hazard in the management of renal cysts, even in a country like Australia where hydatid disease is prevalent.

Bloody cyst aspirate. This may occur because of a traumatic puncture, characterized by initially bloody fluid which clears on further aspiration. It is of no consequence.

A cyst may have bled in the past. It will then contain altered blood. If the walls are lined by irregular clot, a very difficult diagnostic problem arises (Fig. IV.1.H31). There is controversy about whether all such lesions need to be explored in the presence of negative cytological findings. My persuasion is that this is the only safe course. Enzyme estimations (e.g. HBD—hydroxybutyrate dehydrogenase) may be helpful, since these are raised in carcinoma.

Cyst/carcinoma. There are two main presentations of this much vaunted double lesion at renal puncture.

1. The breaking down, necrotic carcinoma containing fluid. This is a not uncommon happening in large renal tumours. The diagnosis is obvious: discoloured, murky fluid is obtained at puncture from a lesion which has shaggy outlines when contrast medium is introduced (Fig. IV.1.H32).

2. The cyst harbouring a tumour in its wall. This is a very rare lesion. Simple cysts may be lined by a sheet of clear cells, and discussion is possible among pathologists whether the diagnosis of carcinoma then made is really sound (Dr R. C. B. Pugh, London—personal communication). Cytology of the cyst fluid offers the possibility of diagnosis in these cases, but they are so excessively rare against the frequency of simple cysts that they should not be allowed to dictate management of a common condition.

The most important safeguard against missing an associated carcinoma is probably to have wary eyes open at each step in the diagnostic pathway. Any even slightly odd finding should raise suspicion, e.g. cyst fluid gelling in the syringe—one of the interesting pointers to a hidden carcinoma which has been encountered.

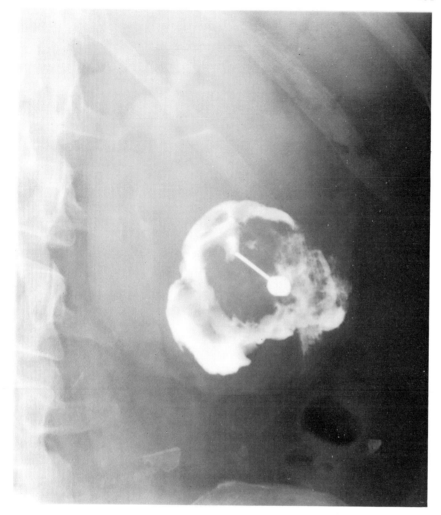

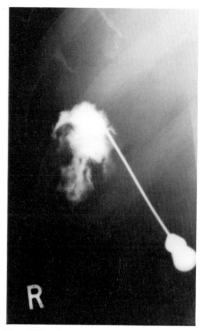

Fig. IV.1.H31 *(left)* Puncture of this avascular lower renal pole mass produced altered blood. A shaggy cavity is outlined, not accounting for the whole of the mass. At operation this was a renal cyst lined with old clot.

Fig. IV.1.H32 *(above)* Necrotic carcinoma—discoloured gritty fluid was obtained at puncture, outlining a grossly irregular cavity.

Ultrasound diagnosis: complex lesion→arteriography

The characteristic angiogram of a renal carcinoma shows a highly vascular lesion of obvious chaotic architecture: the abnormal new vessels of the tumour (Fig. IV.1.H33). There would be no problem if carcinomas alone always produced this image on angiography. Unfortunately this is not so. The main problems are:

1. Avascular carcinomas. A small proportion (about 5%) of renal carcinomas are avascular, with no abnormal vessels for distinguishing a tumour (see Fig. IV.1.H21). There is then an obvious danger of calling the lesion a cyst, though other features (e.g. the ill-defined margin) should help to prevent this mistake.

  If avascular renal tumours present as a diffuse infiltrative process rather

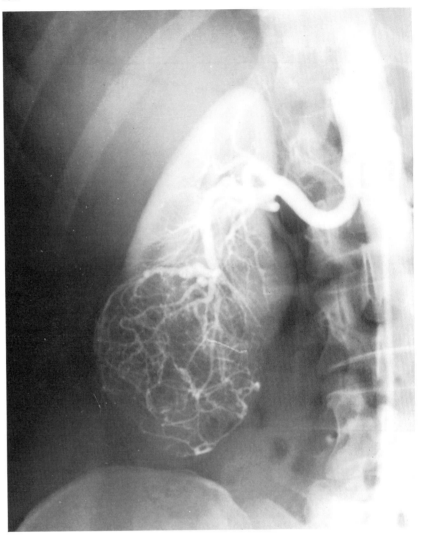

Fig. IV.1.H33 Characteristic selective arteriogram of a renal carcinoma at the lower pole.

than as a discrete lump, then other diagnoses should be considered. The more common possibilities are:

a. Carcinoma of the renal pelvis (i.e. a urothelial tumour). When invading the kidney, these tumours often produce incarceration of the vessels ('cuffing'), with peripheral ischaemia (Fig. IV.1.H34).

b. Metastases, particularly from bronchial carcinoma.

c. Lymphoma.

d. Sarcomatous renal carcinoma.

2. Benign masses with abnormal vessels. Abnormal new vessels are not pathognomonic of renal carcinoma. Inflammatory conditions in particular may show

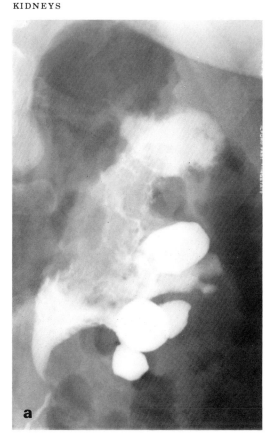

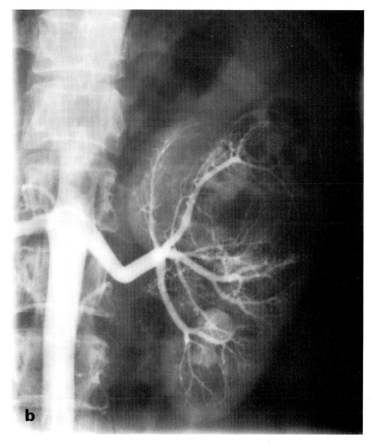

such arteries, though usually in the periphery rather than the centre of the lesion. It is regrettable that abnormal vessels are not a unique marker of malignant states, yet this established fact should help to put into perspective the ingenious attempts made to highlight such vessels. Adrenalin has been used to shut down normal renal vessels, thus casting the abnormal ones into prominence (Fig. IV.1.H35). This makes for attractive arteriograms, but not usually for any critical improvement in diagnostic acumen. Unhappily, the abnormal new vessels found in inflammatory conditions are similarly adrenalin-unresponsive. The place of this technique is therefore increasingly in doubt.

Fig. IV.1.H34a & b   Pyelogram and arteriogram of a renal pelvis carcinoma. Note the ischaemic effects distal to the tumour in the renal parenchyma.

Renal carcinoma investigation

If the IVU and ultrasound point to a likely renal carcinoma why carry out angiography at all, given the above uncertainties of arteriographic diagnosis? Clinical circumstances are indeed met quite often, particularly in the elderly, where a quick nephrectomy of a likely renal carcinoma on IVU and ultrasound appears the best course. Needle puncture of the mass before operation is then

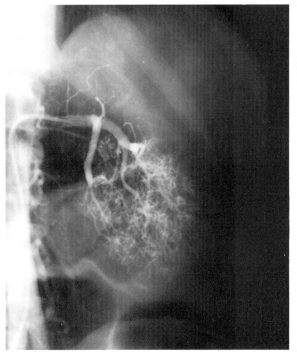

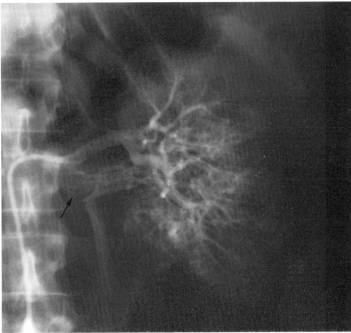

Fig. IV.1.H35 *(left)* Selective arteriogram done immediately after an injection of adrenalin into the renal artery. Only the abnormal vessels in the lower pole carcinoma are shown—the normal upper pole circulation has been shut down.

Fig. IV.1.H36 *(right)* Blocked renal vein shown during selective arteriography. There is a large left renal carcinoma with abnormal vessels. Note reflux down the testicular vein. The arrow points to the blocked renal vein, and also to a leash of abnormal new vessels running into the renal hilum—a sign of tumour extension here.

helpful in confirming the diagnosis and preventing needless surgery of some rare inflammatory lesion like an old abscess.

In most other circumstances arteriography is still the preoperative investigation of choice of a suspected carcinoma. This is because:

1. The diagnosis of renal carcinoma can usually be confirmed/refuted.

2. The contralateral kidney is shown to be normal by the most sensitive technique. An appreciable number of patients with a renal carcinoma have a similar contralateral tumour.

3. The renal vein is shown to be patent or not.

Point 3 is important for surgical management, and can usually be resolved on arteriography. Once a renal tumour circulation has been seen, the unilateral nephrotoxic complications of a large dose of contrast medium are of no concern to a nephrectomy candidate. Selective arteriography should therefore be done with about four times the usual dose (e.g. 15 g iodine). The renal vein and any involvement will then be seen (Fig. IV.1.H36). Failure to see it suggests occlusion, but this needs to be checked with a separate venographic procedure.

It may be noted that arteriography is probably not helpful for staging renal cancer, despite claims to this end (Das *et al,* 1977). In particular, feeding of the tumour by extrarenal arteries is no indication that it has extended outside the renal capsule. Such 'cannibalization' of blood supply happens readily enough because of a carcinoma's avid perfusion needs, making use of existing collateral channels even whilst the tumour remains wholly intrarenal.

Renal carcinoma embolization. At the end of the diagnostic arteriogram the tumour can be infarcted by sending emboli through the selective renal catheter. This can be a very helpful preoperative manoeuvre, making for easier and drier nephrectomy in these highly vascular carcinomas. The method is also used as a palliative measure for inoperable growths. Embolization is a rapidly growing field (*The Lancet,* 1978).

Errors in the diagnostic pathway

The initial ultrasound decision on whether a cyst should be punctured or a possible tumour go to arteriography has an error rate. This is less than 5% in skilled hands. The diagnostic pathway recognizes this possibility. Thus the patient with a renal cyst misread as a complex lesion will have an unnecessary arteriogram, revealing the true diagnosis—costly but not disastrous. More worrying is the tumour misread on ultrasound as a cyst, which will then be needled. As explained above, the hazard of spreading tumour cells by fine needle puncture is very small, and counterbalanced by the advantage of having an unsuspected problem diagnosis lit up in this way. Critical diagnostic pathways like this are trial-and-error exercises: textbook examples of scientific method (Sherwood, 1978).

Other problem ultrasound masses

Renal abscess

This may be within the kidney (renal carbuncle) or without (perinephric abscess). Diabetes is an important predisposing condition. The early stages of abscess formation are now reversible by effective medical treatment. Considerable deformity of the kidney may be seen, but this can still revert to normal without surgery (Fig. IV.1.H37). In gross diabetic renal infection, gas forming organisms may be present to produce gas which may be seen around the kidney, or within the pelvi-caliceal system, ureter or bladder.

Angiomyolipoma

This unusual hamartoma is met in two forms. Multiple renal lesions occur in patients with tuberose sclerosis, and the combined clinico-radiological diagnosis is usually straightforward. In otherwise normal patients with a single renal hamartoma the diagnosis is difficult. The fat content may pinpoint the nature of the angiomyolipoma—the mass is radiolucent (Fig. IV.1.H38). Distinc-

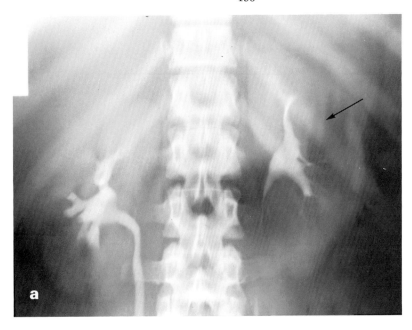

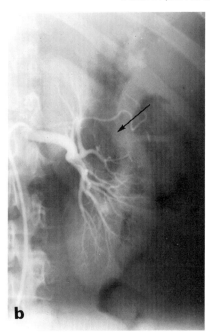

Fig. IV.1.H37a & b IVU and selective
arteriogram in left renal abscess (arrow).
The patient did very well after simple
puncture and aspiration of the pus.

tive angiographic features are described (Barrilero, 1977), but the picture is so
worryingly close to renal carcinoma that most patients come to surgery.

Xanthogranuloma

Xanthogranulomatous pyelonephritis covers a pathological spectrum, beginning with a slight, patchy inflammatory renal reaction to a stone, and ending
with a large mass mimicking a carcinoma. Patients with a large xanthogranuloma are usually sick, anaemic and have lost weight. Renal stones are often
present, together with a urinary infection involving proteus. The picture can
resemble carcinoma very closely. Angiographic features are sometimes helpful
(Gingell *et al*, 1973; Gammill *et al*, 1975) (Fig. IV.1.H39). The best treatment is
probably nephrectomy, so that diagnostic confusion with carcinoma, whilst
inelegant and undesirable, does not lead to mismanagement.

Urinoma

A dissection space filled with extravasated urine is now an increasingly common complication of traffic accidents. Essentially there is a tear of a part of the
pelvicaliceal system, with the formation of a parapelvic urine swelling which
persists ('parapelvic pseudo cyst'—another term best forgotten). Once estab-

lished, the lesion will not resolve spontaneously, and needs surgical attention (Fig. IV.1.H40).

Disappearing cyst

Simple renal cysts may rupture spontaneously (Fig. IV.1.H41). A patient can therefore come for ultrasound examination on the strength of a previous IVU showing a probable cyst, and puzzle the radiologist who cannot now find the lump. If there is obvious discordance between the two examinations, it is better to repeat the IVU than to rush into angiography.

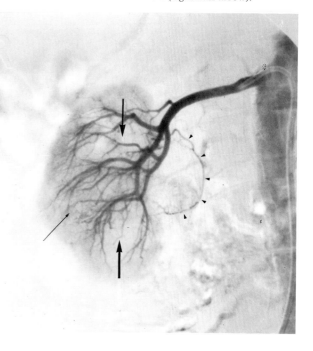

Fig. IV.1.H38 *(left)*   Selective arteriogram in angiomyolipoma—note the black appearance (fat) of the main tumour mass, even though this is clearly a highly vascular lesion. (Courtesy of Dr D. Allison).

Fig. IV.1.H39 *(right)*   Subtraction renal arteriogram in xanthogranulomatous pyelonephritis. Non-excreting kidney blocked by a stone—note the dilated renal pelvis outlined by a stretched artery (arrowheads). The large arrows point to dilated calices, producing avascular areas. Many abnormal new vessels are seen elsewhere (e.g. small arrow).

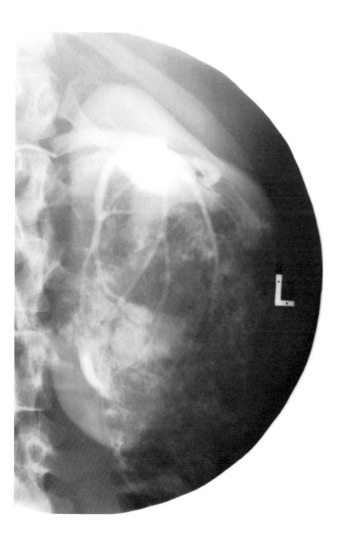

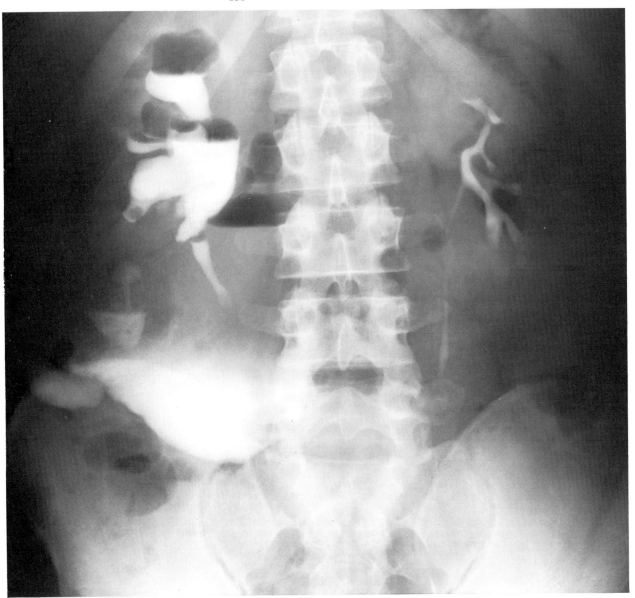

Fig. IV.1.H40 Right urinoma—note
extensive leak of contrast medium into a
large pararenal mass, with additional
fluid levels in calices and also in the
urinoma. A stone is present in the
lowermost calix of this kidney. Attempted
percutaneous drainage of the lesion was
responsible for the air—surgical repair is
the more appropriate treatment.

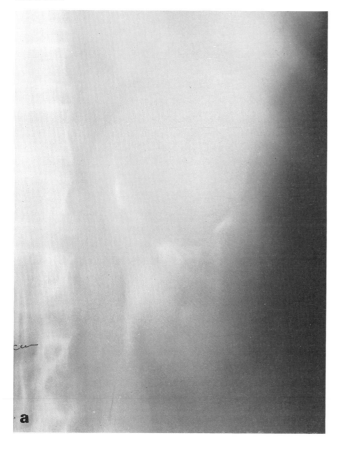

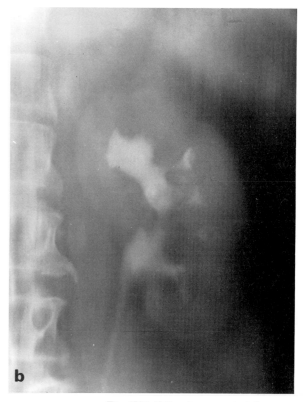

Fig. IV.1.H41a Large cyst at the upper renal pole.
Fig. IV.1.H41b Five months later the lesion has resolved spontaneously—a cyst which has ruptured on its own.

J. TRAUMA

Traffic accidents are now the most common cause of renal injury. Haematuria following flank trauma is the usual presentation. There is controversy about the radiological management of some renal injuries, but probably none about the following three groups of the clinical spectrum:

1. A traffic accident victim is brought into the casualty department with hypotension and obvious clinical signs of brisk intra-abdominal bleeding from renal and/or splenic injuries. Immediate urgent surgery is indicated. If time allows a plain film of the abdomen should be done, but the patient may have to be rushed to the operating theatre at once. It is vital that he should be given an intravenous injection of urographic contrast medium en route to the theatre. On the operating table an abdominal radiograph can then be taken to make sure that the kidney opposite to the injured one is present and of normal size. Hypotension will probably have been corrected by then. In any event, as long as blood pressure is not catastrophically low, a nephrogram will be seen. The importance of this observation is obvious: if the damaged kidney should be the patient's only one, every effort will have to be made to avoid nephrectomy.

2. A fit patient is seen because of haematuria following a flank injury. An immediate IVU is unremarkable, and masterly inactivity is all that is needed.

3. If there is complete unilateral failure of contrast excretion on the IVU, i.e. no nephrogram/pyelogram, or similar results on radioisotope studies, arteriography is indicated—with the exception mentioned below. The renal artery may be completely transected in such a patient, and it is helpful to have full angiographic assessment of the injury before reparative or ablative surgery.

There is one exception to this course of action for a kidney on the side of injury without apparent function on IVU or radioisotope scan. This is when the nature of the injury, the clinical findings and the plain film are all out of keeping with the diagnosis of a severely hurt kidney. The injury may then have fortuitously lit up a long-standing renal functional disorder on that side, e.g. an absent kidney or a hydronephrosis. Under these circumstances an immediate ultrasound scan is very helpful in confirming or refuting these suggestions.

There is dissent about what to do if the IVU shows partial damage to one kidney (Fig. IV.1.J1). This may be seen either as a perirenal/intrarenal haematoma, or as a tear of the renal outline with contrast extravasation. The obvious suggestion is to perform an arteriogram, which will allow full assessment of the extent and site of the injury (Fig. IV.1.J2). However, management of such a fit

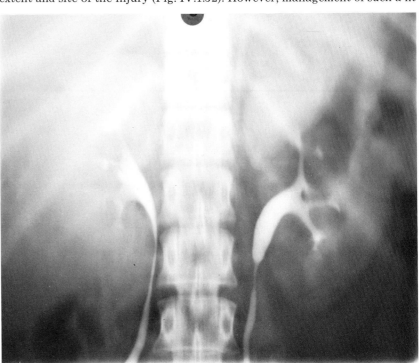

Fig. IV.1.J1 Right perirenal haematoma—note the expanded, ill-defined outline of the right lower renal pole. This was a renal biopsy complication.

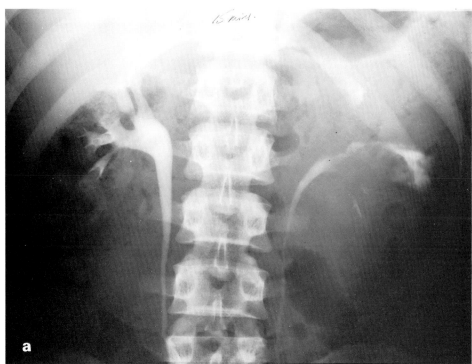

Fig. IV.1.J2a Following trauma to the left flank, the IVU shows contrast medium leaking outside the kidney on this side.

Fig. IV.1.J2b & c Early and late frames on the selective arteriogram—note tear across the middle of the left kidney. (Courtesy of Dr J. J. Stevenson).

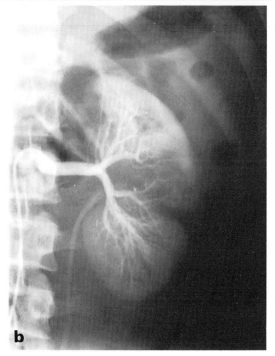

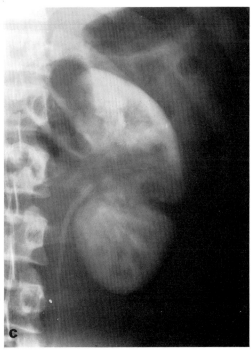

patient with stable blood pressure and pulse rate is generally conservative. Whatever is found angiographically has no important influence on clinical management.

In this country arteriography is therefore not used extensively, and to doves that naturally appears a wise course. The hawks would maintain that good opportunities for conservative, reparative surgery are lost in this way. The question of later hypertension from unevacuated haematomas or ischaemic renal debris is raised, but this seems to be a rare sequel.

Summary note

The non-excreting kidney on the side of injury needs either arteriography, or ultrasound if an irrelevant long-standing disorder is suspected. Every patient with haematuria following flank trauma must have an IVU or radioisotope scan (see Part II section A) to assess the contralateral kidney. This organ cannot be presumed healthy or even present till shown to be so. Enough tragic cases with a 'quick nephrectomy' of a bleeding only kidney are on record to make this an iron first rule of all trauma work.

K. LOIN PAIN AND HAEMATURIA SYNDROME (renal arteritis)

In 1967 Little, Sloper and de Wardener described patients with loin pain and haematuria who had multiple renal cortical perfusion defects on arteriography. These observations have been extended by Higgins and Aber (1974). The patients are predominantly women who show remarkable arteriographic abnormalities of the peripheral renal vasculature (Fig. IV.1.K1) (Guyer, 1978).

The importance of these interesting studies is under debate. We have seen similar patients who have then had normal open renal biopsy findings. Transient perfusion defects can be induced by selective renal artery catheterization and injection alone (Fig. IV.1.K2). Tadavarthy *et al* (1977) have documented spectacular but temporary renal arteriography artefacts which can be put down to vascular spasm. The selective renal arteriogram should always be interpreted with caution—it represents the state of the vasculature at a single unusual moment, which may not be representative of the rest of the 24 hours.

Despite these reservations, the syndrome is clearly of considerable interest, and further studies are awaited. Do these patients have an unusually labile renal circulation in regard to spasm?

Renal arteritis

Polyarteritis nodosa produces the most florid radiological picture under this heading. The angiogram shows multiple renal aneurysms and perfusion defects (Fig. IV.1.K3). Whilst these lesions are frequent and highly suggestive in this

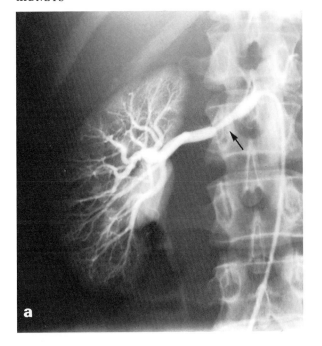

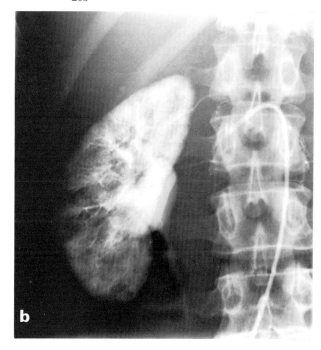

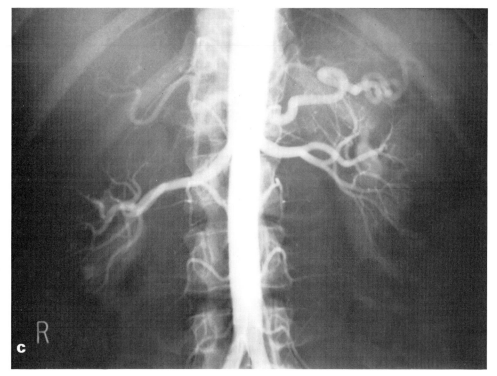

Fig. IV.1.K1a Selective arteriogram in a young woman with loin pain—note that spasm of the main renal artery has been induced (arrow).
Fig. IV.1.K1b On this later arteriogram frame, there are multiple small perfusion defects throughout the renal cortex.
Fig. IV.1.K1c Aortogram—note that the right main renal artery is normal.

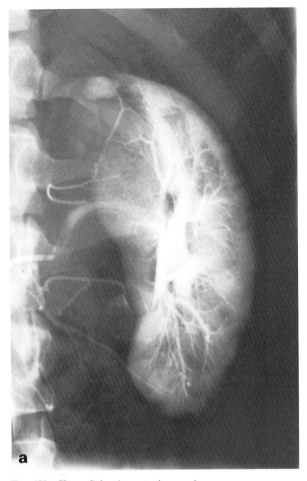

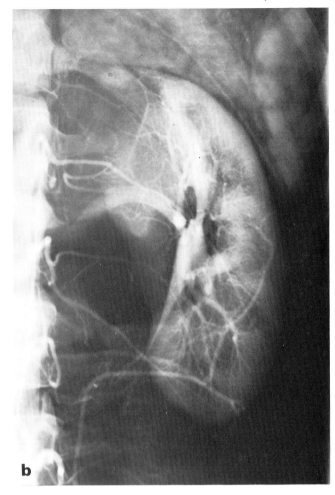

Fig. IV.1.K2a Selective arteriogram in
a patient with a non-excreting upper
moiety of a duplex kidney—she does not
suffer from the syndrome under
discussion. Note multiple small perfusion
defects throughout the renal cortex.
Fig. IV.1.K2b On this frame from the
aortogram done just before selective
catheterization, it is clear that the lower
moiety renal cortex is in fact entirely
normal. (Courtesy of Dr Brenda van
Leuven).

condition, it is possible that any severe arteritis can give rise to similar changes
in the kidney (Robins & Bookstein, 1972). 'Mainline' drug addiction involving
repeated dirty intravenous injections is one example.

Renal arterio-venous fistula

These are now most commonly acquired, not congenital lesions, following renal
biopsy. Most are transient and unimportant, and troublesome haematuria is an
unusual complication (Fig. IV.1.K4). A major fistula is a rare hazard of renal
trauma, or of a careless nephrectomy where artery and vein are tied off together
in one stump (Fig. IV.1.K5).

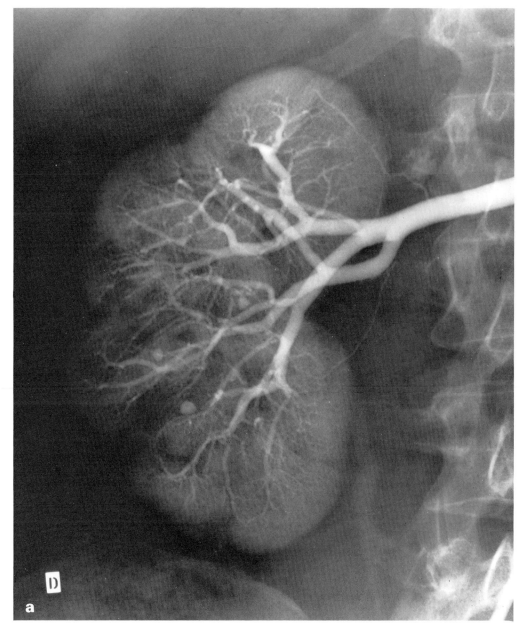

a

Fig. IV.1.K3a *(left)* & **b** *(overpage)*
Polyarteritis nodosa—note multiple large
aneurysms in the kidney and liver on
these selective arteriograms. There are
large ischaemic territories in the kidney.
(Courtesy of unknown French radiologist).

Renal artery aneurysm

Small aneurysms present no great risk in regard to rupture, but may lead to
vascular obstruction and hypertension (Fig. IV.1.K6) (see Part III p. 78).

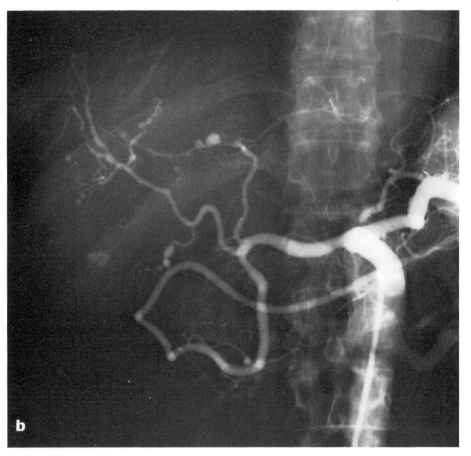

Fig. IV.1.K4 *(facing page—top left)*   Haematuria following renal biopsy. This patient has had several renal biopsies over the years, and the selective renal arteriogram shows an arterio-venous fistula (small arrow), with immediate filling of the inferior vena cava (large arrow). (Courtesy of Dr D. Allison).

Fig. IV.1.K5 *(facing page—top right)*   Post-nephrectomy arteriovenous fistula—on this selective arteriogram contrast medium passes straight from the renal artery stump into a fistulous bag leading to the inferior vena cava.

Fig. IV.1.K6a & b *(facing page—bottom)*   IVU and aortogram in renal artery aneurysm. Note how the aneurysm (large arrows) indents the renal pelvis, and the para-ureteric collaterals (small arrows) the ureter.

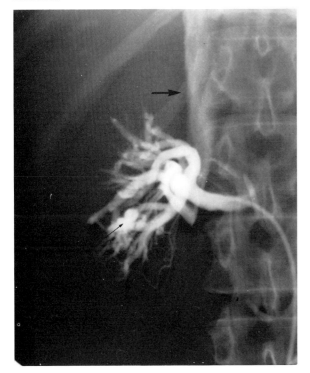

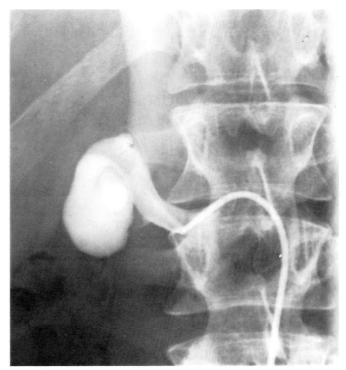

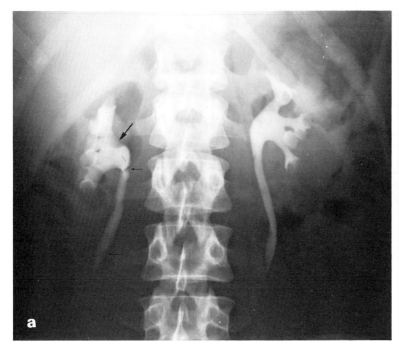

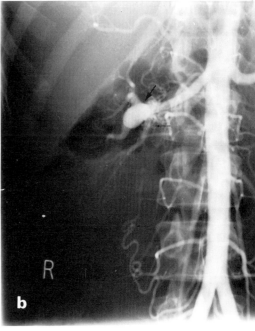

REFERENCES

ALTON D.J. & McDONALD P. (1973) Urographic findings in the Bardet-Biedl syndrome. *Radiology* **109**, 659–663.

ASSCHER A.W. *et al* (1978) Sequelae of covert bacteriuria in schoolgirls. *Lancet* **i**, 889–893.

BARRILERO A.E. (1977) Renal angiomyolipoma. *Journal of Urology* **117**, 547–552.

BLYTH H. & OCKENDEN B.G. (1971) Polycystic disease of the kidneys and liver presenting in childhood. *Journal of Medical Genetics* **8**, 257–284.

BOLANDE R.P. (1974) Congenital and infantile neoplasia of the kidney. *Lancet* **ii**, 1497–1499.

British Medical Journal (1976) Wilms' tumour. **2**, 1166–1167.

BUSH W.H., BURNETT L.L. & GIBBONS R.P. (1977) Needle tract seeding of renal carcinoma. *American Journal of Roentgenology* **129**, 725–727.

CHRISPIN A.R. (1972) Medullary necrosis in infancy. *British Medical Bulletin* **28**, 233–236.

DANIEL W.W., HARTMAN G.W., WITTEN D.M., FARROW G.M. & KELALIS P.P. (1972) Calcified renal masses. *Radiology* **103**, 503–508.

DAS G., CHISHOLM G.D. & SHERWOOD T. (1977) Can angiography stage renal carcinoma? *British Journal of Urology* **49**, 611–614.

DAVIDSON A.J. (1977) *Radiologic Diagnosis of Renal Parenchymal Disease*. W. B. Saunders Co., Philadelphia.

DAVIDSON A.J., BECKER J., ROTHFIELD N., UNGER G. & PLOCH D.R. (1970) An evaluation of the effect of high-dose urography on previously impaired renal and hepatic function in man. *Radiology* **97**, 249–254.

DAVIDSON A.J. & TALNER L.B. (1973a) Urographic and angiographic abnormalities in adult-onset acute bacterial nephritis. *Radiology* **106**, 249–256.

DAVIDSON A.J. & TALNER L.B. (1973b) Lack of specificity of renal angiography in the diagnosis of renal parenchymal disease. *Investigative Radiology* **8**, 90–95.

DE VARGAS A. *et al.* (1978) A family study of vesicoureteric reflux. *Journal of Medical Genetics* **15**, 85–96.

DOYLE F.H., THA AUNG, CARROL R.N.P., WILLIAMS E.D. & SHACKMAN R. (1972) Bone resorption in chronic renal failure. *British Medical Bulletin* **28**, 225–227.

EDWARDS D., NORMAND I.C.S., PRESCOD N. & SMELLIE J.M. (1977) Disappearance of vesicoureteric reflux during long-term prophylaxis of urinary tract infection in children. *British Medical Journal* **2**, 285–288.

EKELUND L. (1977) Radiologic findings in renal amyloidosis. *American Journal of Roentgenology* **129**, 851–853.

FARRANT P. & MEIRE H.B. (1978) Ultrasonic measurement of renal inclination: its importance in measurement of renal length. *British Journal of Radiology* **51**, 628–630.

FELSON B. & CUSSEN L.J. (1975) The hydronephrotic type of unilateral congenital multicystic disease of the kidney. *Seminars in Roentgenology* **10**, 113–123.

FRY I.K. & CATTELL W.R. (1972) The nephrographic pattern during excretion urography. *British Medical Bulletin* **28**, 227–232.

GAMMILL S., RABINOWITZ J.G., PEACE R., SORGEN S., HURWITZ L. & HIMMELFARB E. (1975) New thoughts concerning xanthogranulomatous pyelonephritis. *American Journal of Roentgenology* **125**, 154–163.

GILL W.B., LU C.T. & THOMSEN S. (1973) Retrograde brushing. *Journal of Urology* **109**, 573–578.

GINGELL J.C., ROYLANCE J., DAVIES E.R. & PENRY J.B. (1973) Xanthogranulomatous pyelonephritis. *British Journal of Radiology* **46**, 99–109.

GRIFFITHS G.J., CARTWRIGHT G. & McLACHLAN M.S.F. (1974) Estimation of renal size from radiographs. *Clinical Radiology* **26**, 249–256.

GRIFFITHS G.J., ROBINSON K.B., CARTWRIGHT G.O. & McLACHLAN M.S.F. (1976) Loss of renal tissue in the elderly. *British Journal of Radiology* **49**, 111–117.

GUYER P.B. (1978) Radiology of the loin pain—haematuria syndrome. *Clinical Radiology* **29**, 561–564.

HARE W.S.C. & KINCAID-SMITH P. (1970) Dissecting aneurysm of the renal artery. *Radiology* **97**, 255–263.

HIGGINS P.M. & ABER G.M. (1974) Renal pain and haematuria. *British Journal of Urology* **46**, 601–608.

HIGHMAN W. & SHERWOOD T. (1978) The pre-operative diagnosis of renal masses. *Journal of the Royal Society of Medicine* **71**, 586–590.

HODSON C.J. (1972a) The lobar structure of the kidney. *British Journal of Urology* **44**, 246–261.

HODSON C.J. (1972b) Post-obstructive renal atrophy (nephropathy). *British Medical Bulletin* **28**, 237–240.

HODSON C.J. (1977) Radiology of the renal parenchyma. In *Contributions to Nephrology*, Vol. 5 (Radiology and the kidney), pp. 41–62. Karger, Basel.

HODSON C.J., MALING T.M.J., McMANAMON P.J. & LEWIS M.G. (1975) The pathogenesis of reflux nephropathy. *British Journal of Radiology* Supplement 13.

JOHNSTON J.H. (1973) Megacalicosis: a burnt-out obstruction? *Journal of Urology* **110**, 344–346.

JOHNSTON J.H. & MIX L.W. (1976) The Ask-Upmark kidney: a form of ascending pyelonephritis? *British Journal of Urology* **48**, 393–398.

JUNGHAGEN P. & LINDQVIST B. (1973) Nephroangiography in nephronophthisis. *Acta Radiologica (Diagnosis)* **4**, 106–112.

KINGSTON R.D., SHAH K.J. & DAWSON-EDWARDS P. (1977) Ascending uretero-pyelography in renal failure. *Clinical Radiology* **28**, 483–489.

KOEHLER P.R., TALNER L.B., FRIEDENBERG M.J. & KYAW M.M. (1973) Association of subcapsular haematomas with the non-functioning kidney. *Radiology* **106**, 537–542.

The Lancet (1978) Therapeutic embolization. **i**, 1135–1136.

LEBOWITZ R.L., HOPKINS T. & COLODNY A.H. (1975) Measuring the kidneys—practical applications using a growth and hypertrophy chart. *Pediatric Radiology* **4**, 37–42.

LITTLE P.J., SLOPER J.S. & DE WARDENER H.E. (1967) A syndrome of loin pain and haematuria associated with disease of peripheral renal arteries. *Quarterly Journal of Medicine* **36**, 253–259.

MENA E., BOOKSTEIN J.J. & GIKAS P.W. (1973) Angiographic diagnosis of renal parenchymal disease. *Radiology* **108**, 523–532.

MEYERS M.A., FRIEDENBERG R.M., KING M.C. & MENG C.H. (1967) The significance of renal capsular arteries. *British Journal of Radiology* **40**, 949–956.

PLAINE L.I. & HINMAN F. (1965) Malignancy in asymptomatic renal masses. *Journal of Urology* **94**, 342–347.

POYNTER J.D. & HARE W.S.C. (1974) Necrosis in situ: a form of renal papillary necrosis seen in analgesic nephropathy. *Radiology* **111**, 69–76.

RANSLEY P.G. & RISDON R.A. (1978) Reflux and renal scarring. *British Journal of Radiology* Supplement 14.

RITTER R. & SIAFARIKAS K. (1976) Hemihypertrophy in a boy with renal polycystic disease: varied pattern of presentation of renal polycystic disease in his family. *Pediatric Radiology* **5**, 98–102.

ROBINS J.M. & BOOKSTEIN J.J. (1972) Regressing aneurysms in periarteritis nodosa. *Radiology* **104**, 215–218.

ROYLANCE J., RHYS DAVIES E. & ALEXANDER W.D. (1973) Translumbar puncture of a renal hydatid cyst. *British Journal of Radiology* **46**, 960–963.

RUSIEWICZ E. & REILLY B.J. (1968) The significance of isolated upper pole calyceal dilatation. *Journal of the Canadian Association of Radiologists* **19**, 179–182.

SAXTON H.M. (1969) Urography. *British Journal of Radiology* **42**, 321–346.

SHERWOOD T. (1978) Science in Radiology. *Lancet* **i**, 594–595.

SHERWOOD T., DOYLE F.H., BOULTON-JONES M., JOEKES A.M., PETERS D.K. & SISSONS P.
(1974) The intravenous urogram in acute renal failure. *British Journal of Radiology*
47, 368–372.

SINGH M., CHAPMAN R., TRESIDDER G.C. & BLANDY J. (1973) The fate of the unoperated
staghorn calculus. *British Journal of Urology* **45**, 581–585.

STADALNIK R.C., VERA Z., DASILVA O., DAVIES R., KRAUS J.F. & MASON D.T. (1977)
Electrocardiographic response to intravenous urography. *American Journal of
Roentgenology* **129**, 825–830.

TADAVARTHY S.M., CASTANEDA W. & AMPLATZ K. (1977) Redistribution of renal blood flow
caused by contrast media. *Radiology* **122**, 343–348.

TALNER L.B. & GITTES R.F. (1974) Megacalyces: further observations and differentiation
from obstructive renal disease. *American Journal of Roentgenology* **121**, 473–486.

TEGTMEYER C.J., CAIL W., WYKER A.W. & GILLENWATER J.Y. (1978) Angiographic diagnosis of renal tumours associated with polycystic disease. *Radiology* **126**, 105–109.

TREW P.A., BIAVA C.G., JACOBS R.P. & HOPPER J. (1978) Renal vein thrombosis in
membranous glomerulonephropathy: incidence and association. *Medicine* **57**, 69–82.

VON SCHREEB T., AMER O., SKOVSTED G. & WIKSTAD N. (1967) Renal adenocarcinoma—is
there a risk of spreading tumour cells in diagnostic puncture? *Scandinavian Journal
of Urology and Nephrology* **1**, 270–276.

WHITAKER R.H. (1973) Methods of assessing obstruction in dilated ureters. *British Journal
of Urology* **45**, 15–22.

WHITFIELD H.N. *et al* (1977) The obstructed kidney: correlation between renal function
and urodynamic assessment. *British Journal of Urology* **49**, 615–619.

WRONG O.M. & FEEST T.G. (1976) Nephrocalcinosis. In *Twelfth Symposium on Advanced
Medicine.* Ed. D. K. Peters. pp. 394–406, Pitman Medical, Tunbridge Wells.

DIVISION 2.
THE KIDNEY
AND URETER

A. DUPLICATION

A double (duplex) kidney is a frequent anomaly on the IVU. The division into two moieties involves separation of the upper from the middle + lower caliceal groups (diagram A).

Duplication may be incomplete: there is a wide range in the anomaly, from a bifid renal pelvis to two completely separate ureters. When there are two separate ureters, the one draining the upper renal moiety always enters the bladder in the lower position (diagram B).

Although there are two ureteric orifices in the bladder, the two lower ureteric segments usually travel in a common sheath, making operative separation difficult.

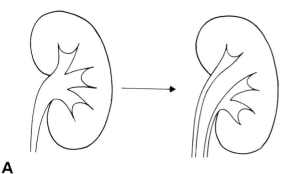

A

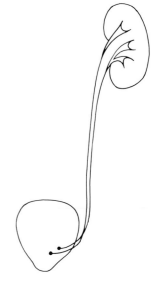

B

Clinical importance

Even a minimal duplication anomaly, e.g. bifid renal pelvis/upper ureter, is often said to predispose to urinary infection hazards. There is no good evidence for this statement. Uncomplicated duplication anomalies are of little clinical moment. They are usually chance findings on the IVU.

At the other end of this spectrum are severe urinary tract deformities impairing ipsilateral renal function, or even the integrity of the opposite kidney. The main clinical problem groups are:

1. Incomplete duplication: yo-yo reflux

2. Complete duplication:
  a. ectopic drainage of upper renal moiety
  b. ectopic ureterocele with destruction of the upper renal moiety
  c. vesico-ureteric reflux with destruction of the lower renal moiety.

211

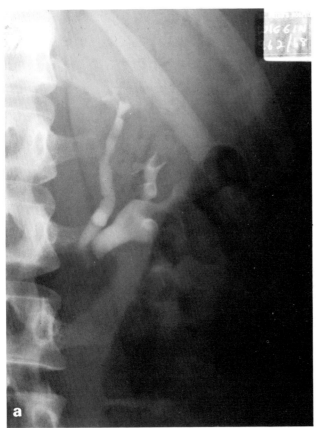

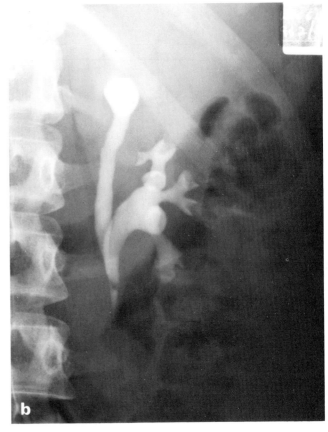

Fig. IV.2.A1a Duplex left kidney with normal upper moiety.
Fig. IV.2.A1b A moment later the upper moiety has become distended because of yo-yo reflux from the lower moiety.

1. Incomplete duplication with yo-yo reflux

When the two ureters join somewhere along their course, the possibility exists that a bolus of urine will be propelled down one of them and immediately up the other. This neat idea has attracted more attention than it merits clinically. The upper ureter may indeed by distended for a moment in this way (Fig. IV.2.A1). It is very rare for this to give rise to symptoms, though pain (distension) and infection (inefficient urinary drainage) are always touted. The anomaly should only be accepted with caution as an explanation for symptoms. Very many individuals have it with no trouble whatever.

2. Complete duplication

a. Ectopic drainage of upper urinary tract

The most important clinical presentation is as a wetting problem in girls, so this is further discussed in the lower urinary tract section (Division 4 section A). In

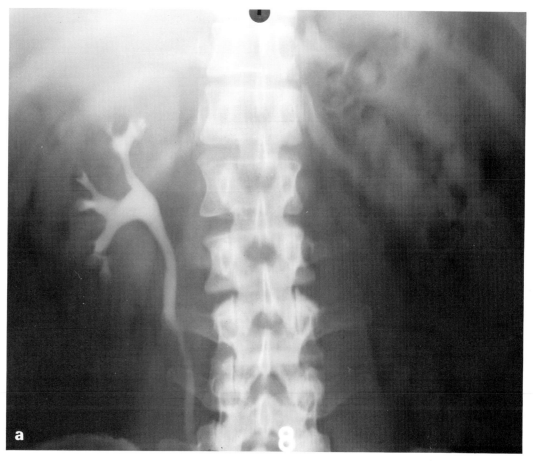

girls (but not in boys) an ectopic ureter is usually part of a duplex anomaly, and involves the ureter draining the upper renal moiety. The ureter may end in the genital tract, leading to incontinence in girls and complex deformities in boys (Fig. IV.2.A2). Other sites include the urethra: if the opening is below the pelvic floor, incontinence will result.

The single ectopic ureter is more commonly seen in boys. Bilateral single ectopic ureters are a great rarity, and always associated with a severe deformity of the whole bladder neck; hence its alternative name 'absent bladder neck syndrome' (Williams & Lightwood, 1972).

Fig. IV.2.A2a Young man with urinary infections and non-excreting left kidney.

b. Ureteroceles

These lesions generally obey certain simple rules which make them delightful radiological diagnostic exercises. Rule one concerns proper spelling, deriving from the idea that these are congenital hernias into the bladder ($\kappa\eta\lambda\eta$ = hernia).

The best division of ureteroceles is into *orthotopic* (= 'simple' or 'adult') and

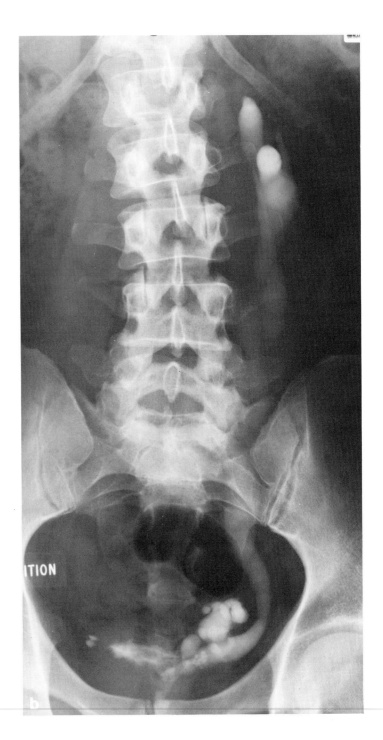

Fig. IV.2.A2b On cystography there is reflux into the ectopic left ureter via the seminal vesicle.

ectopic (= 'complex' or 'child'). The alternative names point to the common clinical presentation. Orthotopic ureteroceles are usually unimportant chance findings when adults come to have IVUs for some other reason. Ectopic ureteroceles are troublesome and therefore present in childhood.

Orthotopic ureteroceles: these are bulbous congenital deformities of the lowermost ends of single ureters. The IVU shows a characteristic 'cobra-head' picture —a radiolucent halo where the ureteric + bladder mucosa separates contrast medium in the lesion from that already in the bladder (Fig. IV.2.A3). They may be uni- or bilateral (Fig IV.2.A4). If very large they may give rise to trouble by distortion, causing obstruction in the parent or even the opposite ureter.

Ectopic ureteroceles: these are always part of a duplex anomaly, involving the lower end of the upper-renal-moiety ureter. The 'ectopic' label of the lesion refers to its opening. Because the lower-renal-moiety ureter already occupies the normal position for opening into the bladder on the trigone, a ureterocele

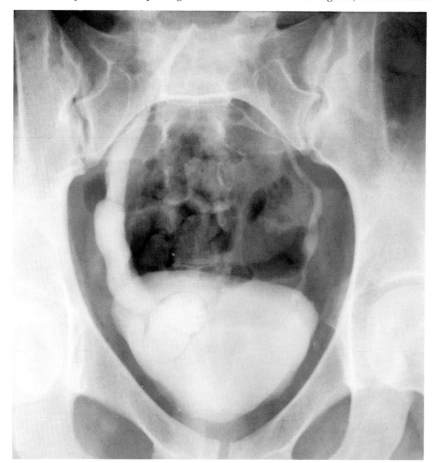

Fig. IV.2.A3 Orthotopic ureterocele on the right. Note dilatation of the ureter above.

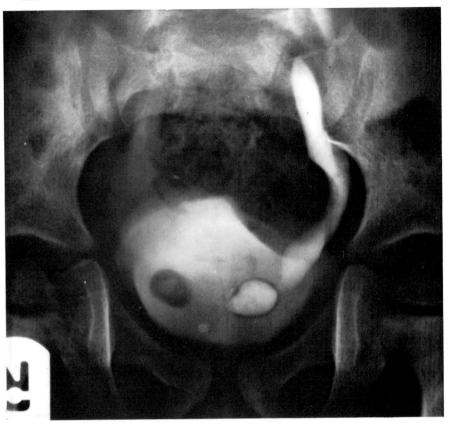

Fig. IV.2.A4 Bilateral orthotopic ureteroceles.

deformity of the upper-moiety ureter usually means an abnormal, displaced opening of this ureter. The opening may be into the bladder neck or urethra.

The ectopic ureterocele is associated with a badly made ('dysplastic') upper renal moiety, which will always appear abnormal on the IVU. Worse, the lesion distorts the trigone, and so leads very readily to severe obstruction of the ipsilateral or contralateral ureters (Fig. IV.2.A5). Infection is an obvious complication of such events (Table IV.2.1).

Rule-of-thumb: in practice a normal IVU picture of the upper renal moiety of a duplex kidney *excludes* the possibility of an ipsilateral ectopic ureterocele or ectopic ureter.

Dynamic aspects of ectopic ureteroceles: the voiding cystogram can provide valuable information here. Is the ureterocele tense or floppy, i.e. does it alter shape as bladder pressure rises on voiding? Tense ureteroceles support the ipsilateral (lower moiety) ureter, whereas floppy ones allow reflux to occur into this ureter (Fig. IV.2.A6) (Williams *et al*, 1972). Is there defective backing by the bladder wall behind the ureterocele, so that the lesion bulges beyond the vesical

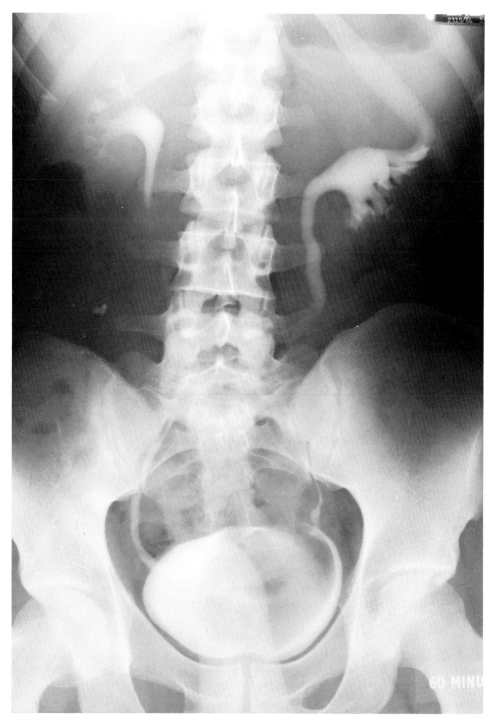

Fig. IV.2.A5 Distended non-excreting left upper renal moiety, with large ureterocele in the bladder. Because the ureterocele shadow is wholly within the bladder, ectopia is probably minimal here.

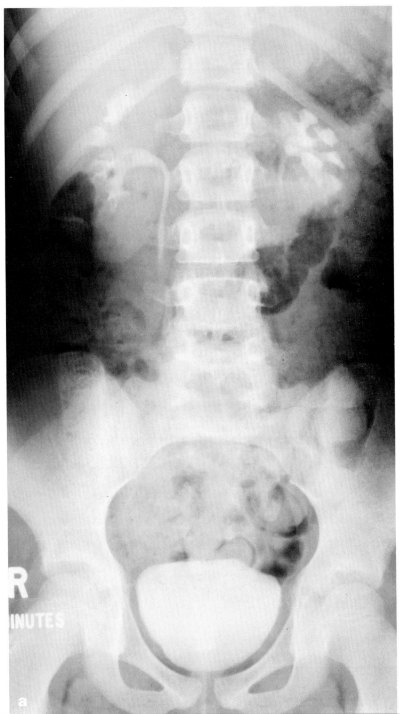

Fig. IV.2.A6a IVU showing a
non-excreting left upper renal moiety, and
rather distended lower renal moiety.

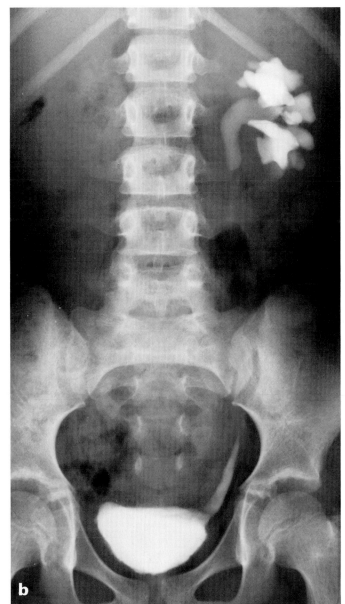

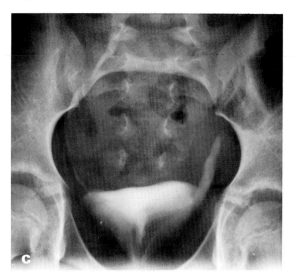

Fig. IV.2.A6b *(left)* On cystography there is reflux into the left lower renal moiety. Taken together with the IVU findings, a floppy ectopic ureterocele ought to be present, but has not been seen so far.

Fig. IV.2.A6c *(below)* The floppy, largely extra-vesical ureterocele is seen as a crescentic impression on the left border of the bladder, but only when the bladder is no longer tense.

contour on voiding, rather like a bladder aneurysm (Fig. IV.2.A7)? Then operative repair of the feeble bladder patch will be needed at the time of heminephrectomy, not just simple uncapping of the ureterocele. Spontaneous rupture of an ectopic ureterocele may occur.

Summary comment. The diagnosis of ectopic ureterocele is often straightforward, but can be very hard indeed. It is worth remembering as a last-ditch explanation for the occasional child with baffling urinary tract deformities.

c. Vesico-ureteric reflux into the lower renal moiety

Rule-of-thumb: when the *upper* moiety of a duplex kidney shows no contrast excretion on the IVU, ectopic drainage or an ectopic ureterocele is the likely explanation, i.e. *dysplasia/obstruction.* This is not so with a non-excreting *lower* moiety, where *reflux* is the probable offender.

Fig. IV.2.A7a *(right)*   Large ectopic ureterocele in the bladder, obstructing the right kidney, with a non-excreting left upper renal moiety.

Fig. IV.2.A7b *(below)*   Oblique projection at the end of voiding—note how the ureterocele (marked out) has been squeezed a little way beyond the bladder contour, taking a sulcus of contrast medium with it.

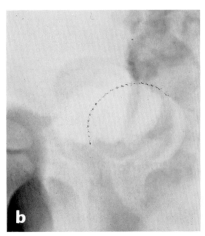

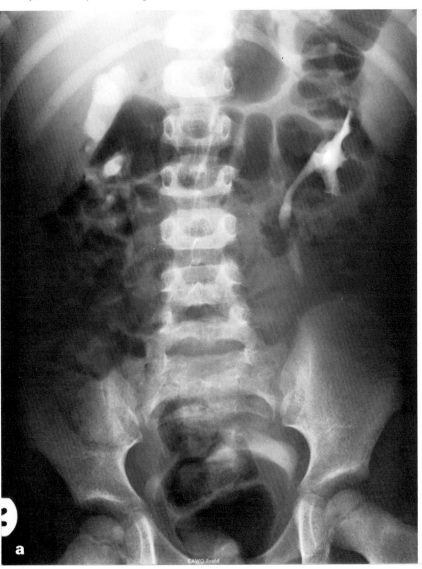

Fig. IV.2.A8a *(facing page)* Non-excreting left lower renal moiety.
Fig. IV.2.A8b *(facing page)*   Gross reflux into the left lower moiety on cystography.

Table IV.2.1 *Differences between ureteroceles*

	Orthotopic	*Ectopic*
Parent ureter	single system	duplex system: upper-renal-moiety ureter
Site of opening of ureter	normal (trigone)	abnormal—below normal ipsilateral (lower moiety) ureter: bladder neck or urethra
Kidney above lesion	usually normal, rarely obstructed	upper renal moiety abnormal (dysplastic); ipsilateral lower moiety and contralateral kidney often obstructed
Common clinical background	chance finding	urinary infection
IVU bladder picture	lesion wholly within bladder outline	lesion based on bladder wall; ureterocele may be largely outside bladder outline, with only a crescentic defect in vesical contour

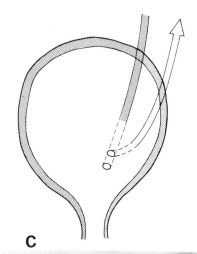

C

Reflux occurs into the lower-renal-moiety ureter in complete duplication because of the short, transverse course of this ureter through the bladder wall (Fig. IV.2.A8). The longer, oblique course of the upper-renal-moiety ureter is similar to the normal anatomy, preventing reflux (diagram C).

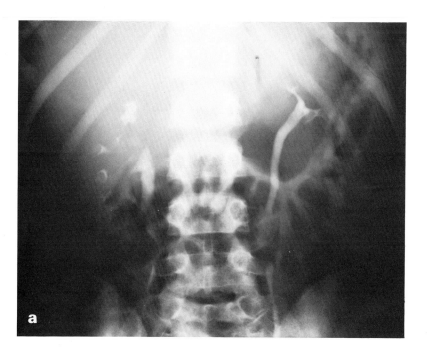

a

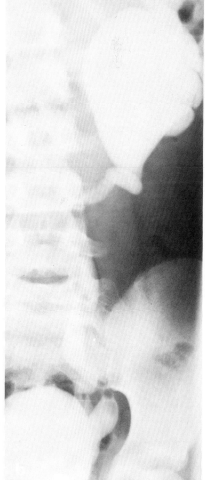

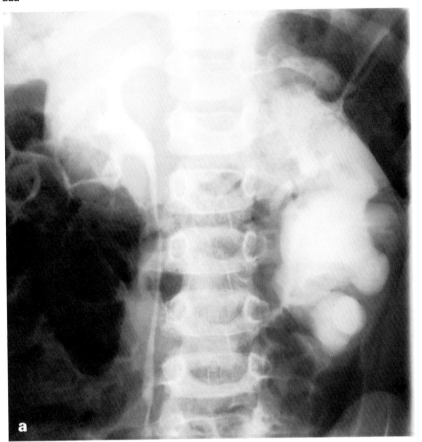

Fig. IV.2.A9a *(right)* Markedly
distended left lower renal moiety.
Fig. IV.2.A9b *(below)* Frame from a
pressure/flow study on the lower
moiety—the perfusing cannula can be
seen in position. This moiety is obstructed
at the pelvi-ureteric junction.

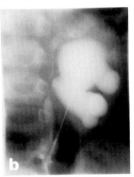

Dilatation of the lower renal moiety by reflux may be severe enough to call
for heminephrectomy rather than ureteric reimplantation. Pelvi-ureteric junction obstruction can sometimes occur, with gross dilatation (Fig. IV.2.A9).

B. DILATED URETER: OBSTRUCTION

Acute vs chronic obstruction

  Sudden obstruction of a kidney—pain
    IVU: increasingly dense nephrogram, and ureter dilated down to site of
    obstruction
    Kidney: continuing glomerular filtration and water reabsorption, i.e. very
    active traffic into and out of proximal nephron.
  Gradual or long-standing renal obstruction—often painless
    IVU: nephrogram unremarkable in onset and disappearance but may out-
    line dilated non-opacified calices (soap-bubble nephrogram).

Kidney: nephron loss, i.e. comparable with chronic renal failure states—too few nephrons coping with too large a load.

Acute obstruction by stone—Casualty IVU

In the patient presenting with ureteric colic, only a very short (two film) examination is needed to make or break the diagnosis. A plain film of the abdomen is commonly the only X-ray investigation done in these patients, but this approach has serious shortcomings. Any opacity in the line of the ureter might or might not be the offending stone on this plain film. The additional contrast film of the casualty IVU will sort this out (Fig. IV.2.B1). There are two advantages to this practice:

1. Diagnosis: however characteristic a patient's ureteric colic may appear, other causes may mimic a ureteric stone. Examples are acute appendicitis in right-sided symptoms, or the repeated attacks of the drug addict craving an opiate injection. The make-or-break diagnostic value of the casualty IVU is obvious.

2. Management: any patient presenting with ureteric colic and an obstructed kidney must be followed carefully through the obstruction episode. A possible underlying metabolic disorder will have to be investigated. The severity and duration of obstruction will determine how the acute episode is managed: does the patient need surgical intervention because the stone is too large, or because he has been severely obstructed for too long? Certainty about the presence and functional importance of the ureteric stone on the casualty IVU puts further management on a sound footing.

Technique. Full-length plain and 20–30 min contrast films are generally all that is required. The second film should be done immediately after micturition, so that the contrast-filled bladder is not allowed to obscure the lower ureters. If only a dense nephrogram is seen on the side with symptoms, severe acute obstruction is likely (Fig. IV.2.B2). In less acute cases, the nephrogram may be a soap-bubble picture, with distended non-opacified calices presenting as regular round spaces against the opacified renal parenchyma (see Fig. IV.1.B4). The patient can then be admitted, and follow-up films at 6 and 24 hours will usually show the distended ureter down to the site of obstruction.

a. Stone

This is the commonest cause of ureteric obstruction. Most stones are radio-opaque, but a low kV radiographic technique is important for picking out the less dense ones. Guesswork about the chemical make-up of the stone from its radiographic picture is not usually very rewarding. The characteristic triangular stone with a denser rim than centre is a very important exception: it is of course really a necrotic papilla (see Figs. IV.1.B2 and IV.1.G9).

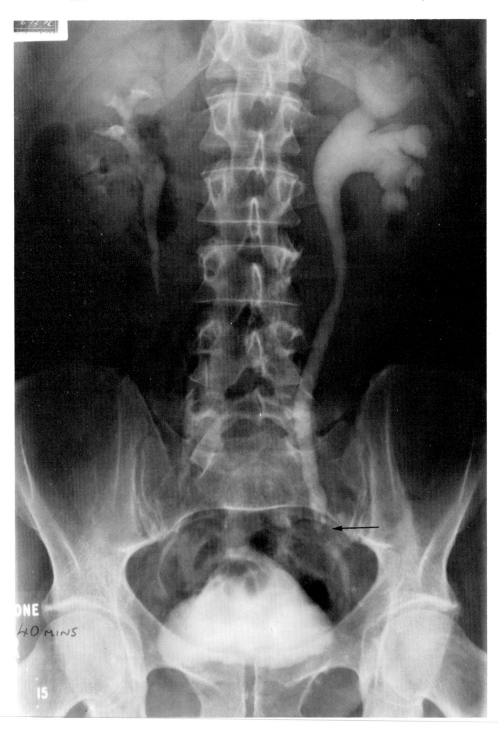

Fig. IV.2.B1 Acute obstruction—a prone film shows the dilated left upper urinary tract down to the responsible stone (arrow).

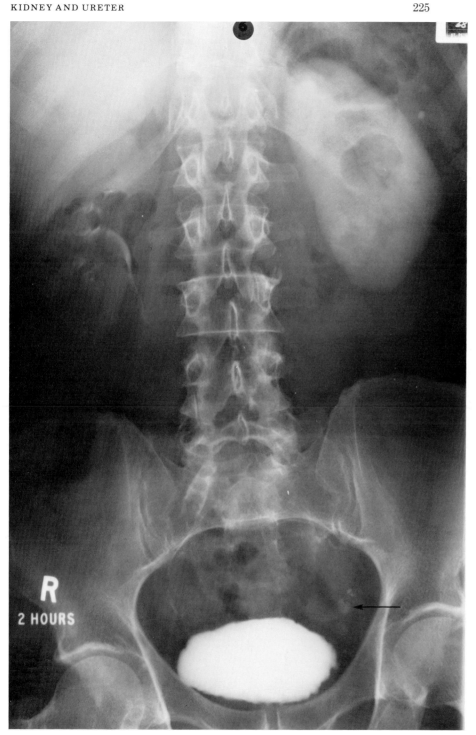

Fig. IV.2.B2 Increasingly dense nephrogram in the left kidney points to severe acute obstruction by the stone in the lower left ureter (arrow). This is the same patient illustrated in Fig. IV.2.B1, having a new IVU one month later. The ureteric stone has moved down, causing more severe obstruction.

Radiolucent stones. When a ureter is obstructed by a radiolucent filling defect, it is helpful to have a stand-by list of common causes at the ready. This will include:

1. radiolucent stone
2. blood clot
3. ureteric (urothelial) tumour
4. necrotic papilla.

Notes:

1. Uric acid is the commonest radiolucent stone. *Matrix* stones are soft deformable structures based on an organic groundwork, and always associated with urinary infection, often proteus. *Cystine* stones are faintly radio-opaque. Other radiolucent stones are very rare, e.g. xanthine.

Fig. IV.2.B3a   Stone in the left upper ureter (arrow).

Fig. IV.2.B3b   Idle, dilated left ureter below the stone, without any lower obstruction.

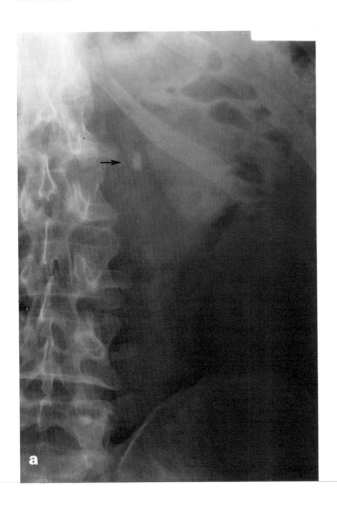

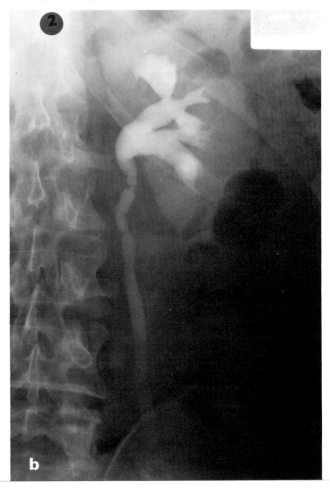

2. In the ureter obstructed by *clot* there is often either an obvious clinical cause, e.g. renal biopsy, or a helpful history of haematuria. Further clot may be seen in the renal pelvis above. A repeat examination days or weeks later may be needed to sort out the diagnosis: the changing picture of the filling defects will confirm that clot was present (see Fig. IV.1.D5). *Rule-of-thumb:* bleeding may affect the upper urinary tract IVU picture in three main ways: *a.* renal haematoma with the appearance of a renal mass or subcapsular haematoma compressing the kidney; *b,* filling defects in renal pelvis or ureter; *c.* retroperitoneal bleeding, seen as a mass displacing the ureter. Peri-ureteric fibrosis leading to ureteric obstruction is a late sequel to repeated retroperitoneal bleeding, as in haemophilia or an abdominal aortic aneurysm.

Sites of obstruction. Ureteric stones are commonly arrested at one of three sites: (1) in the upper ureter in the pelvi-ureteric junction; (2) in mid-ureter at L3/4 level; (3) in the lower ureter at ischial spine level. It is fortunate that they are not usually held up over the sacrum, where they can be extremely hard or impossible to recognize.

The dilated ureter below a stone. It may happen that a ureter is seen to be considerably dilated below a stone (Fig. IV.2.B3). This need not lead to an

Fig. IV.2.B4 *(below left)* This child has a non-opaque stone in the right renal pelvis (arrow). The ureter below it is dilated and tortuous, but returned to normal after stone removal.

Fig. IV.2.B5 *(below right)* There is a stone in the lower left ureter (arrow). Note the marked oedema deforming the ureteric orifice.

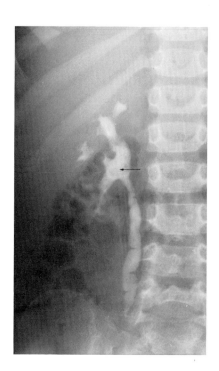

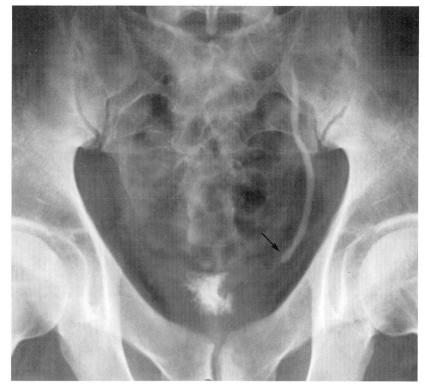

anguished search for a further obstructing stone lower down, but can be accepted as a sick ureter, which will recover when the stone above is removed. This state occurs at its worst in children with infected stones, where gross 'corkscrew' ureteric deformities may be seen below the stone (Fig. IV.2.B4). *Ureteritis* appears an unexceptionable label for this disorder, and emphasizes that it is a reversible lesion.

Ureteric oedema. A stone arrested in the lower ureter close to the bladder wall can give rise to spectacular bladder deformity on the IVU. This is because of local oedema, seen as an impression on the bladder mucosa, often at its best on the post-voiding film (Fig. IV.2.B5).

b. Megaureter

This term might clearly refer to a ureter enlarged for any reason, but is usually reserved for a badly made ureter, i.e. a congenital anomaly. At its most characteristic there is a short tapering normal-calibre segment to the lower-most ureter, with dilatation above (Fig. IV.2.B6). This is a picture which has naturally suggested obstruction. 'Primary obstructive megaureter' is a common label, putting the notion of congenital obstruction. An obstructive lesion, however, may not be present on dynamic tests (see section D p. 244), and obstruction as a necessary ingredient of the syndrome is under debate (Whitaker & Johnston, 1976). 'Primary wide ureter' may be a better term, if less incisive. Much of the difficulty over the megaureter lies in the absence of any consistent histological or abnormal functional criteria for making the diagnosis.

Despite these difficulties 'megaureter' is necessary and useful shorthand for a clinico-radiological entity. There is a wide spectrum from a minor megaureter deformity, discovered as a chance finding in an adult, to severe ureteric dilatation presenting as urinary infection in a child. The natural history varies accordingly, from wholly benign to destruction of a kidney's function by an obstructive ureter. The diagnosis is made on the characteristic IVU ureteric deformity, in the absence of ureteric stricture, stone or reflux. These last three are important exclusions as alternative (and treatable) causes of a dilated ureter. They usually cause no difficulty, but note:

1.   A megaureter may contain stones in its lower half. These are secondary to urinary stasis and/or infection. An IVU showing freely mobile stones lying in a baggy ureteric segment will make plain that they are not the primary cause of ureteric distension (Fig. IV.2.B7).

2.   Vesico-ureteric reflux may sometimes occur in a megaureter. The severity of ureteric distension and of reflux are then out of step, so that reflux alone cannot be responsible for the deformity.

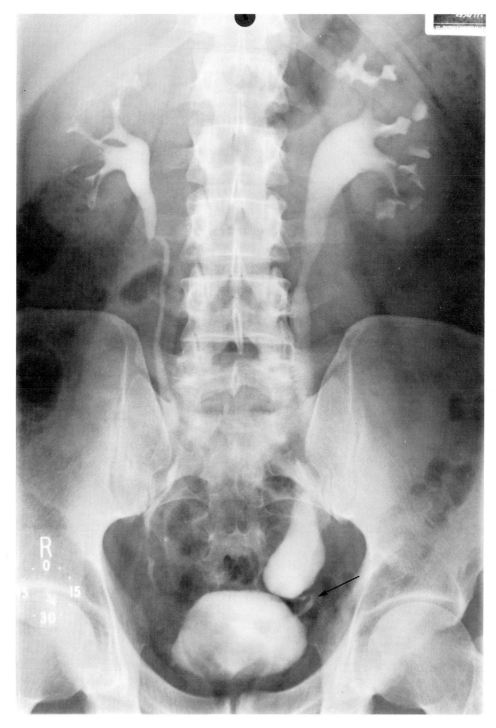

Fig. IV.2.B6 Left megaureter—note the distended left upper urinary tract, and the normal calibre of the lowermost ureter (arrow).

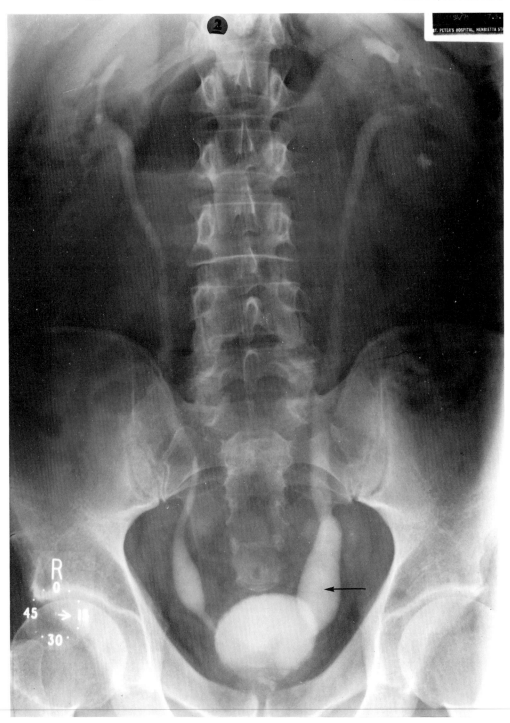

Fig. IV.2.B7 Mild
bilateral megaureters—
several small mobile
stones are present in the
static left lower ureter
(arrow).

c. Tumour

Ureteric tumours are just one expression of urothelial neoplastic disease. Disease of the renal pelvis (see Division 1 section D) and of the bladder (Division 3 section D) are more familiar examples. The notion of an unstable urothelium explains why new primary tumours may arise even after complete excision of an initial tumour elsewhere in the urinary tract. A patient who has already had a bladder carcinoma may thus develop a later ureteric tumour (Fig. IV.2.B8). The frequency of this complication is not known. With the bladder tumour under control, regular (perhaps yearly) short IVUs are probably a worthwhile exercise for keeping a watch on the upper urinary tracts.

The IVU diagnosis of a ureteric tumour is made on the signs of either (1) an irregular filling defect; or (2) obstruction (Fig. IV.2.B9).

In a narrow tube like the ureter it might be thought that obstruction would be an early and obvious sign of a tumour. In practice this is not always so, and it is unfortunately easy to miss a tumour in still normal-calibre ureters.

d. Stricture

Ureteric tumour is very much a part of the differential diagnosis when ureteric narrowing is found. 'Look on every stricture as a tumour till proven otherwise' is sometimes preached, though hardly as a helpful maxim for the radiologist, for

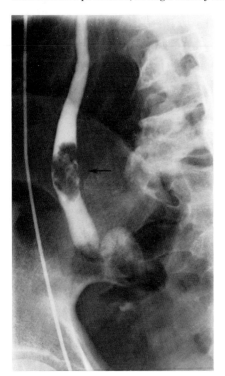

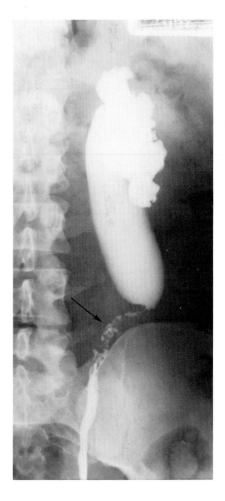

Fig. IV.2.B8 *(left)* This patient's bladder carcinoma has obstructed both lowermost ureters so severely that a percutaneous nephrostomy was done on the right. Part of the draining catheter is projected alongside the ureter, but a large new ureteric tumour has also been found (arrow).

Fig. IV.2.B9 *(right)* The left upper urinary tract is badly obstructed by the irregular growth in the left ureter (arrow). This is a rare benign ureteric tumour—a polyp. (Courtesy of Mr J. P. Williams).

how do you prove otherwise? In general, inflammatory strictures are *smooth, tapering* lesions whilst tumours present as *rough, irregular* ureteric defects. This simple mechanical guide can be put to good clinical use (Fig. IV.2.B10).

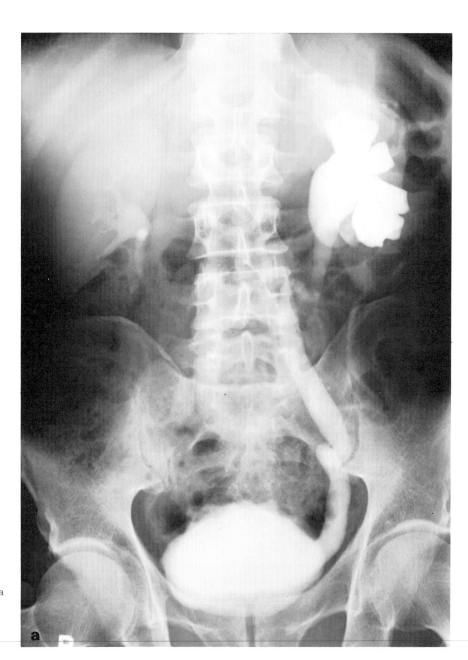

Fig. IV.2.B10a Following resection of a bladder tumour near the left ureteric orifice, this patient's left upper urinary tract is dilated, raising the question of tumour invasion of the lower ureter.

Usual causes of stricture

Tb.
Bilharzia.
Following surgery.
Following lodgement of a ureteric stone.

Tb. Other abnormalities will usually be found on the IVU: erosion/cavitation/fibrosis/calcification in the kidney, and contraction/mucosal irregularity in the

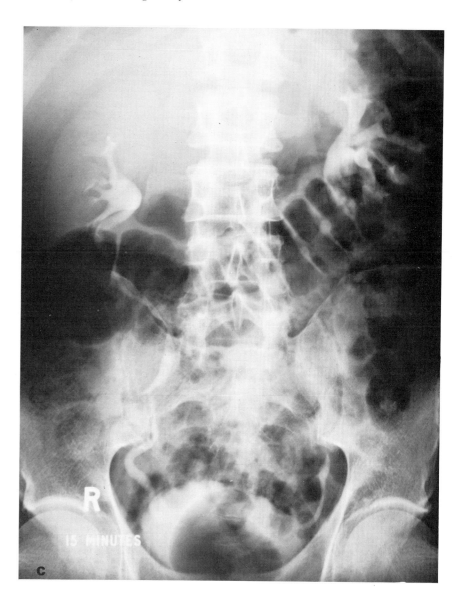

Fig. IV.2.B10b An oblique view of the lower left ureter shows a smooth, tapering stricture. This is the picture of a benign lesion, probably a complication of bladder diathermy.

Fig. IV.2.B10c Six weeks later all is well, confirming the diagnosis.

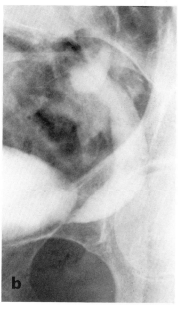

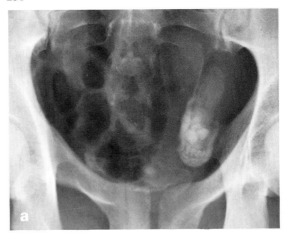

Fig. IV.2.B11a Calcification of the bladder and the lower left ureter in bilharzia—note additional stones in the left ureter. (Courtesy of Dr A. A. Salem).

bladder. The occurrence of ureteric narrowing is a particular hazard during the early weeks of anti-tuberculous medical treatment (see Fig. IV.1.G14). The danger is such that short (one film) follow-up IVUs should be done twice in the first 3 months of treatment. All being well then, wider intervals can be chosen for follow-up.

Bilharzia. This involves the lower ureter in particular, and may be accompanied by calcification in the bladder as well as the ureter (Fig. IV.2.B11). It is a very important cause of obstructive renal atrophy and of stone formation in the endemic areas of the Middle East, Africa and South America.

e. Extrinsic lesions incarcerating the ureter

Retroperitoneal fibrosis is the prime example of this state. Retroperitoneal tumour masses, particularly involving para-aortic lymph nodes, may also be troublesome (Fig. IV.2.B12). The ureter can be strangled in the bony pelvis by tumour (e.g. carcinoma cervix) or by a gynaecologist's inadvertent ligature. Endometriosis is another example.

Retroperitoneal fibrosis (RPF) may be benign or malignant. Malignant lesions causing this peritoneal reaction may arise in the pelvis, e.g. rectal, sigmoid or female genital tract carcinomas. Or they may be distant tumours, e.g. breast, bronchus, pancreas. Depending on local hospital referral patterns, they make up 10–30% of all RPF. They also put up a strong case for surgery, on one ureter at least, in all cases of RPF, in order to obtain material for a histological diagnosis. Steroids are now a quite effective medical treatment of RPF (Fig. IV.2.B13).

Benign RPF can result from drugs. Methysergide (used in migraine) is well known in this regard. Analgesic abuse has also been implicated. Benign RPF can also arise by a reaction to foreign material in the retroperitoneum: blood

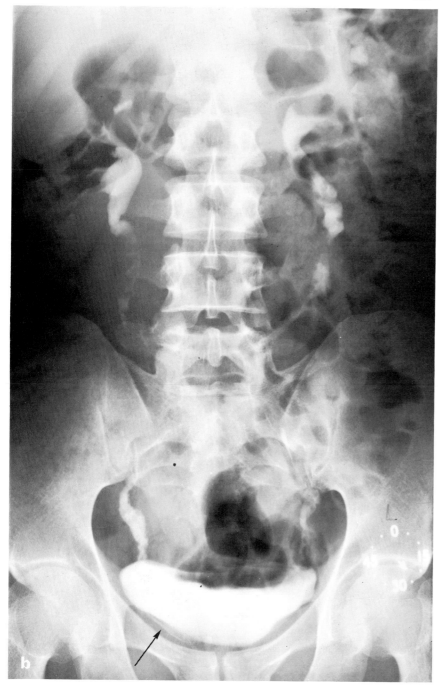

Fig. IV.2.B11b Another patient who also has bilharzia—note the bladder calcification (arrow). Multiple filling defects in both ureters point to extensive ureteritis.

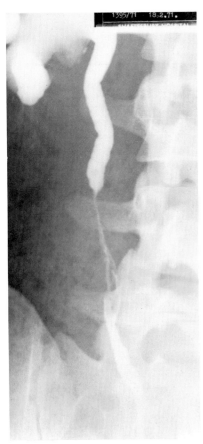

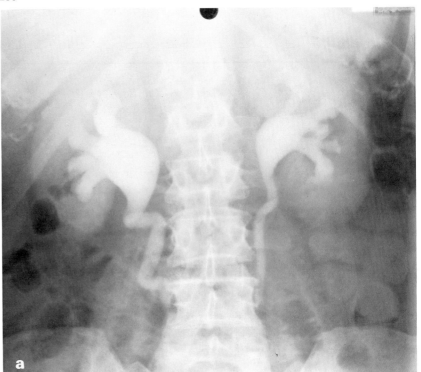

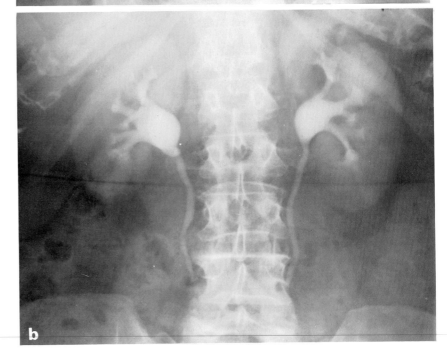

Fig. IV.2.B12 *(above)*   This young man
suffering from a teratoma of the testis has
involved para-aortic nodes incarcerating
the right ureter. Note the difficulty of
distinguishing extrinsic from intrinsic
lesions of the ureter here.

Fig. IV.2.B13a   Retroperitoneal
fibrosis—both upper urinary tracts are
dilated.
Fig. IV.2.B13b   This patient has been
treated with steroids alone, and 6 years
later all is well.

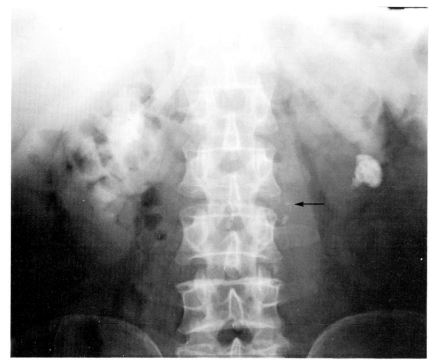

Fig. IV.2.B14 Retroperitoneal fibrosis, with severe obstruction of both kidneys, worse on the left. Note the tell-tale calcification in the abdominal aortic aneurysm (arrow)—the disease here is secondary to blood leaking into the retroperitoneum.

Fig. IV.2.B15 *(below)* Retroperitoneal fibrosis shown during an antegrade pyelogram—note the sharp medial hitch of the ureter.

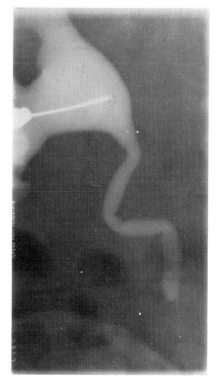

from a leaking aortic aneurysm (Fig. IV.2.B14), or urine following renal rupture from any cause.

Diagnosis: RPF is characterized by ureteric obstruction, not necessarily ureteric deviation. It may be unilateral at first. The fibrous plaque usually begins sharply across the upper ureter at L2/3 level, and ends equally abruptly at the upper sacrum. The ureter will therefore appear obstructed over this segment, with variable dilatation above. Pelvi-caliceal distension may be quite slight. *Medial deviation* of the ureter is an overrated finding in this disease. Seeing a sudden (right angle) medial hitch can indeed be helpful (Fig. IV.2.B15), but a gentle drift of the ureter toward the midline as it descends is a common normal variant (Saxton *et al*, 1969).

In this disorder the IVU always alerts to the presence of obstruction; retrograde studies may be needed to define the site and make the diagnosis.

Note that the ureters are often deliberately displaced laterally in the surgery of RPF (ureterolysis). Follow-up IVUs may therefore look strange (Fig. IV.2.B16).

Retrocaval ureter is a rare, spectacular cause of the incarcerated ureter. This congenital anomaly affects the right ureter. Patients may present with right-sided loin symptoms because of obstruction, but the lesion can also be an unimportant chance finding. The IVU picture is highly characteristic. Descending from a dilated pelvicaliceal system, the distended upper ureter reaches the

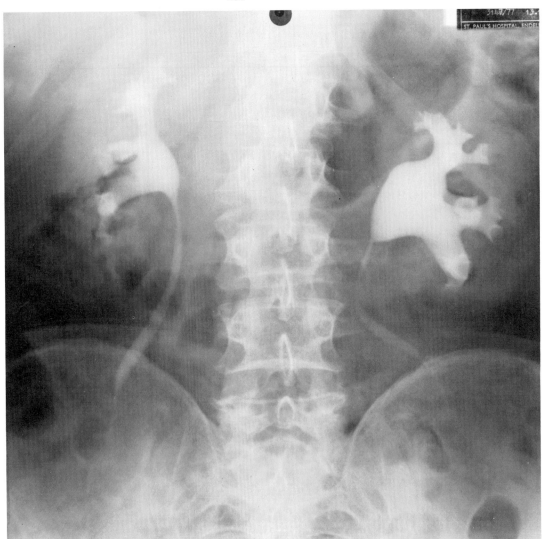

Fig. IV.2.B16 This is the same patient as in Fig. IV.2.B15. Following ureterolysis, both ureters have been placed laterally.

L3 level, then takes a distinct medial and upward bend to reach a position behind the cava. From there it descends close to the midline, no longer dilated (Fig. IV.2.B17). Special manoeuvres have been recommended to confirm the diagnosis, e.g. simultaneous ureteric catheterization and a vena cavagram. They are made unnecessary by a good IVU, which is pathognomonic.

C. DILATED URETER: REFLUX

Vesico-ureteric reflux and chronic pyelonephritis are terrible twins: everyone realizes they are related, but no-one knows who the parents are. Possible

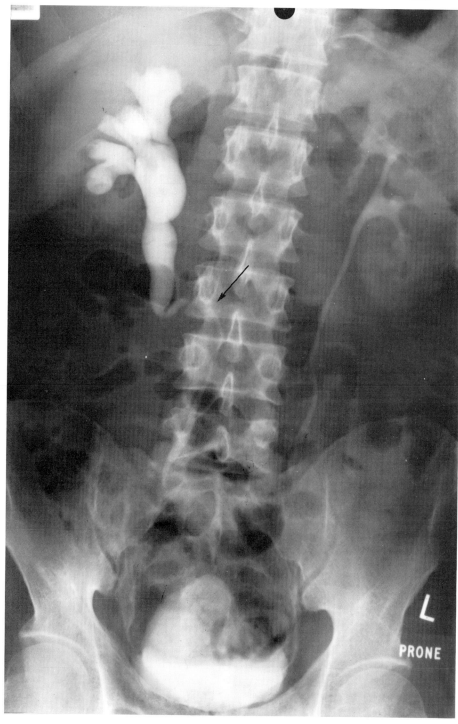

Fig. IV.2.B17 Retrocaval
ureter. Characteristic sweep of
the ureter behind the cava at L3
(arrow).

mechanisms of renal damage in vesico-ureteric reflux have been considered in Division 1 section G p. 143. In this section we are concerned with the recognition of reflux itself.

Rule-of-thumb: Reflux threatens the growing kidney of the young child, where it may lead to chronic pyelonephritic scarring or renal atrophy. It hardly ever endangers the integrity of the adult kidney, except for the special circumstances of a neuropathic bladder, or surgical diversion of the ureters as in uretero-sigmoid anastomosis.

The recognition of reflux is therefore specially important in children. Grading of reflux on the MCU can be done in various ways. Obvious reflux occurring at once as the empty bladder is filled with opaque medium might be classed as severe, by contrast with intermittent, transient reflux seen only during voiding. The importance of such factors in the behaviour of reflux is not known. The simplest grading scheme ignores them. It recognizes three steps:

Grade I: reflux into lower ureter only

Grade II: reflux reaching the kidney without distending (ballooning) the pelvicaliceal system

Grade III: caliceal distension, and possibly intra-renal reflux.

The growing kidney is probably damaged only by grade III reflux (Rolleston *et al*, 1970). This means that finding children with grade I or II reflux is a signal for initial conservative management. Such reflux is likely to cease as the child and the vesico-ureteric junction mature (Edwards *et al*, 1977). Whilst mild reflux is an intermittent phenomenon, not always reproducible between different MCUs, there is usually no important worsening in grades with time. In particular, children seen with grades I or II reflux will not deteriorate toward grade III reflux.

Severe reflux can exist in the presence of a normal upper urinary tract, i.e. a normal IVU. This examination is therefore not an adequate screening test for reflux. However, grade III reflux does often have IVU clues:

1. There may be obvious ureteric dilatation, or even renal scarring.

2. The post-micturition film may bring out transient ureteric dilatation.

3. Longitudinal ureteric folds may be seen on the IVU as evidence of reflux (see Figs. IV.1.F1 and IV.1.G25). These imply a collapsed ureter seen on the IVU only, the redundant wrinkles stretching out as the refluxing ureter becomes distended during voiding (MCU). This simple mechanical explanation of such folds is probably better than the one linking them with ureteric inflammation.

A small *bladder diverticulum* or *saccule* is quite often associated with a badly refluxing ureter at its orifice (Fig. IV.2.C1). This small para-ureteric hernia is generally a sign that ureteric reimplantation will be necessary since reflux is unlikely to stop when severe enough to cause this lesion.

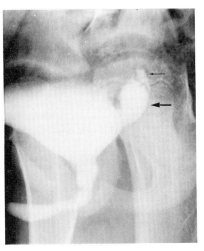

Fig. IV.2.C1   Para-ureteric saccule (large arrow) associated with ureteric reflux (small arrow). Note how the saccule has prolapsed through the faulty ureteric tunnel—it is not the primary lesion.

Investigative strategy

The child presenting with a proven urinary infection needs careful, alert clinical follow-up, even after the presenting episode has been treated successfully. The following programme only applies to such close clinico-radiological teamwork.

IVU:

a. If the IVU is normal, a first infection in girls usually needs no further radiological investigation. Grade I and II reflux will be missed, but this is unimportant given careful follow-up.

b. A normal IVU in boys is best followed by an MCU except in the most experienced clinical hands. This is because bladder outflow obstruction is a particular worry in boys over and above the reflux question. The MCU will answer both queries.

c. An abnormal IVU, or recurrent infections with a normal IVU, are indications for an MCU in both sexes.

d. Follow-up examinations to monitor known reflux are best done as radionuclide cystograms. Resolution for seeing reflux may be poorer, but usually adequate for clinical management (Rothwell *et al*, 1977). The radiation dose is of course much less than in an MCU—see Part II section A p. 55.

Less common reflux problems

As children grow older, reflux becomes much less common. This is probably because the adult vesico-ureteric junction is more oblique, with a longer intramural course of the terminal ureter, discouraging reflux. Looking for adult reflux as an explanation for a dilated ureter is therefore not very rewarding. It may have to be done to exclude a correctable, troublesome disorder. However, even in the setting of a urinary infection clinic for women, reflux does not appear a frequent or important entity.

Reflux in ureteric diversion is mainly of two sorts. When the ureters drain into a conduit like an *ileal loop,* reflux can commonly be demonstrated by filling the loop retrogradely ('loopogram'). Since this reflux only occurs under such conditions of artificial stasis, and not during the everyday function of the loop as a conduit, it is of little clinical importance. Where the ureters drain directly into a reservoir, e.g. the colon in *uretero-sigmoid anastomosis,* reflux can be a serious problem. In this case constant reflux of infected faecal material can give rise to the typical scars of pyelonephritis (see Fig. IV.1.G3). The development of such scars in adult life is very rare in any other circumstances.

Reflux may also occur in the *neuropathic bladder,* leading to ureteric dilatation. The cause of such reflux will usually be obvious from the clinical, urodynamic and radiographic findings pointing to an abnormal bladder.

D. DILATED URETER: NO OBSTRUCTION OR REFLUX

Traditionally the dilated ureter seen on an IVU has two possible causes: reflux or obstruction. The two may coexist—this is rare. Reflux can be readily excluded by a cystogram, so that we are left with the equation 'ureteric dilatation (no reflux) = obstruction'.

This idea cannot cope with a primary defect in ureteric muscle as a cause for dilatation, and is therefore inadequate. A number of non-refluxing dilated ureters are seen as chance findings in adult life, with no evidence of progressive structural or functional deterioration. Obstruction appears an unlikely explanation in such patients on clinical grounds. This suspicion can be confirmed in selected cases by dynamic measurements.

The 'raped ureter'

The commonest unobstructed, non-refluxing wide ureter seen in adults is the result of some past insult, no longer operative or important. A good example is the wide right ureter seen in women who have been pregnant. The upper urinary tracts become distended during pregnancy, the right more so than the left. Obstruction and an altered hormonal environment are the explanations put forward. Even years later, the right ureter may remain overdistensible, with characteristic dilatation down to the level of the right common iliac artery (Fig. IV.2.D1). It is important to recognize this deformity as a clinically unimportant scar of battles fought long ago. Similarly ureters that have been severely obstructed by stone or stricture may never return to normal dimensions, even when the responsible obstruction has been relieved. A particularly worrying instance of this post-obstructive change is the wide ureter above a bladder with treated outflow obstruction because of an enlarged prostate. Even after successful prostatectomy, such ureters may remain wide: no longer obstructed, but overstretched and rather ineffective (Fig. IV.2.D2).

The notion of a non-refluxing, unobstructed wide ureter is of particular importance in paediatric urology, where quite grossly dilated but unobstructed ureters are met. Careful dynamic investigation of these children will help to sort out those who do and do not need surgery.

Investigation of suspected upper urinary tract obstruction

1. IVU. The standard examination with a contrast medium dose of about 300 mg iodine/kg produces a mild osmotic diuresis. Most upper urinary tract obstructions will be lit up without much difficulty in this way.

2. Diuresis IVU. Where doubt remains, an IVU under the stress of a brisk diuresis can be helpful. A water load of 1 litre by mouth during the examination might appear the simplest method, but it is not always effective. Drinking so much is uncomfortable, and variable absorption times make the timing of films

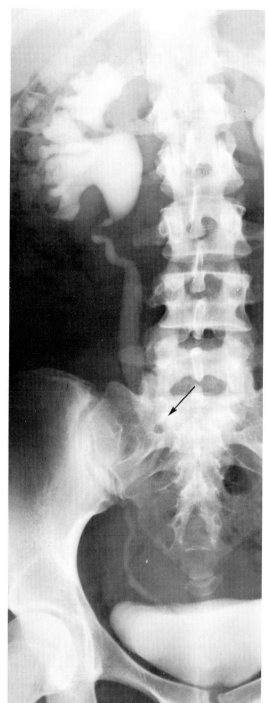

Fig. IV.2.D1 *(left)* Characteristic dilatation of the right upper urinary tract following pregnancy—this will now be life-long, but not associated with symptoms. The arrow points to the right common iliac artery.

Fig. IV.2.D2 *(below)* This man with prostatic bladder outflow obstruction has had continuous bladder drainage for over a month, but his ureters remain idle and dilated. There is no ureteric reflux—this is a picture during bilateral antegrade pyelography.

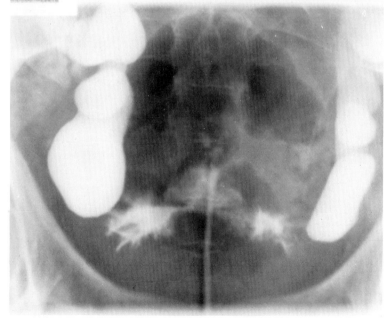

difficult. Faced with a challenging clinical problem, it is not uncommon to end up with a persisting question mark instead of a solution. In the process the patient will probably have had too many films taken. The intravenous injection of a fast diuretic, e.g. frusemide 20–40 mg, makes for a shorter and much more certain examination. The diuretic is best given some minutes after the contrast medium, so that a base-line pyelogram can be obtained first. The effect of the diuresis can then be followed over the next few minutes by intermittent fluoroscopy or radiography. The examination is particularly apt for resolving doubts about possible pelvi-ureteric junction obstruction in patients with unexplained loin pain.

3. Pressure/flow studies by antegrade pyelography. This is the only way of establishing a cast-iron diagnosis of obstruction. In the difficult case, too much time should not be wasted over other procedures. It is tempting but unhelpful to ask for repeat standard IVUs in the hope of resolving such problems. Retrograde catheter studies are also inappropriate, since they involve mechanical interference with the very lesion in question. The diuresis IVU has considerable limitations: it is best suited to investigating the wide renal pelvis or upper ureter, i.e. where a high obstructive lesion is suspected. With the mid or lower ureter involved, it is often best to move straight from the standard IVU to the pressure study, instead of wasting time and radiation on less decisive procedures.

Demonstrating obstruction

Three forces transport urine from the kidney to the bladder:

a. end-filtration pressure in the nephron

b. hydrostatic pressure in the erect position

c. ureteric peristalsis.

In the standard procedure carried out in the horizontal position, a high urine flow rate (via antegrade perfusion) replaces the variable final nephron flow, and gravity plays no part. The study is specifically on the look out for a local correctable lesion which might be causing obstruction. Definition of such a lesion involves:

1. Structure: demonstration of the lesion, e.g. a narrowing.

2. Function: raised pressure proximal to the lesion, or a pressure drop across it.

3. Flow: reduced across the lesion.

Method. The standard study is concerned with 1 and 2 above. The kidney is punctured (see Part I section D p. 15) and perfused at 10 ml/min. Upper tract pressure is continuously measured through a side-arm in the perfusion system. Pressure below the suspected lesion is measured via a perurethral bladder catheter. The normal upper tract is able to cope with this fast perfusion rate, mimicking a very high urine flow rate. It shows no progressive pressure rise, or pressure drop from kidney to bladder (normal range up to 20 cmH$_2$O for both). A mounting pressure in the upper tract together with a large kidney/bladder pressure drop spells obstruction (Fig. IV.2.D3). Fluoroscopy during the examination will pinpoint the site of hold-up.

Results. We have performed the procedure most often in children. Wide non-refluxing ureters of sufficient severity to demand such investigation fall into two groups here:

1. Suspected primary megaureter, i.e. a badly made ureter with defective musculature. Most of these patients can be diagnosed and managed on the information from a standard IVU. In the problem case, dynamic studies can be very helpful to answer the important question: is this an obstructed system? The most florid example in this group is the prune belly syndrome, where grossly dilated but unobstructed ureters are met (Fig. IV.2.D4).

2. Suspected obstruction at abnormal bladder wall, secondary to bladder outflow obstruction, neuropathic bladder etc. The boy who has had his urethral valve resected may still be left with distended ureters. As the years go by, this upper tract dilatation may even worsen. He no longer has bladder outflow obstruction, and never suffered from reflux. Are these just tired, overstretched ureters, no longer able to cope (i.e. untreatable), or is there an obstruction at bladder wall

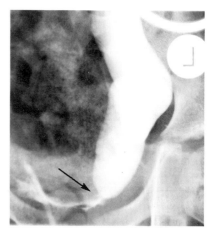

Fig. IV.2.D3 Obstructed left lower ureter during pressure/flow antegrade pyelogram. This boy has had his urethral valve resected, but there is additional obstruction at the vesico-ureteric junction, shown by a pressure drop across it of 25 cm water.

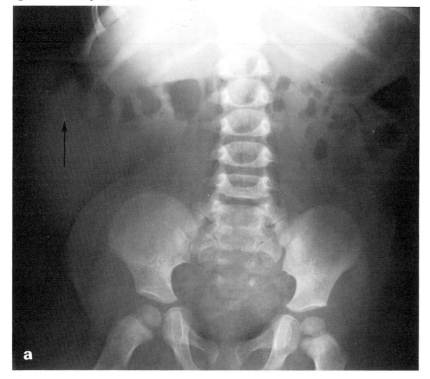

Fig. IV.2.D4a Prune belly syndrome— note that the diagnosis can be made by the radiologist on this plain film because the deficient anterior abdominal wall allows lateral spread of abdominal contents (arrow points to hepatic flexure).

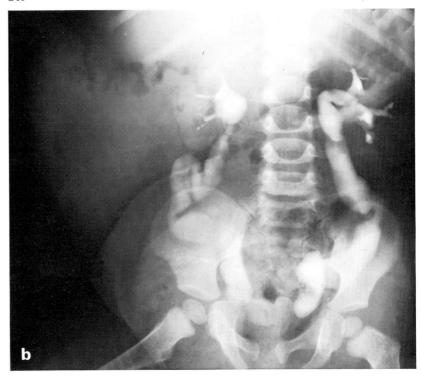

Fig. IV.2.D4b The IVU shows characteristic dilated, laterally placed ureters, but these are not obstructed. The kidneys are also badly made.

level (i.e. correctable)? The dynamic study can help with this vital distinction, though it would be silly to pretend that easy answers are always obtained in these complex patients (Fig. IV.2.D5).

We have found that obstruction can be excluded in many wide ureters, so saving patients needless surgery. The proportion found obstructed or not in such studies will depend on local referral patterns of patient selection. Among our children with wide ureters having antegrade pyelograms, we find about two thirds are unobstructed, one quarter obstructed, and about 10% remain problem cases even after investigation (Whitfield *et al*, 1976).

Summary comment

Why is there stasis in dilated, unobstructed and non-refluxing ureters? Our present investigations do not answer this question. Primary or secondary im-

Fig. IV.2.D5 Pressure trace during an antegrade pyelogram, reading from right to left. This boy who has had his urethral valve resected was suspected of additional ureteric obstruction. Perfusion of the upper urinary tract at first leads to a progressive pressure rise, suggesting obstruction. However, there is no obstruction when the bladder pressure is dropped to atmospheric level. Bladder pressure and volume are important in these problems.

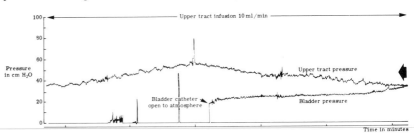

pairment of ureteric musculature is the obvious suggestion, but it is proving remarkably difficult to nail such defects in precise structural and functional terms. Such acknowledged ignorance should not discourage radiologists from carrying out dynamic studies. The aim is to separate a surgically correctable state (*obstruction*) from a disorder where surgery is usually irrelevant (*dilatation ± stasis*). At present we may not understand either, but we can try to find the right course of action for the patient.

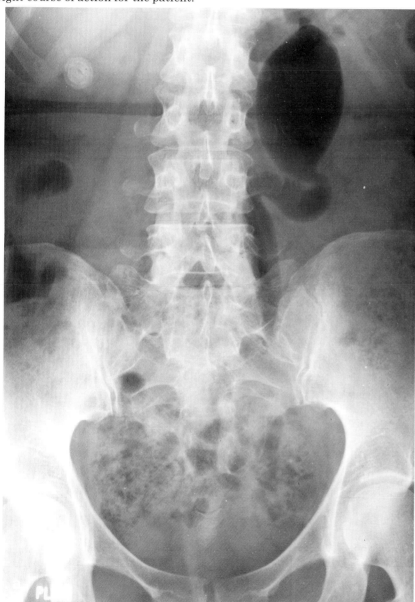

Fig. IV.2.E1a *(left)* & **b** *(overleaf)* Gas pyelogram in uretero-colic diversion. A gallstone is also present.

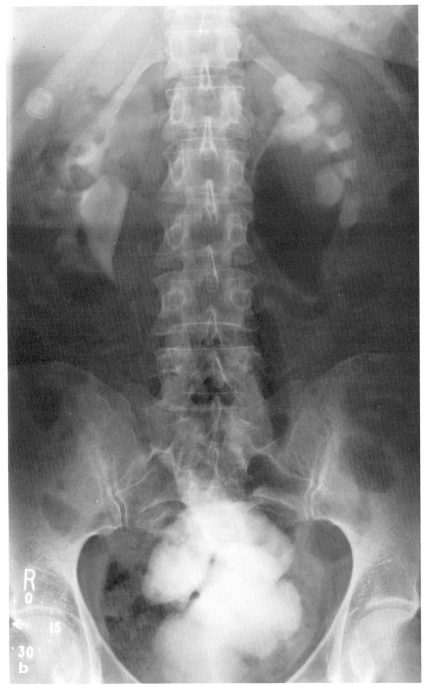

E. DIVERTED URETER

Even without clinical information the radiologist may sometimes spot at once that a patient has a diverted ureter: by a *gas pyelogram* on a plain abdominal film (Fig. IV.2.E1). Ureteric diversion is much the commonest cause of this picture. Others are:

—vesico-colic fistula secondary to carcinoma or diverticulitis of the colon
—severe urinary infection in diabetics.

Acute problems

In the immediate postoperative period, breakdown of the anastomosis between ureter and bowel may be suspected. Retrograde injection studies of the bowel may then be necessary, or the answer may be quite clear on the intravenous urogram (Fig. IV.2.E2).

Chronic problems

1. Reflux/infection: This is a particular hazard of uretero-colic diversion, and has already been considered in section C p. 241. It can then lead to quite gross renal scarring, looking like characteristic chronic pyelonephritis on the IVU (see Fig. IV.1.G3).

2. Obstruction: The anastomosis may become narrowed by fibrosis. If the diagnosis is not complete on the IVU, an antegrade pyelogram will usually be needed (Fig. IV.2.E3).

3. Tumour: Where the ureteric diversion was done because of a bladder carcinoma (total cystectomy), new tumour can arise in the upper urinary tract. This is because the urothelium lining the whole tract may be unstable in the sense of malignant transformation. Follow-up IVUs in these patients need careful scanning of calices, pelvis and ureter for any tell-tale filling defects (Fig. IV.2.E4). Antegrade pyelography can be very helpful for such suspect lesions, since it allows cytological examination of urine collected nearby. Cytology of ileostomy urine mixed with the cells always shed from an ileal loop is difficult or impossible (see Fig. I.5 p. 15).

In long-standing diversion a different and much rarer tumour problem can arise. A small number of patients have developed a carcinoma at the anastomosis between ureter and bowel, probably originating from intestinal mucosa. Diversion has usually been established for many years and involves colon, e.g. a childhood operation for bladder exstrophy (Fig. IV.2.E5). The tumour may possibly represent a response to the abnormal environment of urine washing over gut. This well-publicized lesion is uncommon.

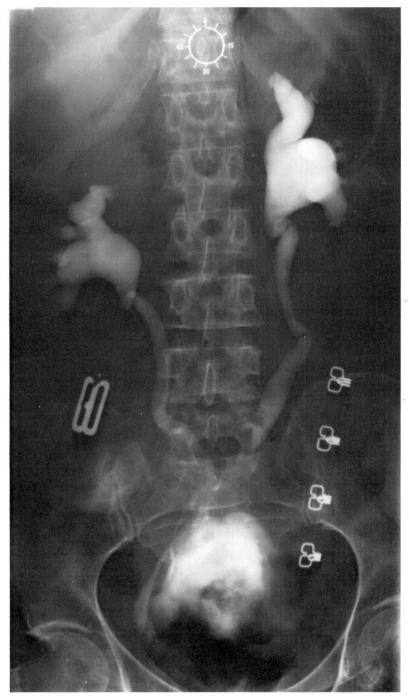

Fig. IV.2.E2 This patient has had an ileal loop diversion, but postoperatively all is not well. The IVU shows contrast leaking into a cavity which is obviously not the ileal loop.

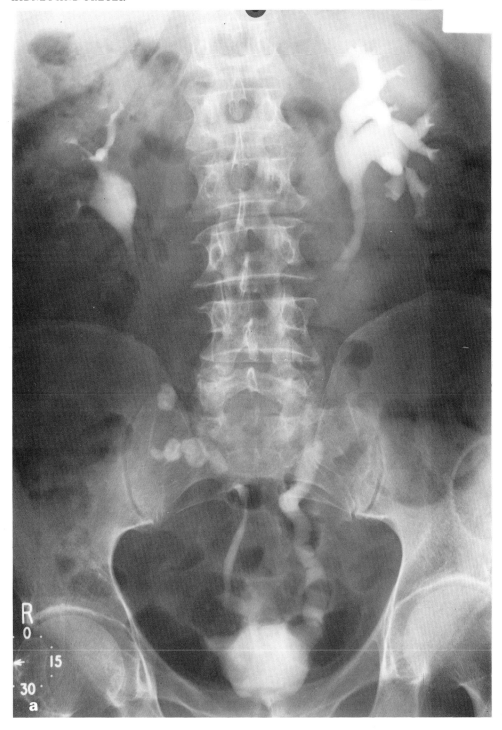

Fig. IV.2.E3a This patient has had an abdomino-perineal resection because of a rectal carcinoma. Note the characteristic medial position of the lower ureters following this operation.

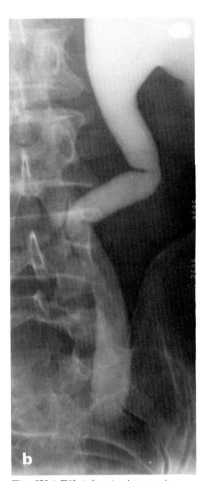

Summary comment

The complications of ureteric diversion have been highlighted in the section— most diversions in fact work very well indeed. This needs saying in particular about uretero-colic diversion, at present out of favour. In properly selected patients this can still give excellent results, avoiding the need for urinal appliances (Fig. IV.2.E6).

REFERENCES

EDWARDS D., NORMAND I.C.S., PRESCOD N. & SMELLIE J.M. (1977) Disappearance of vesicoureteric reflux during long-term prophylaxis of urinary tract infection in children. *British Medical Journal* **2**, 285–288.

ROLLESTON G.L., SHANNON F.I. & UTLEY W.L.F. (1970) Relationship of infantile vesicoureteric reflux to renal damage. *British Medical Journal* **1**, 460–463.

ROTHWELL D., CONSTABLE A.R. & ALBRECHT M. (1977) Radionuclide cystography in the investigation of vesicoureteric reflux in children *Lancet* **i**, 1072–1074.

SAXTON H.M., KILPATRICK F.R., KINDER C.H., LESSOF M.H., McHARDY-YOUNG S. & WARDLE D.F.H. (1969) Retroperitoneal fibrosis. *Quarterly Journal of Medicine* **38**, 159–181.

WHITAKER R.H. & JOHNSTON J.H. (1976) A simple classification of wide ureters. *British Journal of Urology* **47**, 781–787.

WHITFIELD H.N., HARRISON N.W., SHERWOOD T. & WILLIAMS D. INNES (1976) Upper urinary tract obstruction: pressure/flow studies in children. *British Journal of Urology* **48**, 427–430.

Fig. IV.2.E3b *(above)* A ureteric diversion had to be carried out later because of extreme frequency, followed 1 year later by bilateral renal obstruction. This antegrade pyelogram shows the left upper urinary tract distended down to the anastomosis—the cause was fibrosis only.

Fig. IV.2.E4 *(right)* New urothelial tumour in the left kidney (arrow) arising in a patient who has already had a total cystectomy for bladder cancer.

Fig. IV.2.E5 *(facing page)* This young man with exstrophy had a uretero-colic diversion. His right kidney was destroyed by pyelonephritis, but 20 years later his remaining left kidney has become enlarged because of severe obstruction. He has a frozen pelvis because of tumour at the anastomosis.

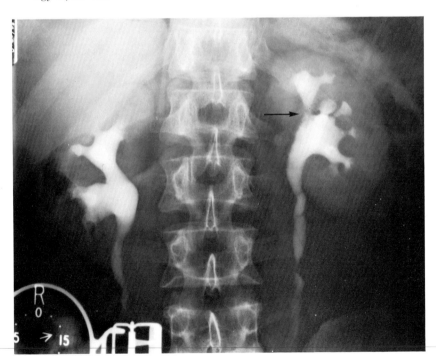

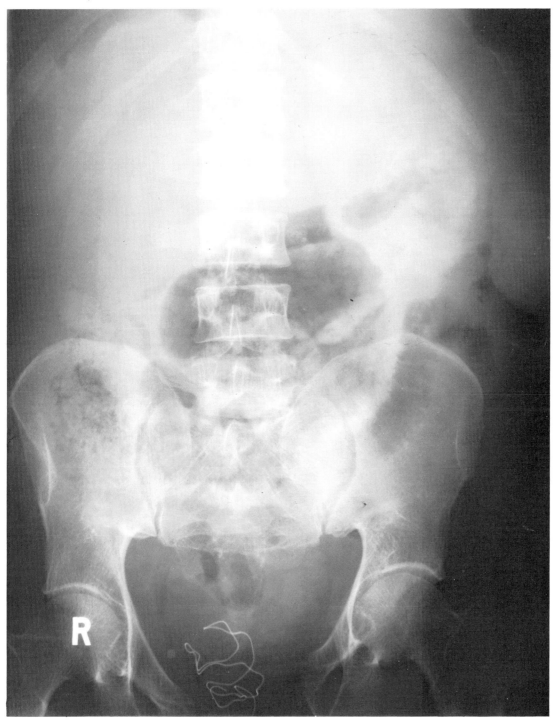

Fig. IV.2.E6 This young man with exstrophy also had a uretero-colic diversion, but 20 years later his kidneys remain entirely normal.

WILLIAMS D. INNES, FAY R. & LILLIE J.G. (1972) The functional radiology of ectopic ureterocele. *British Journal of Urology* **44**, 417–433.

WILLIAMS D. INNES & LIGHTWOOD R.G. (1972) Bilateral single ectopic ureters. *British Journal of Urology* **44**, 267–273.

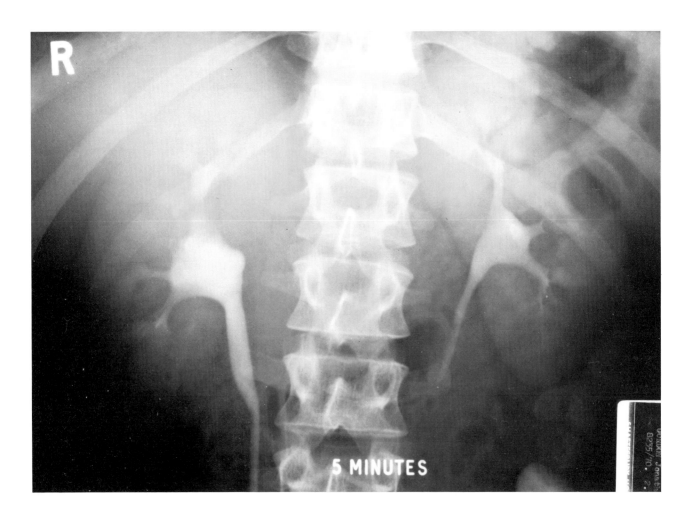

DIVISION 3.
THE BLADDER
AND URETHRA—
ADULT

A. OBSTRUCTION

Bladder outflow obstruction linked with prostatic enlargement is so common that 10% of the male readers of this book are likely to need surgical attention on this account in their later years. Disorders of micturition like frequency, urgency and nocturia are usually put under the heading of 'prostatism'. Whilst this is useful shorthand, it is important to understand that these symptoms often point to abnormal bladder behaviour induced by the prostatic obstruction: the 'unstable bladder' further discussed below.

Obstruction—prostate

Prostatic enlargement—adenoma or carcinoma?

These are still sometimes regarded as being benign or malignant varieties of the same disease, which is a misunderstanding. Benign prostatic hypertrophy, the usual cause of bladder outflow obstruction in elderly men, affects the inner part of the prostate surrounding the urethra. Prostatic carcinoma is entirely different, arising from the peripheral component of what is too often thought of as one uniform gland. Carcinoma hurts the patient by local invasion around the bladder base (Fig. IV. 3.A1), and by metastases, particularly in lymph nodes and bone (Fig. IV.3.A2). However, malignant foci in the peripheral prostate are a frequent chance finding at prostatic resection for central, benign adenomatous enlargement. They may be quite silent clinically, and indeed the probability of harbouring such a silent focus rises steeply with advancing years.

The prostate and the IVU—residual urine

An IVU is traditionally requested for the patient with suspected bladder out-flow obstruction. This can be quite informative, but has limitations which are not always well understood.

The IVU can assess any effect of the obstructed bladder on each upper urinary tract, and it can also usefully look at the state of the bladder wall. The second point is important where obstruction is so severe that the bladder wall has been damaged by local blow-outs—saccules (small) or diverticula (large). In their presence the outlook for the patient is markedly worse, even if obstruction is relieved.

The IVU *cannot* determine whether bladder outflow obstruction exists in the

255

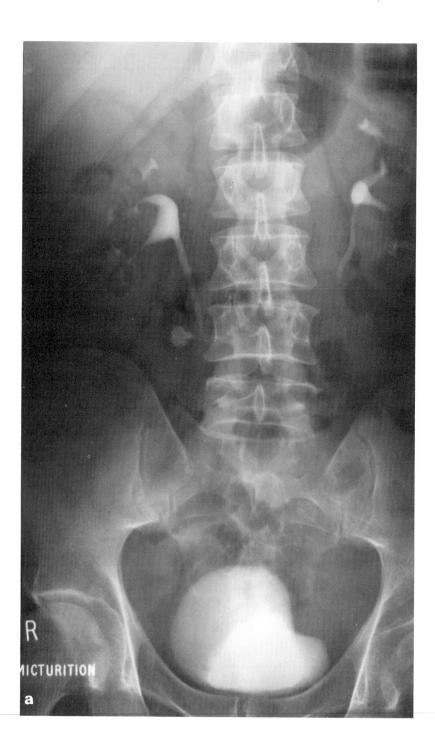

Fig. IV.3.A1a This IVU from a patient with prostatic carcinoma looks normal enough, though in retrospect there is already bladder deformity.

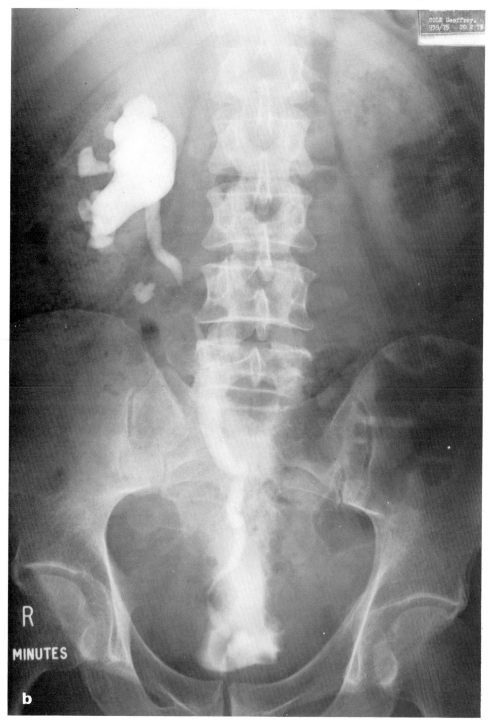

Fig. IV.3.A1b Four months later the bladder has become very severely distorted because of tumour extension and lymph node spread. There is also bilateral ureteric obstruction, much worse on the left. These gross deformities may be expected to improve if the tumour responds to treatment.

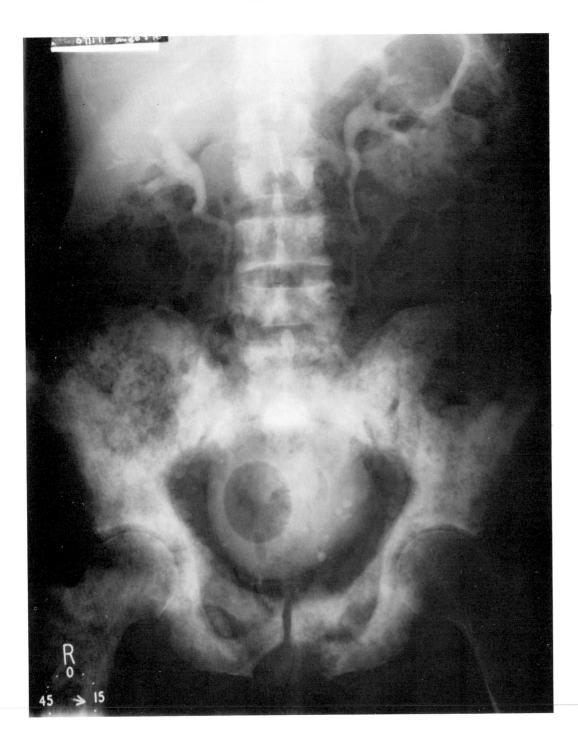

first place. In particular the question of any *residual urine* seen after voiding is much overrated. If there is no residual urine, all may of course be well. But it is equally possible that there is severe bladder outflow obstruction: like any muscular pump which runs into obstruction problems, the bladder is at first able to cope with the additional load by work hypertrophy. During this phase of *compensated obstruction*, voiding pressures are raised and flow rate reduced, but there is still complete bladder emptying (Fig. IV.3.A3). Eventually bladder failure supervenes, voiding pressure is no longer markedly raised, and residual urine is seen *(decompensated obstruction)*.

If the IVU does show residual urine, it may of course be a pointer to the bladder failure stage in obstruction. This conclusion will be strengthened if the sign is constant, remembering that there are two post-micturition films on the IVU—the preliminary plain film as well as the last contrast one. Inadequate bladder emptying may of course occur very easily just in the unfamiliar setting of the X-ray department. If the lavatory is far from the X-ray table, the bladder may be refilling again fast by the time the patient arrives back for his post-micturition film. For these reasons the residual urine found in the absence of symptoms or signs is usually best ignored.

Fig. IV.3.A2 *(facing page)* Massive bone involvement by secondary deposits in prostatic carcinoma.

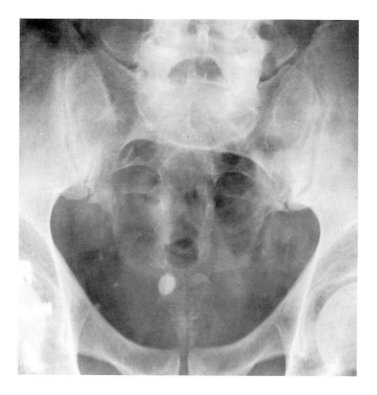

Fig. IV.3.A3a This man already has a bladder stone because of his severe bladder outflow obstruction.

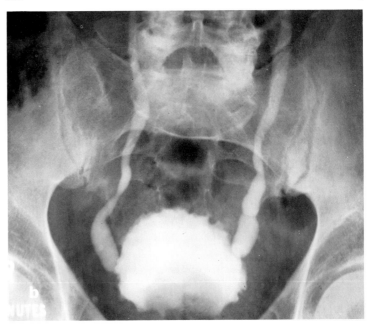

Fig. IV.3.A3b His bladder wall is trabeculated and his ureters are mildly obstructed.

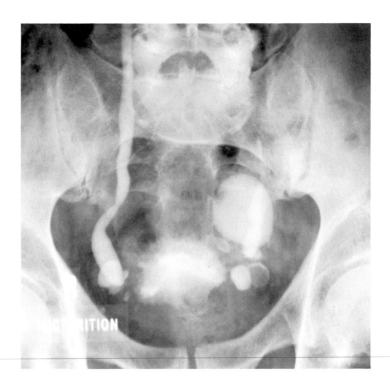

Fig. IV.3.A3c Nevertheless he is still able to empty his bladder almost completely, blowing up a number of diverticula.

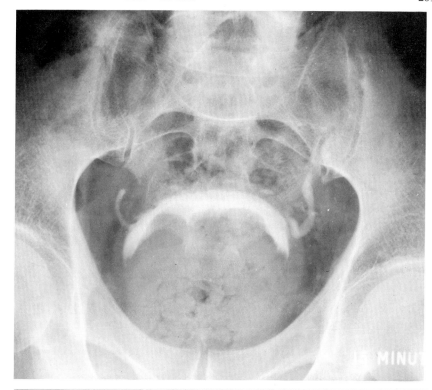

Fig. IV.3.A4 Very large prostate indenting the bladder base.

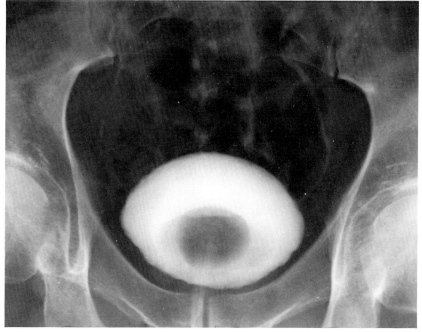

Fig. IV.3.A5 Island prostate making a filling defect in the middle of this bladder projection.

The prostate and the IVU—specific signs

Basal deformity of the bladder on the IVU and prostatic enlargement are obviously related. (Fig. IV.3.A4). However, this relation is not close, and guessing the size of the prostate from the IVU is an unrewarding endeavour. The 'island prostate' presenting as an apparently intravesical filling defect is worth remembering (Fig. IV.3.A5). The IVU is good at assessing ureteric involvement. The ureters may be hooked up because of elevation of the bladder base by the prostate (Fig. IV.3 A6). Or there may be dilatation of both upper urinary tracts secondary to bladder outflow obstruction (Fig. IV.3.A7).

If upper tract involvement is markedly asymmetric, local invasion by a carcinoma of the prostate must be considered (see Fig. IV.3.A1).

Prostatic calcification or calculi are unhelpful signs, barely worth comment in X-ray reports. They occur in normal and abnormal states, and are of no clinical relevance as a rule.

Osteitis pubis is a rare complication of urethral instrumentation (Fig. IV. 3. A8).

Obstruction—urodynamics

Pressure/flow studies during voiding cystography have provided splendid insights into the natural history of bladder outflow obstruction. Most patients suspected of this disorder will not need them. They are most useful when patients present with complex problems.

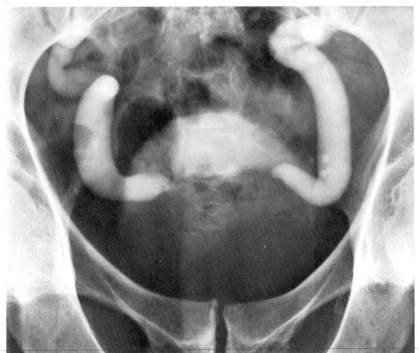

Fig. IV.3.A6 Both lower ureters are hooked up by the enlarged prostate.

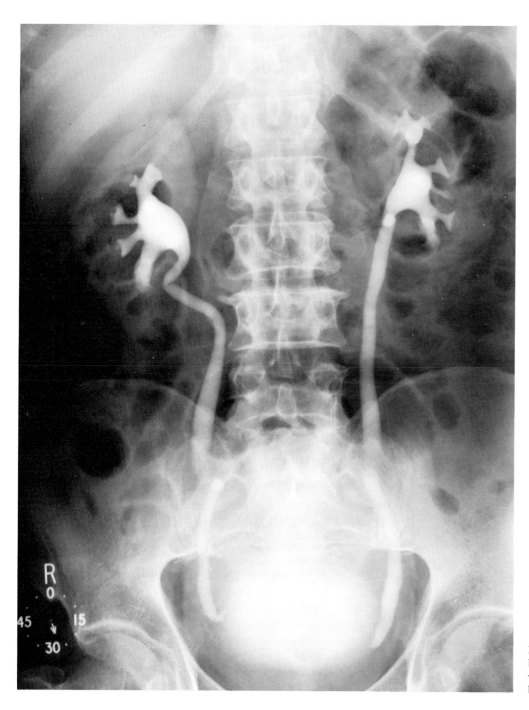

Fig. IV.3.A7 Severe bladder outflow obstruction, with secondary dilatation of both upper urinary tracts.

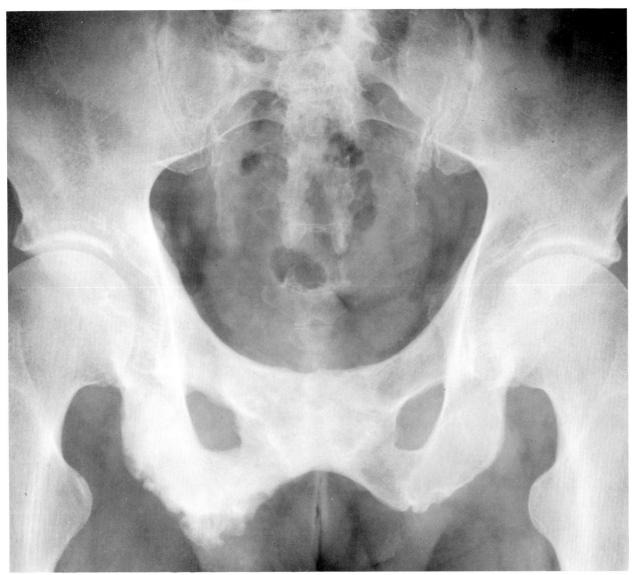

Fig. IV.3.A8   Osteitis pubis—note new bone growth and bridging of the symphysis.

The urodynamic diagnosis of obstruction is based on raised voiding pressure and reduced flow rate. As a rough guide, adult voiding pressure is normally less than 50 cm water, and flow rate at least 20 ml/sec. The young child can generate considerably higher voiding pressures as a normal event. Detrusor pressure should always be interpreted in the light of flow rate. In severe long-standing obstruction, for instance, the bladder will eventually fail, no longer able to generate a raised voiding pressure (see Decompensated Obstruction above). In this late stage of obstruction normal voiding pressure may be found, but flow rate will be grossly reduced.

Voiding flow rate is the single most helpful measurement in suspected obstruction, and many clinical problems can be solved by coupling it with the standard clinico-radiological approach of history, examination and IVU. Clinical sense is needed, of course: in a young man with impaired flow rate and unremarkable history a urethrogram should be an early investigation, to look for the likely stricture.

The unstable bladder

During bladder filling inappropriate, unwanted bladder contractions may be seen. They are discernible only by their kicks on the detrusor pressure trace (see Part I section B) and are not reflected by any change in the cystographic image. Such contractions are never a feature of the normal adult bladder, however hard it is stretched by overfilling. They make up the sign of the unstable bladder (Fig. IV.3.A9). Sometimes they are only brought out by provocative manoeuvres: standing up or coughing.

The unstable bladder may be an acquired sign, induced by outflow obstruction. Symptoms like frequency, urgency and nocturia are common parts of 'prostatism'. Their explanation is often uninhibited bladder contractions, arising as a complication of obstruction. Successful surgical relief will cure the instability in most of these patients. A few will return with persisting symptoms after operation. A dynamic cystogram study will then distinguish between those with persisting obstruction, and those who are now unobstructed, but still have an unstable bladder as source of their symptoms. Clearly further surgery is out

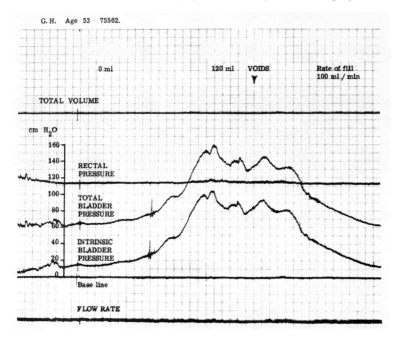

Fig. IV.3.A9 On this extract from a dynamic study, only the scale for the detrusor (intrinsic bladder) pressure is shown. This is an unstable bladder with an unwanted detrusor contraction during bladder filling. This was so severe that the patient voided uncontrollably after only 120 ml.

of place in the second group. In these problem patients with post-prostatectomy symptoms the combined study comes into its own for indicating proper management (Turner Warwick *et al*, 1973a).

Obstruction in young men

Urethral stricture is an important cause here, discussed further in the next section. An additional group of men, often young, has recently been identified, with a different and interesting cause for their bladder outflow obstruction. They present with symptoms such as hesitancy, urgency, frequency and dysuria, and these have often driven them to various doctors and diagnoses, including 'prostatitis'. They suffer from an obstructive bladder neck which does not open normally during voiding (Turner Warwick *et al*, 1973b). Considerable bladder wall hypertrophy may occur in time, leading to a compensated obstruction state with no residual urine. The dynamic cystogram is diagnostic; there is failure of the bladder neck to open properly during voiding, together with impaired flow rate and raised detrusor pressure. Unstable bladder contractions may be seen as an acquired phenomenon (Fig. IV.3.A10).

The condition can be treated very successfully by judicious bladder neck incision. Symptoms are relieved, and the secondary bladder instability disappears. It is therefore well worth referring patients for the combined study when this diagnosis is suspected, rather than resting content with a vague label like 'chronic prostatitis'.

Fig. IV.3.A10a Normal study—note fast flow rate.

Fig. IV.3.A10b On this study there is reduced flow rate and increased detrusor pressure—the signs of obstruction. The fluoroscopic image pinpoints the site—the bladder neck does not open properly.

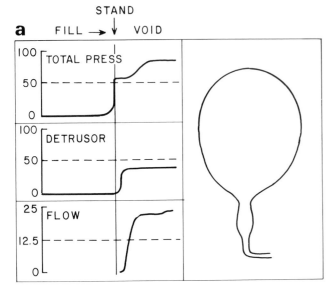

VIDEO FRAME FROM NORMAL VOIDING STUDY

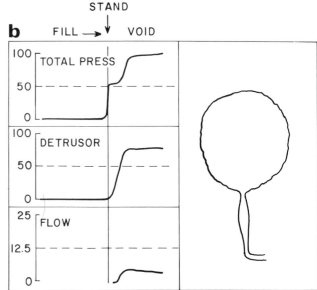

VIDEO FRAME : FAILURE OF BLADDER NECK OPENING
WITH OUTFLOW OBSTRUCTION

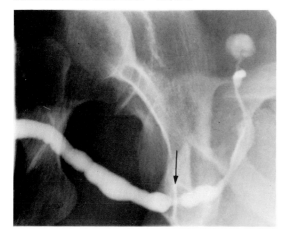

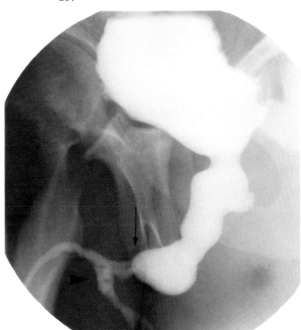

Fig. IV.3.A11 *(above)*   Urethrogram with a bulbar stricture (arrow).

Fig. IV.3.A12 *(right)*   A voiding cystogram in a patient with a urethral stricture (small arrow). There is also a sinus tracking to the skin (large arrowhead). Note how dilatation above the lesion demonstrates the severity of obstruction on this voiding study.

Obstruction—urethral stricture

The conventional division of this subject is into congenital and acquired strictures. It is hard to pin down the true congenital stricture, though some young adults presenting with a short stenotic segment in the bulbar urethra may be examples of this entity.

Most urethral strictures are acquired, with gonococcal infection as the important cause. Urethrography generally allows a beautiful demonstration of the site and extent of the stricture (Fig. IV.3.A11). It is of course by design a test of structure, and does not provide any information about the functional importance of any stricture. To this end voiding flow rate or voiding cysto-urethrography are needed (Fig. IV.3.A12).

There are two radiological pictures of *gonococcal stricture*. The more common is a sharply localized lesion in the bulbar urethra (Fig. IV.3.A13). If the disease has come to involve the anterior urethra, it does not usually result in such short, well-defined stenoses. Instead there is extensive narrowing of the lumen of the urethra by diffuse fibrosis (Fig. IV.3.A14). The failure of distension of the anterior urethra on urethrography can therefore be an important pointer to the presence of a long stricture.

Fistula formation is a complication of urethral stricture, and may advance to the awful, grotesque picture of multiple fistulae, the 'watering can perineum' (Fig. IV.3.A15).

Traffic accidents are now the common background to the development of *traumatic strictures,* further discussed in section F p. 307.

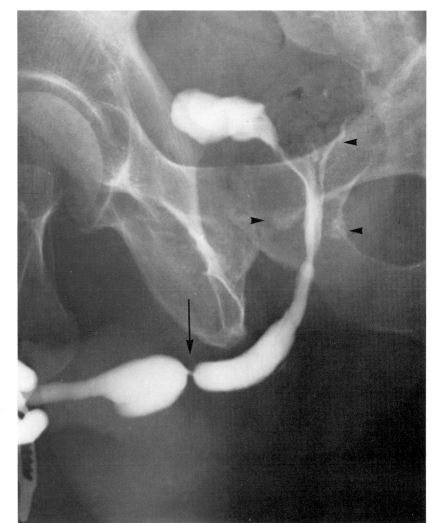

Fig. IV.3.A13 (*right*) Urethrogram with a local stricture (arrow). The arrowheads point to reflux into prostatic and ejaculatory ducts.

Fig. IV.3.A14 (*below*) On this urethrogram there is extensive fibrosis throughout the anterior urethra, marked out by irregular narrowing.

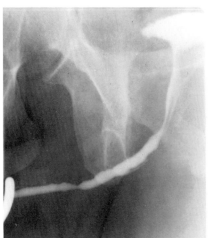

Obstruction—bladder diverticula

Acquired blow-outs of the bladder wall are important for the increased hazard they impose on patients with bladder outflow obstruction. This hazard is largely that of infection, because of inadequate bladder emptying. Posterior bladder diverticula near the trigone can give rise to marked ureteric displacement (Fig. IV.3.A16). Congenital bladder diverticula are considered in the children's section (Division 4 section B), but may also be seen in the adult (Fig. IV.3.A17).

Obstruction—bladder stones

Outflow obstruction is the usual background to bladder stones, and they are

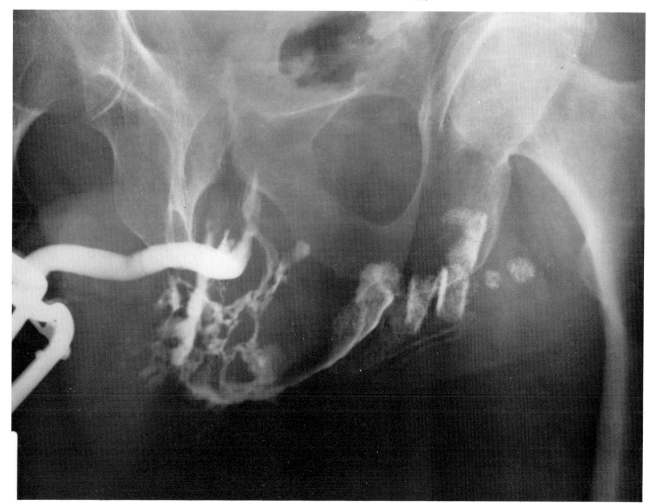

therefore extremely uncommon in women. They may grow to very large size (Fig. IV.3.A18) or be multiple and small (Fig. IV.3.A19).

Fig. IV.3.A15 Multiple urethral fistulae—the 'watering can perineum'.

Summary comments

1. Prostatic bladder outflow obstruction can usually be well assessed on the basis of history, examination and voiding flow rate. An IVU is useful for looking at any secondary blow-out effects on the upper urinary tracts and on the bladder wall (diverticula). The absence of residual urine does not exclude obstruction.

2. Instability may be provoked by obstruction, and is usually cured by its relief. In patients with persisting post-prostatectomy symptoms the unstable bladder takes on particular importance. These patients are best referred for pressure/flow video-cystography.

Fig. IV.3.A16 Large right-sided bladder diverticulum. Note how this has displaced the lower ureter medially (arrow).

3. Urethral stricture is an important cause of obstruction in younger men, and the urethrogram should be an early investigation here. Bladder neck dysfunction is a less common but interesting cause of obstruction, also seen in this age group. It needs full urodynamic assessment.

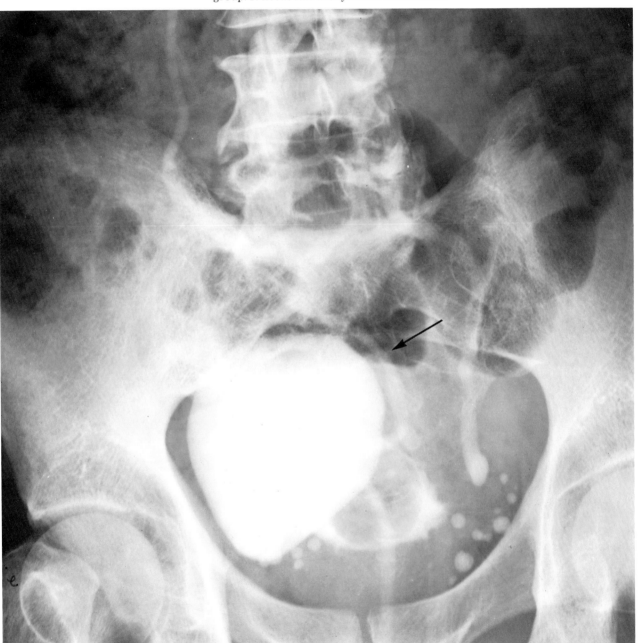

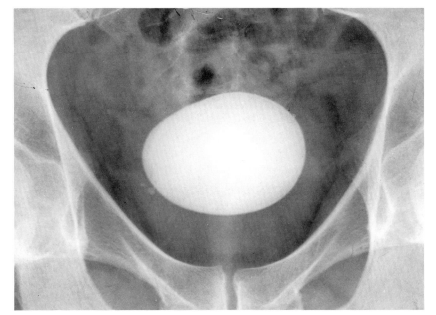

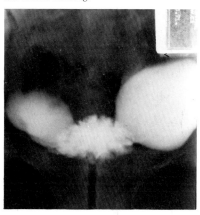

Fig. IV.3.A17 *(below)* An adult with symmetrical bladder diverticula, one on each side of the midline. The small central structure is the nearly empty bladder at the end of voiding.

Fig. IV.3.A18 *(left)* Large bladder stone.

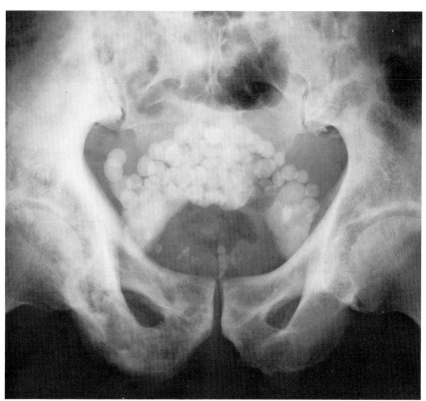

Fig. IV.3.A19 Multiple small bladder stones. Note how they outline the enlarged prostate. This patient also has Paget's disease.

B. INFECTION

Urinary infection is common in children and adults. The need for radiological investigation, however, is sharply different between the two age groups. It can be reasonably argued that every child with a proven urinary tract infection should have an IVU. The position in adults is the reverse. They need to be protected from useless radiological investigation.

Recurrent cystitis in women

This can be such a troublesome problem that with some despair all available diagnostic help is sought. Unhappily the pay-off from routine IVUs in this condition is very poor indeed. So many women will have unnecessary radiation exposure under this régime, not to speak of the cost, that any routine radiological investigation can be seriously questioned.

The occasional find of an important lesion will be used to justify the practice. *Renal stones* may be discovered, apparently unsuspected. Or a *pelvi-ureteric junction obstruction* with a hydronephrotic kidney is seen for the first time.

The question to be asked is how such near-chance findings could be anticipated on the clinical presentation of recurrent urinary infection. The identity of the infecting organism can help. Proteus infections should always raise the alarm about a possible stone, and are a good indication for radiological studies. Plain film tomography of the renal areas may be needed before the IVU in order to look for a poorly calcified stone. It is much better to investigate the small minority of patients with likely lesions intensively than to cast a general superficial radiological look, missing the very abnormalities sought.

Loin symptoms may point to a hydronephrosis, and it is probably right to investigate such adults. Most of them will have normal IVUs. Apart from hydronephrosis, renal papillary necrosis is worth remembering as a cause of unexplained infection having an upper urinary tract flavour. Women with recurrent infection need to be quizzed about possible analgesic abuse. Any clinical suspicion in this direction, perhaps supported by a story of 'passing bits in my water' is a good indication for an IVU (Fig. IV.3.B1).

A small kidney with reflux may occasionally be found in adults presenting with cystitis and loin pain (Fig. IV.3.B2). Whilst the renal damage was clearly done long ago, persisting troublesome pain and infection on the side of the abnormality may add up to a good reason for surgical intervention.

Urethral diverticula are sometimes discovered in women during recurrent cystitis investigations (Fig. IV.3.B3). They may even be multiple (Fig. IV.3.B4). The voiding cystogram is the easiest but arguably not the most reliable way of detecting them. Urethrography may be done (Bretland, 1973), if there is strong clinical suspicion of a hidden diverticulum. The frequency and importance of these lesions is debated—at present they do not amount to any good indication for routine screening.

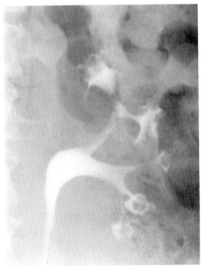

Fig. IV.3.B1 Characteristic papillary necrosis—note how the pyelogram outlines the abnormal papillae, with multiple dissection tracks within them.

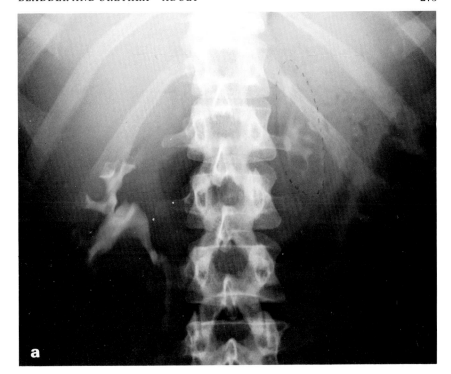

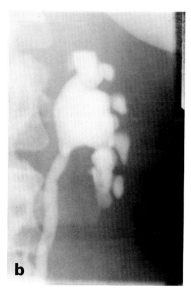

Fig. IV.3.B2a *(left)* IVU in a woman with recurrent urinary infections—the left kidney is tiny.

Fig. IV.3.B2b *(below)* A cystogram shows gross reflux into the scarred kidney.

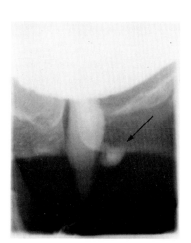

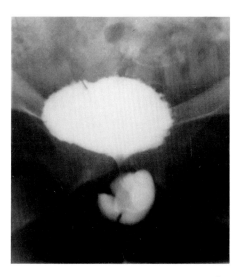

Fig. IV.3.B3 *(left)* MCU—the arrow points to a small urethral diverticulum in this woman.

Fig. IV.3.B4 *(right)* MCU in a woman with multiple urethral diverticula.

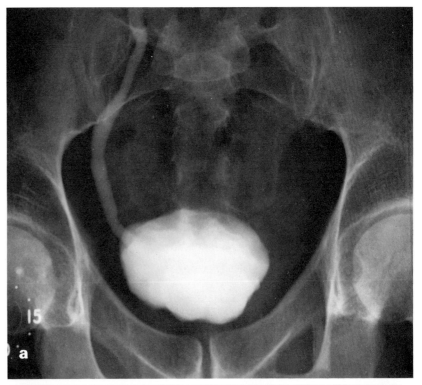

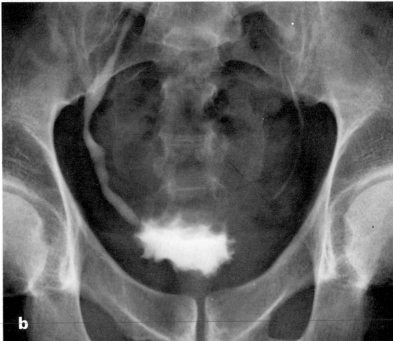

Fig. IV.3.B5a & b IVU before and after
voiding in a young man with acute
cystitis. Note the deformed, oedematous
bladder wall, with hold-up in the right
lower ureter. See also Fig. IV.3.D6.

Cystitis in men

This topic is closely linked to the question of bladder outflow obstruction, and a voiding flow rate will be of help in resolving it. Quite severe obstruction may first present with infection.

Acute cystitis in young men is sometimes seen in venereal disease clinics. The bladder wall is markedly deformed and oedematous, and this may be severe enough to give rise to ureteric hold-up (Fig. IV.3.B5). A tuberculous cystitis may be suspected, but often no plausible organism of any sort is found. However, the condition responds to antibiotics, and the bladder then returns to normal (Fig. IV.3.B6).

Urethral diverticula are rare congenital lesions which may collect stones (Fig. IV.3.B7). They usually present in childhood (see Division 4 section B).

Summary comments

1. Recurrent cystitis in women is generally not a problem for radiological help. The radiologist with his clinical colleagues should try to select for study those women to be suspected of upper urinary tract lesions, particularly stones, papillary necrosis, and hydronephrosis.

2. Whilst renal stones etc. may also occur in men, bladder outflow obstruction is

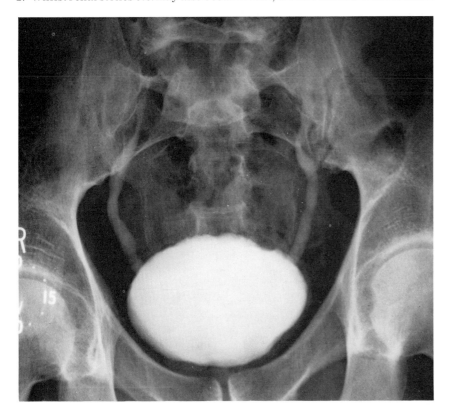

Fig. IV.3.B6 The same patient as in Fig. IV.3.B5, after resolution of the cystitis—all is well now.

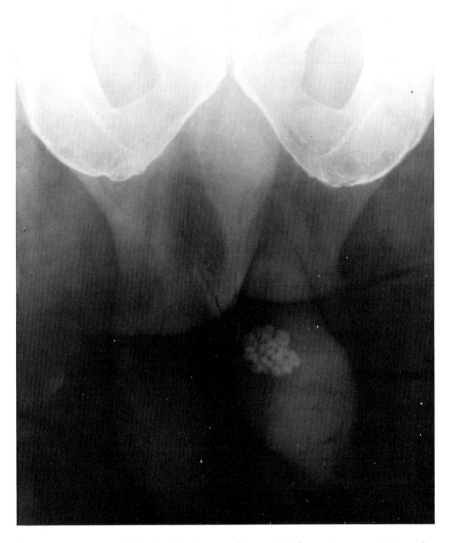

Fig. IV.3.B7 Stones in a urethral diverticulum.

the more common aetiological background to cystitis here. Acute cystitis can be a venereal infection.

3. Tuberculosis is not to be forgotten.

Pneumaturia—fistulae

'Bubbles in my water' is a story clearly indicating either a fistula from bowel to urinary tract, or a roaring urinary infection. Infections with gas forming organisms, severe enough to cause this symptom, usually spell diabetes. Gas may then be seen not just in the lumen of the bladder, but also dissecting into its wall, and within or without the upper urinary tract.

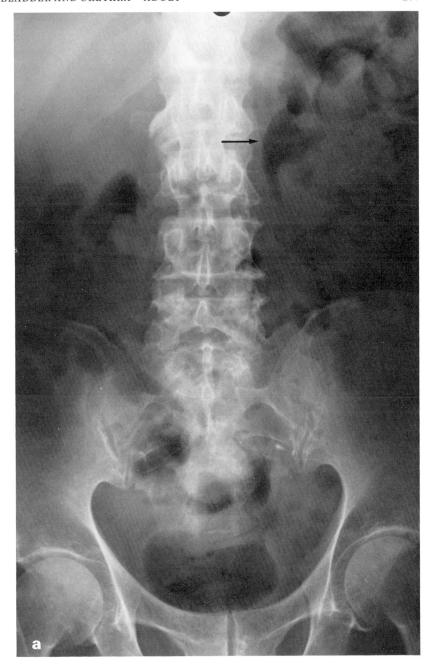

a

Fig. IV.3.B8a *(left)* & **b** *(overleaf)* Plain film and later IVU in a patient with a sigmoid carcinoma invading the bladder. The arrow points to the gas pyelogram, and there is also gas in the bladder. Note the invasion of the bladder by the tumour, mimicking a bladder carcinoma.

Fistulae are almost always the result of primary bowel disease. This may be either inflammatory, e.g. diverticulitis or Crohn's disease, or neoplastic, e.g. sigmoid carcinoma (Fig. IV.3.B8). Fistulae are not a complication of primary

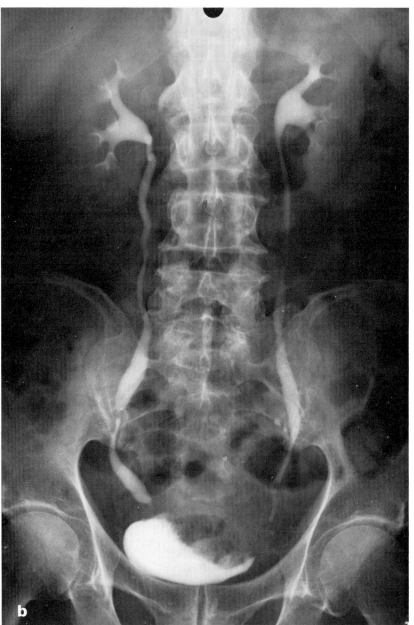

bladder tumours. Rarely a prostatic carcinoma may erode into the rectum (Fig. IV.3.B9).

When an entero-vesical fistula is suspected, it will be found more readily on investigation of the bowel rather than the urinary tract. A barium enema is therefore a useful first step (Fig. IV.3.B10).

These paragraphs have dealt with the patient complaining of pneumaturia. The commonest cause of gas seen in the upper urinary tract by the radiologist is a different matter. This is brought about by surgical ureteric diversion: a uretero-colic anastomosis, or sometimes an ileal loop diversion (see Fig. IV.2.E1). Such a gas pyelogram is of course evidence of reflux into the diverted ureter. It is a more sensitive index than contrast examinations (Fig. IV.3.B11).

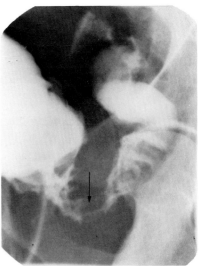

Fig. IV.3.B9 *(above)* Cystogram in a patient with a prostatic carcinoma, which has eroded into the rectum. A balloon catheter is seen in the bladder, and the arrow points to the fistula.

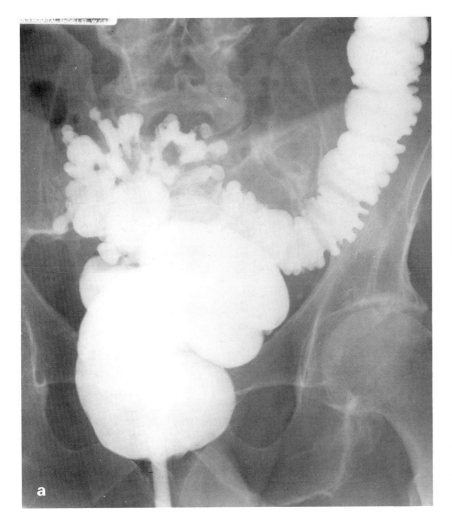

a

Fig. IV.3.B10a *(left)* & **b** *(overleaf)* AP and lateral projections of a barium enema in a patient with diverticular disease. Note that the bladder is filled through a fistula.

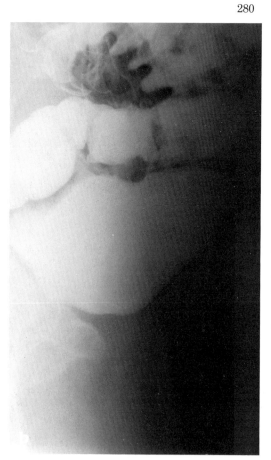

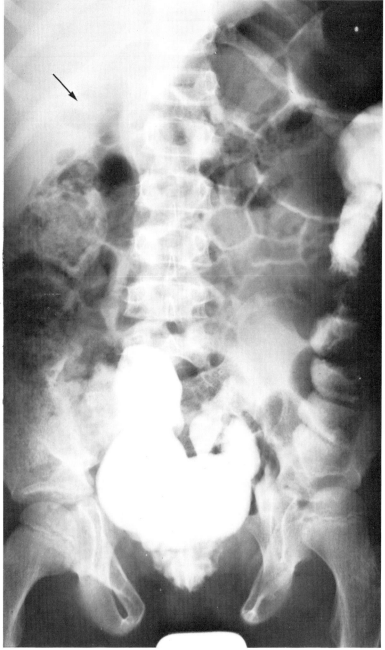

Fig. IV.3.B11 *(right)* This boy with
exstrophy has had a uretero-colic
diversion. The arrow points to the gas
pyelogram, indicating reflux from the
colon into the right kidney. However, this
reflux cannot be shown with the contrast
medium instilled into the colon on this
film.

C. INCONTINENCE

'Wet pants' make up a large fund of human misery, often rather neglected by doctors in general and research workers in particular. At the same time it is important to get the subject in perspective. Pilot work suggests that the majority of British adults have minor micturition symptoms. Women occasionally wet themselves on coughing. Men have a slight post-micturition dribble (vulgar reminder: 'if you can't wait to shake your peg, you'll have it running down your leg'). This may not be a state of perfect health, but it is normal. Investigation of such slight symptoms is not in the best interests of the 'patients'.

Stress incontinence

Women who wet themselves on coughing, straining, laughing, running etc. come to the radiologist in two broad groups: symptoms have either arisen for the first time, or there is already a history of surgical intervention.

Most women first presenting with stress incontinence will have a mechanical disarray alone. The bladder behaves normally, but its sphincters are weak. The bladder neck may already be open at rest, and a rise in intra-abdominal pressure brought about by coughing or laughing is enough to overcome the distal (or urethral) sphincter mechanism as last resistance: incontinence results.

On cystography the open incompetent bladder neck will be seen, accentuated by coughing. This observation alone has no discriminative value for distinguishing simple sphincter incompetence from other causes of incontinence. The same can be said of structural measurements like the posterior urethro-vesical angle, which we have not found at all helpful. Cystography is sometimes advocated just for excluding unusual chance findings such as urethral diverticula in these patients—a poor justification for a cystogram.

It is worth proposing that routine cystography has nothing to offer the woman presenting with apparent stress incontinence. The important endeavour here is to detect the patient whose bladder is at fault not because of sphincter incompetence, but as the result of inappropriate detrusor contractions, i.e. *bladder instability* (see section A p. 265). We have to understand that her bladder neck too will appear incompetent, having been opened by the unwanted contraction. Cystography cannot distinguish between the two, but seeing an abnormal wave on the detrusor pressure recording will nail the unstable bladder. To make matters more difficult, it may be coughing in particular which fires the unstable bladder into inappropriate activity (Fig. IV.3.C1), so that incontinence on coughing is not necessarily a sign of sphincter incompetence.

This distinction is vital. There is everything to be said in favour of careful surgery for troublesome sphincter incompetence, but operations will do no good for the patient with primary bladder instability. Most women presenting with a story of stress incontinence will fall into the first group, and in the straightforward patient any further studies may be quite unnecessary before surgery. If

Fig. IV.3.C1 Two episodes of coughing are shown on these extracts from a dynamic study in a woman with supposed stress incontinence. The coughs are reflected by kicks on the total bladder and rectal pressure traces. They also cause artefacts on the detrusor (intrinsic bladder) pressure trace, for which a scale and baseline are shown. Note that the mean detrusor pressure rises from 20 to 40 cm with each coughing episode: the bladder has been stimulated into inappropriate contraction. Bladder instability is bad enough to cause incontinence, registered on the voiding flow rate trace during the second episode (arrow). At the end of this trace the patient begins to void voluntarily, with an additional normal rise in detrusor pressure.

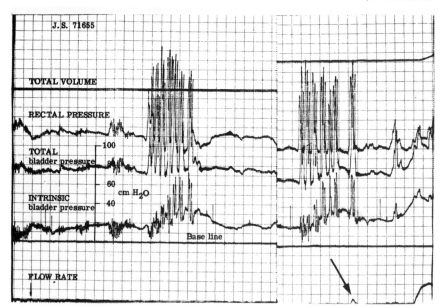

there is additional urgency or nocturia in the history, however, these may be pointers to instability. This is particularly so if urge incontinence is described by the patient: she begins to void uncontrollably if she does not reach a lavatory at once on the call to micturition. Such motor urge incontinence as the result of an unstable bladder is to be distinguished from sensory urgency brought about by inflammatory vesical disorders. Sensory urgency and cystitis are not accompanied by instability.

Patients with complicating symptoms such as urgency will benefit from a urodynamic study to exclude instability. This will apply with much greater force to those who have already had surgery, but are still troubled by bladder symptoms. Second and third operations may have been done. When such patients are investigated there is naturally a much higher yield of finding an unstable bladder. This may either have been present from the start, accounting for operation failure, or even induced by an obstruction worsened at surgery. Should simple sphincter incompetence with a stable bladder predominate after surgery, a further operation may be worthwhile. The combined study comes into its own in these often difficult patients, with the cystographic image particularly important for pointing out urethral distortion.

Summary comments

1. Women presenting with a story of simple stress incontinence are likely to have sphincter imcompetence with a stable bladder. In experienced clinical hands preoperative investigation has little to offer, and certainly routine cystography nothing at all.

2. Additional symptoms such as urgency are danger signals that a more complex disorder may be present, which will not benefit from surgery: the unstable bladder. These patients should generally have a urodynamic study. A full pressure/flow videocystogram is ideal, but the essential distinction between the stable and unstable bladder can be accomplished by simpler pressure recordings in this group.

3. Patients whose incontinence has already failed to improve with surgery deserve a full combined study. The pressure/flow data are needed to test for instability and obstruction, the synchronous cystogram to look at the bladder neck and urethral distortion.

Prostatic problems

Incontinence following prostatectomy can be a troublesome complaint. Continence is maintained in normal men by two powerful, independent sphincter mechanisms: the bladder neck (or internal sphincter), and the distal mechanism (or external sphincter). The distal mechanism is made up of two elements: the pelvic floor muscles, and the membranous urethra itself. During a prostatectomy the bladder neck is of course resected, but patients remain continent thanks to the intact distal mechanism. If the membranous urethra has already been hurt by some earlier insult, e.g. trauma, then resection of the bladder neck will remove the last bastion of continence available to that patient.

The *unstable bladder* is of particular importance in post-prostatectomy incontinence. As explained in section A above, uninhibited bladder contractions may occur as a complication of obstruction, but usually recede after successful surgery on the prostate/bladder neck. If they do not, there may be incontinence, with the distal mechanism unable to cope on its own. A pressure/flow video-cystogram will then be needed to sort out the cause of incontinence. The bladder neck will of course be found wide open in anyone after prostatectomy.

If prostatic surgery has been ineffective in relieving obstruction, or prostatic regrowth occurs, incontinence may arise by overflow from a distended bladder.

Ectopic ureters

These problems present in childhood, and are considered in Division 4 section A p. 316. However, the true diagnosis may have been missed for far too long, so that it has to be made in adult life. The tell-tale clinical story is of course of a woman complaining that she has always been damp, day and night (Fig. IV.3.C2). This is different from an acquired uretero-vaginal fistula (Fig. IV.3.C3)!

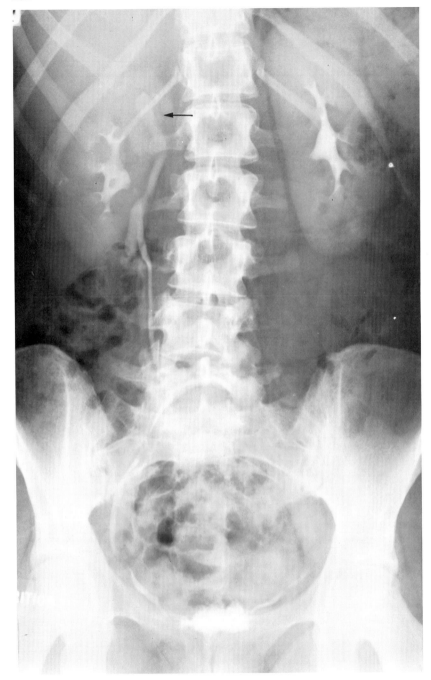

Fig. IV.3.C2 A young woman with
lifelong incontinence who has already
had several (inadequate) IVUs. The arrow
points to the abnormal upper moiety of
her duplex right kidney, draining into the
vagina.

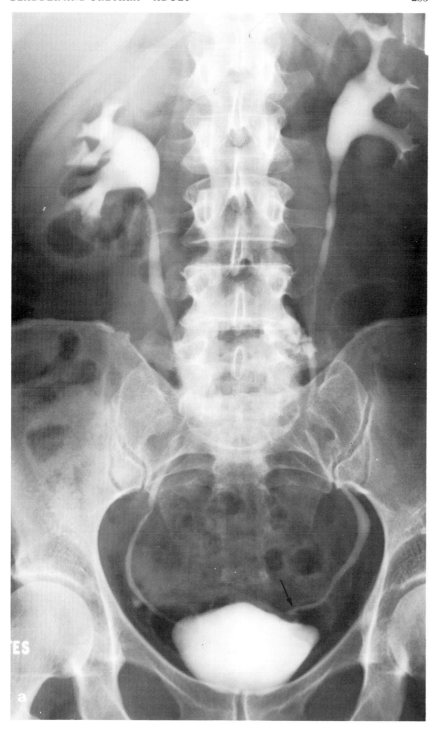

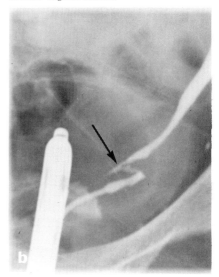

Fig. IV.3.C3a *(left)*   This woman is continually damp after a gynaecological operation—note the asymmetry of her lower ureters (arrow). The main task of the IVU in these problems is to disclose such asymmetry.

Fig. IV.3.C3b *(below)*   Retrograde examination—the arrow points to the uretero-vaginal fistula.

Neuropathic bladder

This is a subject of such ready confusion that using the right words seems doubly important. 'Neurogenic bladder' is a nonsense term, since all normal micturition is neurogenic.

A further difficulty is that radiological teaching on the neuropathic bladder is often set in a rigid framework copied from one authority to the next. This scheme is mentioned here for brief summary and dismissal. The argument is that there are distinctive X-ray pictures of the neuropathic bladder dependent on the level of the neuronal lesion. In its simplest form, it points to the thick-walled, trabeculated bladder as a typical upper motor neurone lesion, contrasted with the thin-walled, flaccid bladder characteristic of lower motor neurone lesions. In practice the radiological pictures are very mixed. Neuropathic bladders can be thick-walled just because of associated infection/inflammation. The shape of the bladder is no reliable indicator of neuropathy. As an example, the obstructed bladder can give a 'typical neuropathic' picture (Fig. IV.3.C4). Using the cystographic image for characterizing the neurological lesion is a barren endeavour.

Fig. IV.3.C4a *(left)* This picture has the appearance of a neuropathic bladder—note elongated shape and trabeculated wall (see also Fig. IV.4.A10).
Fig. IV.3.C4b *(right)* The explanation is obstruction, not neuropathy—note how the enlarged prostate stretches the posterior urethra (arrow).

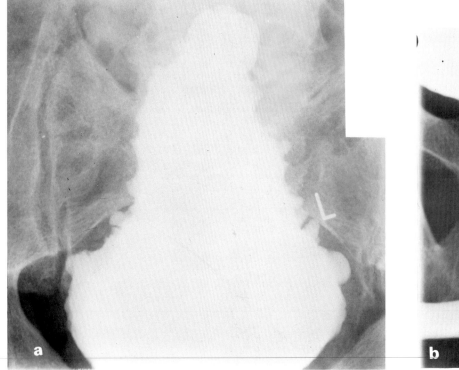

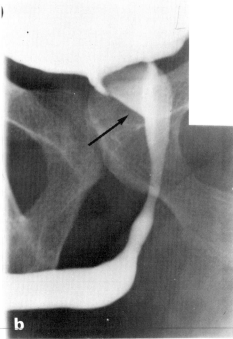

There are much more cogent reasons for radiological studies in the patient
with a neuropathic bladder. These are:

1. Discovering a cause in the spinal canal.

2. Monitoring the state of the upper urinary tracts.

3. Assessing bladder outflow obstruction.

4. Judging residual urine.

1. The cause

Congenital or acquired spinal lesions play a large part in the neuropathic
bladder problem. The diagnosis of congenital lesions will often be perfectly
obvious, as in a myelomeningocoele, and the important contribution of radiology is to uncover the hidden ones. An example is the deficient sacrum, usually
presenting with childhood incontinence. If there is gross pelvic deformity, this
will be obvious on the AP view (Fig. IV.3.C5). However, this projection can be
quite deceptive for checking on the sacrum. In any unsolved incontinence
problem, it is always worth taking a lateral view (Fig. IV.3.C6).

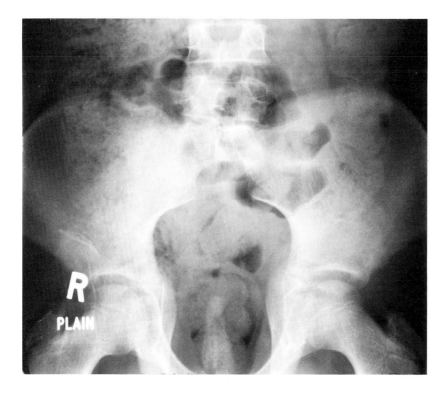

Fig. IV.3.C5 Absent sacrum, with gross,
characteristic pelvic deformity.

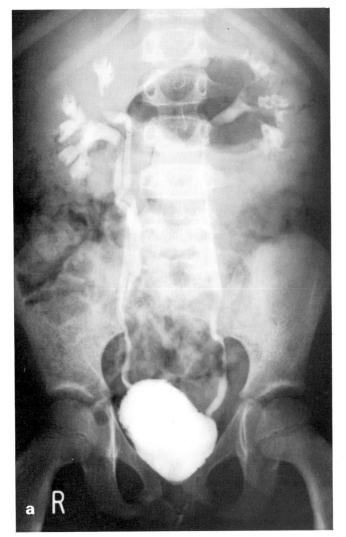

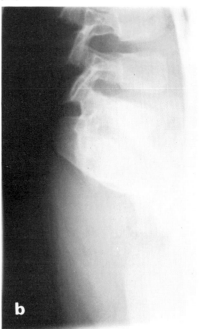

Fig. IV.3.C6a *(left)* In AP projection this incontinent child looks normal enough.
Fig. IV.3.C6b *(below)* She has an absent sacrum, revealed by this lateral projection.

The importance of some acquired spinal lesions is under debate. Obvious cord problems like tumour or compression need no further comment, but the question of degenerative skeletal disorders does. Can incontinence in the elderly have a neuropathic cause, with degenerative hypertrophic changes in the lumbar and sacral spine pressing on nerve roots or cauda equina (Sharr *et al*, 1976)? There are convincing examples where surgery of the offending spinal lesion (decompression laminectomy) has led to satisfactory improvement. This is a subject for exploration: degenerative joint changes are of course very common with advancing years, and in most patients with incontinence problems they are probably unimportant chance findings.

Summary comment. Anyone suspected of a neuropathic bladder needs careful plain film study of the lumbar and sacral spine in the absence of neurological signs pointing to a higher lesion.

2. Upper urinary tracts

The kidneys of a patient with a neuropathic bladder are always under threat. This comes about not through the urinary infections which many of these patients suffer, but by the mechanical insults of either ureteric obstruction or reflux. Obstruction arises particularly in the high pressure obstructed bladder with a thickened wall (see below), when the ureter can no longer empty its contents.

The tell-tale sign of important obstruction or reflux is dilatation of the upper urinary tracts on the IVU (Fig. IV.3.C7). This sign is in advance of functional impairment such as glomerular filtration rate. Upper urinary tract drainage needs careful monitoring therefore, and this is particularly important once

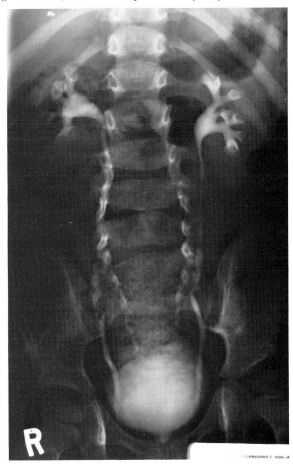

Fig. IV.3.C7 Neuropathic bladder—note severe spinal defect. There is stasis in both ureters—the early sign of obstruction or reflux. This child went on to rapid deterioration of both upper urinary tracts.

there is suspicion of early trouble. Deterioration may then advance quickly. Conservative ureteric surgery (e.g. reimplantation) is often unrewarding in the neuropathic bladder, and a urinary diversion may have to be done.

3. Bladder outflow obstruction

This is a common problem in neuropathy, and important not only because of inefficient bladder emptying, but also for the ureteric hold-up it may cause (see above). Assessment of ureteric reflux and bladder outflow obstruction are good indications for cystographic study of the neuropathic bladder. The usual site of urethral obstruction is the external sphincter, though bladder neck obstruction may occur. In the gross example the cystogram can differentiate between the two, but in general combined dynamic studies (pressure/flow video-cystography) are most helpful in directing management. If obstruction is found, further measures will be dictated by the state of the upper urinary tracts, and by the clinical background. If a male patient is already incontinent because of his neuropathy, it is often right to make him wholly incontinent by surgery to the urethral obstruction. In this way infection and ureteric obstruction risks are lessened. In women, urinary diversion may have to be advised.

Neuropathic bladders are usually grossly unstable, i.e. they show uninhibited contractions during bladder filling (Fig. IV.3.C8). These may rise to high levels of 100 cm water or more.

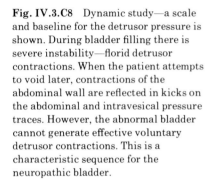

Fig. IV.3.C8 Dynamic study—a scale and baseline for the detrusor pressure is shown. During bladder filling there is severe instability—florid detrusor contractions. When the patient attempts to void later, contractions of the abdominal wall are reflected in kicks on the abdominal and intravesical pressure traces. However, the abnormal bladder cannot generate effective voluntary detrusor contractions. This is a characteristic sequence for the neuropathic bladder.

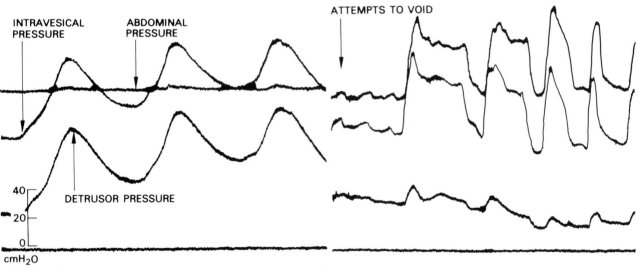

INTRAVESICAL PRESSURE   ABDOMINAL PRESSURE   ATTEMPTS TO VOID

DETRUSOR PRESSURE

40
20
0
cmH₂O

FLOW RATE

It is worth remembering one rare but important complication of cystography in patients with a high cord lesion (above mid-thoracic level). This is sudden severe hypertension during bladder filling, sometimes called autonomic dysreflexia (Barbaric, 1976). If this occurs, the bladder should be emptied at once.

4. Residual urine

Infection is very difficult or impossible to control in the presence of a large residual urine. The problem is clearly related to that of bladder outflow obstruction. It can be attacked in suitable cases by drug treatment, e.g. adrenergic blockade. The residual urine must then be monitored, and ultrasound is a quick, painless and repeatable method of doing this, even in children (Harrison *et al*, 1976).

D. HAEMATURIA

Bladder tumour

The adult patient presenting with haematuria traditionally has an IVU to look at possible renal causes. A kidney tumour may of course be discovered in this way. However, the explanation of adult haematuria is commonly in the bladder. It could therefore be argued that cystoscopy should precede the IVU. Against this is the fact that an IVU will still be needed whatever is seen by the surgeon. If a patient has a bladder tumour, proper management will demand knowing the state of the upper urinary tracts (ureteric hold-up, further urothelial tumours etc.). If cystoscopy is normal, an IVU will again be needed.

There is therefore much to be said for beginning with the IVU, as long as it is clearly understood that cystoscopy must follow. The danger is that an 'IVU normal' report will be misunderstood in the sense of 'bladder tumour excluded'. The IVU cannot do this. Indeed, the multiple bladder views sometimes advocated to look for such lesions are really misdirected efforts. The bladder cancer suspect, i.e. the adult with haematuria, needs a cystoscopy.

There *is* value in judging IVU bladder filling defects accurately. This applies particularly where a possible bladder tumour is a chance finding, on an IVU done for some quite different reason. Whether such a patient then needs a cystoscopy is determined by the radiologist's confidence in differentiating unimportant overlying gas shadows from the real thing. The white-line sign described by Simpson *et al* (1974) can be very helpful here. A 2 mm white line can often be seen outlining gas shadows projected over the contrast filled bladder: the bowel wall (Fig. IV.3.D1). This sign should not be used if the bladder is incompletely opacified, or for a much thinner white line. Filling defects without their white line will not all turn out to be bladder tumours. But when the proper sign is present, a bowel shadow can be confidently diagnosed where this is a chance worry, not prompted by haematuria.

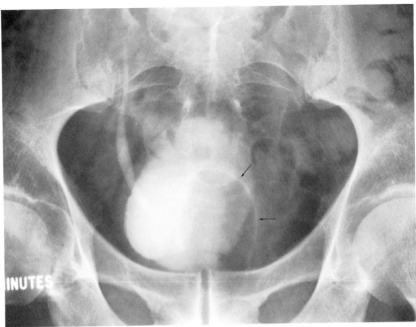

Fig. IV.3.D1 The bladder is deformed, but not by the rectum projected over it! Arrows outline the bowel wall—note how this white line continues over the bladder filled with contrast medium.

There is no difficulty about recognizing the large bladder tumour (Fig. IV.3.D2). The radiologist's task is to look where the urologist cannot see through the cystoscope: at possible obstruction of one or other ureter, and at new urothelial tumours that may arise in the upper tracts. When one non-excreting kidney is found above a bladder carcinoma, an antegrade pyelogram

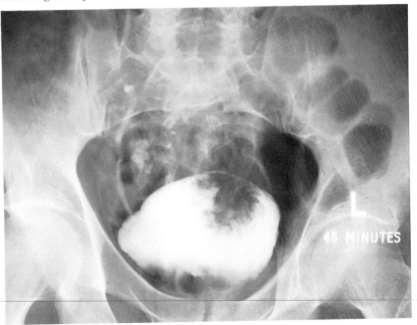

Fig. IV.3.D2 Irregular bladder filling defect—a characteristic bladder tumour.

can be very helpful. The important distinction is between complete obstruction because of the bladder lesion (Fig. IV.3.D3), and growth extending up the ureter, at worst converting the whole upper urinary tract into a solid tumour structure (Fig. IV.3.D4).

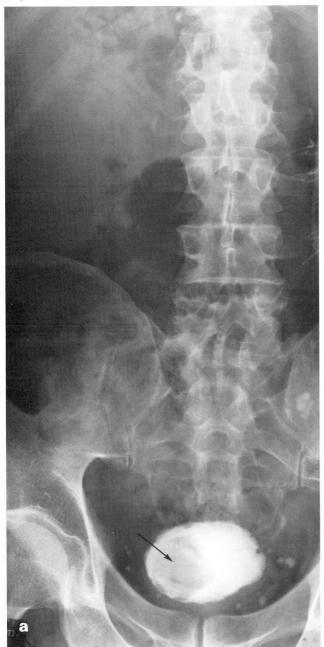

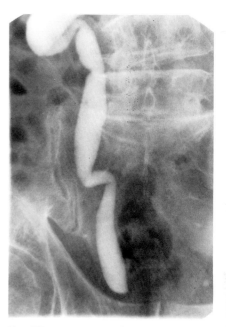

Fig. IV.3.D3 *(above)* This patient had a non-excreting right kidney because of his bladder tumour. An antegrade pyelogram shows that this is simple obstruction at the lower end of the right ureter, with a dilated but clear upper urinary tract above.

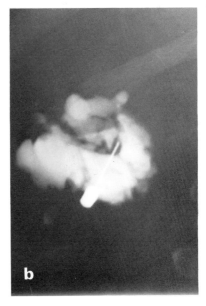

Fig. IV.3.D4a *(left)* This patient also has a non-excreting right kidney—note the right-sided bladder tumour (arrow).
Fig. IV.3.D4b *(right)* An attempted right antegrade pyelogram only shows dissection spaces in the right kidney—the whole right upper urinary tract is solid with tumour from the bladder upwards.

Once a bladder tumour has had successful local treatment, ureteric hold-up may still be seen at follow-up IVUs. The natural suspicion is that there is ureteric involvement by growth, but the answer may be much less serious: minor ureteric stasis can be a simple complication of surgery near the ureteric orifice (see Fig. IV.2.B10). However, the task of follow-up IVUs is certainly to keep a check on the upper urinary tracts. The question of new upper urothelial tumours arising in the natural history of the disease has already been mentioned in Division 1 section D above. The desirable frequency of follow-up examinations is not known. Upper urothelial tumours following bladder cancer are not a frequent problem, but often very troublesome once they occur. Local resection can then be followed by recurrence or new tumour elsewhere (Fig. IV.3.D5).

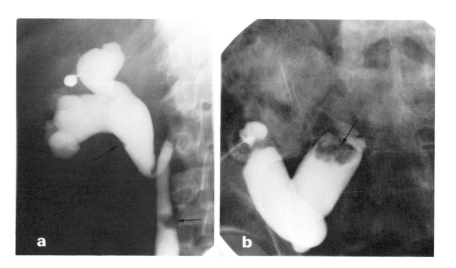

Fig. IV.3.D5a This patient has already had a total cystectomy for his bladder cancer. A follow-up right antegrade pyelogram shows multiple new tumours in the upper urinary tract (arrows).

Fig. IV.3.D5b One year after right nephro-ureterectomy, further new tumour has grown into the ileal loop from the lower left ureter (arrow).

Summary comment. The radiologist competing with the urologist in the diagnosis of bladder carcinoma is wasting his time and effort. By contrast, monitoring the state of the upper urinary tracts is a particular radiological responsibility. Staging the tumour is usually done by palpation and biopsy, and can be unreliable. CT probably has an important part to play here.

Acute cystitis

Pain, frequency and haematuria are pointers to a condition not obviously in the radiologist's court. Although acute cystitis is not a good indication for radiological studies, it is as well to be familiar with its X-ray characteristics. The bladder wall can be very markedly thickened and irregular. At worst, this may lead to ureteric hold-up. This is seen at its most florid in young men as a venereal infection of unknown cause (Fig. IV.3.D6). The picture could be mistaken for tuberculous cystitis, but resolves quickly on standard antibiotic treatment.

Fig. IV.3.D6 *(facing page)* Acute cystitis as a venereal infection in a young man—note the deformed bladder wall, and stasis in the right upper urinary tract. See also Fig. IV.3.B5.

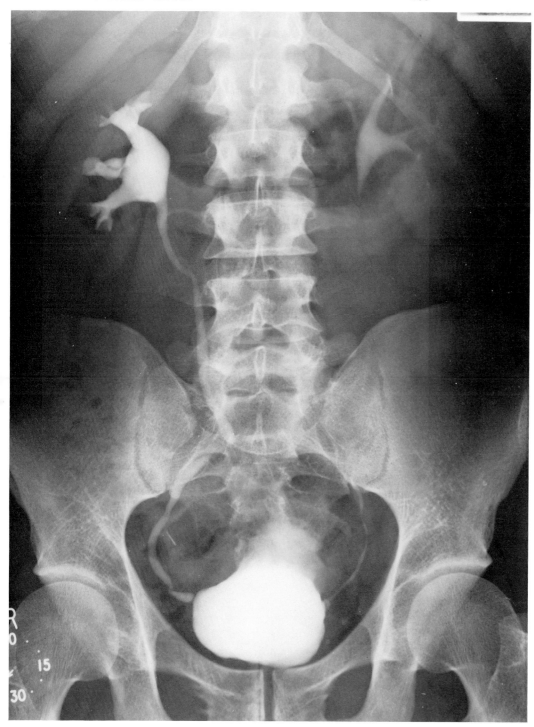

Recurrent urinary infections in adults, particularly women, are of course a different story. There is very little useful place for radiological investigations here. If there are leading symptoms such as consistently unilateral loin pain, an IVU may be helpful in disclosing a hydronephrosis or renal stone. If recurrent cystitis is the clinical diagnosis, the routine IVU is a waste of resources and an unnecessary radiation burden on the patient. In short: to be avoided.

A vicious, rare form of acute cystitis can be induced by cyclophosphamide. Haematuria may be of life-threatening severity here. Cyclophosphamide can also lead on to a chronic cystitis with severe bladder wall thickening and rigidity, inducing ureteric reflux (see Division 4 section E).

Chronic cystitis

Tuberculous bladder involvement leads to a small contracted bladder, already illustrated in Division 1 section G (Fig. IV.1.G15). It will be accompanied by renal and perhaps ureteric lesions.

There is a chronic, intractable state of uncertain aetiology under the name of chronic interstitial cystitis. It was first described in women by Hunner, and is therefore also called Hunner's ulcer. Symptoms can be very disabling, particularly if the patient ends up with a small contracted bladder. A urinary diversion may then be considered. The condition is also seen in men, always accompanied by very proper anxiety whether a bladder carcinoma is not being missed.

Bladder stone

This condition may present with haematuria rather than obstruction symptoms, but is considered in section A p. 268. It is much more common in men than women.

Bilharzia

This is a topic of huge importance in the Middle East, Africa and South

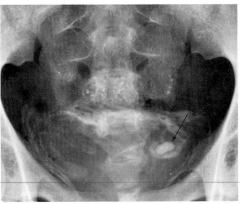

Fig. IV.3.D7 Bladder calcification in bilharzia. The arrow points to a stone in the left lower ureter. (Courtesy of Dr A. A. Salem).

America, the cause of widespread chronic ill health. The best known X-ray sign is calcification in the bladder wall (Fig. IV.3.D7). This does not make the bladder a rigid organ, and so the calcification ring will change shape depending on the state of bladder filling.

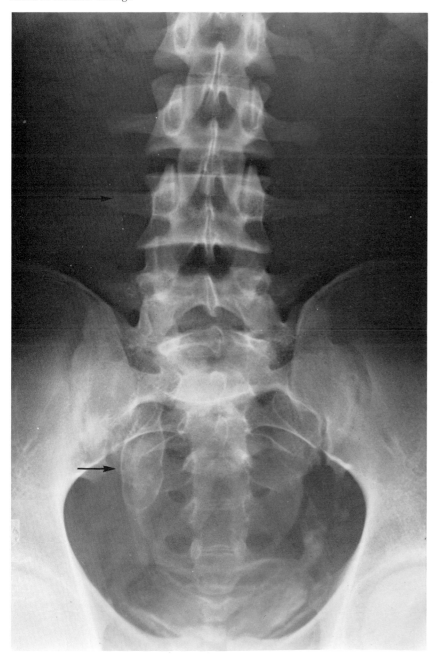

Fig. IV.3.D8 Bilharzia—calcification in bladder and ureters (arrows). (Courtesy of Dr A. A. Salem).

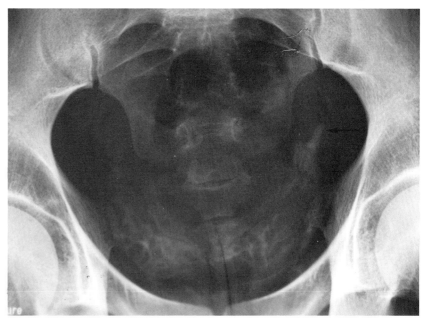

Fig. IV.3.D9 Bilharzia has caused calcification of the seminal vesicles as well as the bladder here. The arrow points to a stone in the left lower ureter. (Courtesy of Dr A. A. Salem).

Other parts of the urinary and genital tracts are attacked by bilharzia. The lower ureters are frequently involved, so that granulomas will be seen as filling defects here as well as in the bladder. Later there will be ureteric strictures, perhaps with associated calcification (Fig. IV.3.D8). The seminal vesicles are another site of calcification, so that a florid genito-urogram may be seen on the plain film (Fig. IV.3.D9). The best memorandum for making the diagnosis is simply to be aware of the condition in its many forms. Any bladder or ureteric lesion or unexplained hydronephrosis in anyone from the bilharzia belt falls under suspicion. It is important to have these suspicions early on in the disease when treatment offers a chance of reversing ill effects. There is no diagnostic difficulty, only clinical despair, by the time gross X-ray calcification signs are apparent to everyone (Fig. IV.3.D10).

Urethral carcinoma and warts

Urethrography is helpful in pinpointing these lesions. A urethral carcinoma is seen as a single irregular filling defect (Fig. IV.3.D11). Venereal warts (condyloma acuminata) may invade the urethra, with a characteristic picture of multiple filling defects (Fig. IV.3.D12).

Fig. IV.3.D10 *(facing page)* Bilharzia with bladder and ureteric calcification. The ureteric stricture has resulted in a huge staghorn calculus of the right kidney. (Courtesy of Dr A. A. Salem).

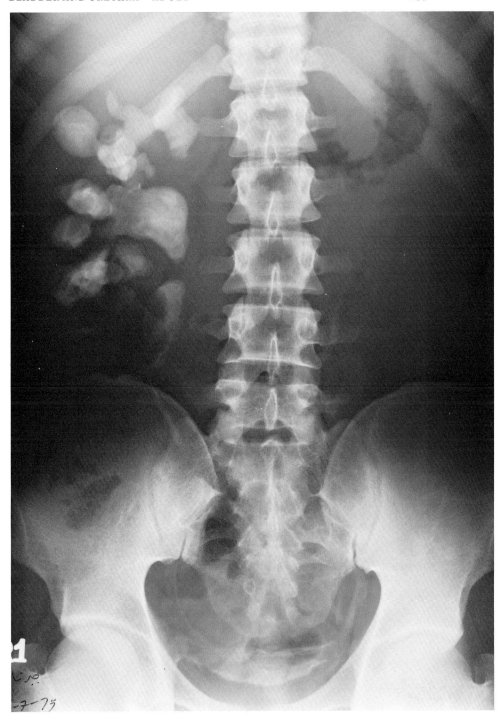

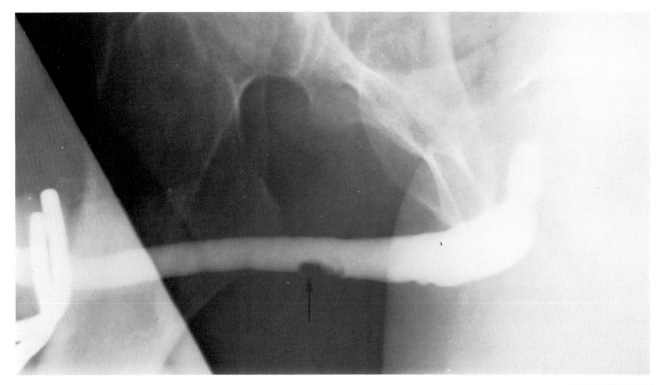

Fig. IV.3.D11 Urethral carcinoma.
(Courtesy of Dr R. Eban).

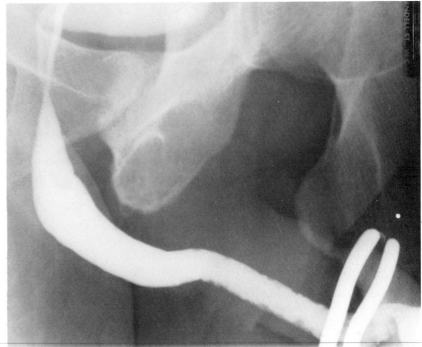

Fig. IV.3.D12 There are multiple
irregular filling defects in the anterior
urethra on this urethrogram—venereal
warts.

E. ODD BLADER SHAPES

The bladder may obviously be deformed by masses arising near it, for instance in the pelvic bone (Fig. IV.3.E1). It can be involved in hernias (Fig. IV.3.E2). Several more symmetric oddities of bladder shape are discussed below. There is no common pathological thread connecting them. They are grouped together here because they present as a radiological problem on the IVU.

1. Pelvic lipomatosis

This is an interesting condition where fat is laid down within the bony pelvis as a tightly packed mass, surrounding the bladder and recto/sigmoid colon (Moss *et al*, 1972). It is not an invasive disease in the sense of malignancy, but can become troublesome because of obstructive effects, on the ureters in particular. Its aetiology is not understood.

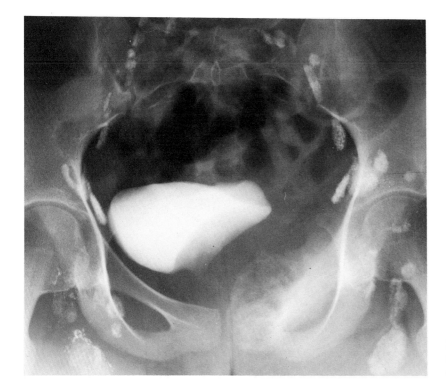

Fig. IV.3.E1 A child with a Ewing's tumour—note how the bone lesion has deformed the bladder.

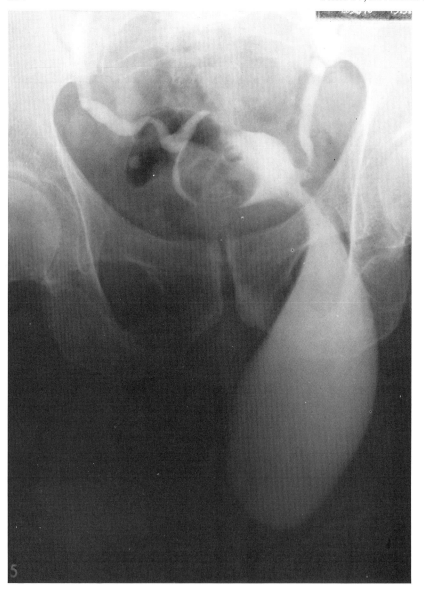

Fig. IV.3.E2 Bladder in inguinal hernia.

The IVU findings are characteristic. On good plain films the radiolucent nature of the fat may give a clue, with too much 'black' in the pelvis. The contrast films show a bladder squashed from side to side (Fig. IV.3.E3). The most helpful supporting evidence is a brief barium enema. The rectum and sigmoid

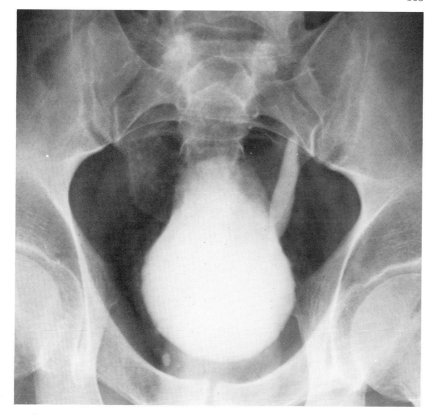

Fig. IV.3.E3 Pelvic lipomatosis—note how the bladder is squashed by the fat.

will be seen similarly affected, rising straight up out of the pelvis, displaced by the fat (Fig. IV.3.E4).

In most patients pelvic lipomatosis will be an unimportant chance finding, though bladder symptoms like frequency are sometimes put down to it. Occasionally more severe problems arise (Fig. IV.3.E5) (Pepper *et al*, 1971).

2. Lymph nodes

Involvement of iliac nodes by lymphoma can cause a symmetrical deformity of the bladder (Fig. IV.3.E6). Extensive carcinoma deposits are occasionally seen with a similar picture (see Fig. IV.3.A1).

3. Inferior vena cava obstruction

The squashed bladder is an interesting feature of this disorder (Fig. IV.3.E7). The natural explanation is that venous collaterals in the pelvis are responsible, but this evidence about the internal iliac system is not easy to come by.

Fig. IV.3.E4 (*overleaf—left*) Barium enema in the same patient as Fig. IV.3.E3—the sigmoid is displaced out of the pelvis by the fat.

Fig. IV.3.E5 (*overleaf—right*) Pelvic lipomatosis—bladder distortion is so severe that both upper urinary tracts have become obstructed at the lower ureters, much worse on the left.

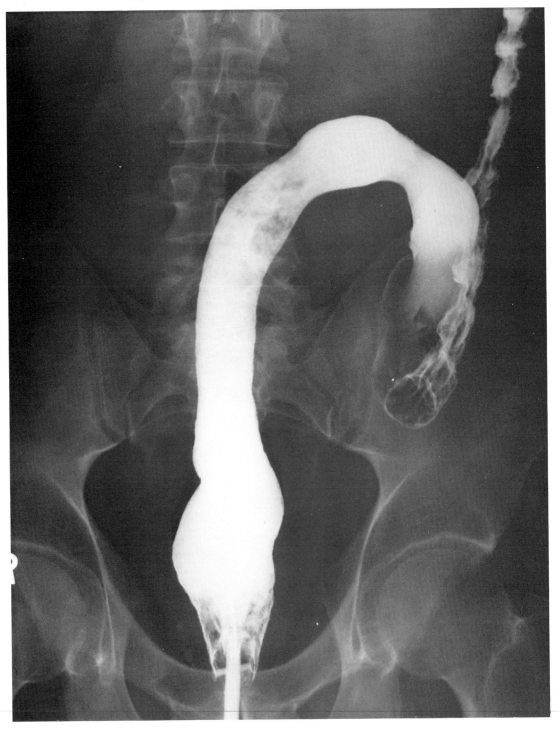

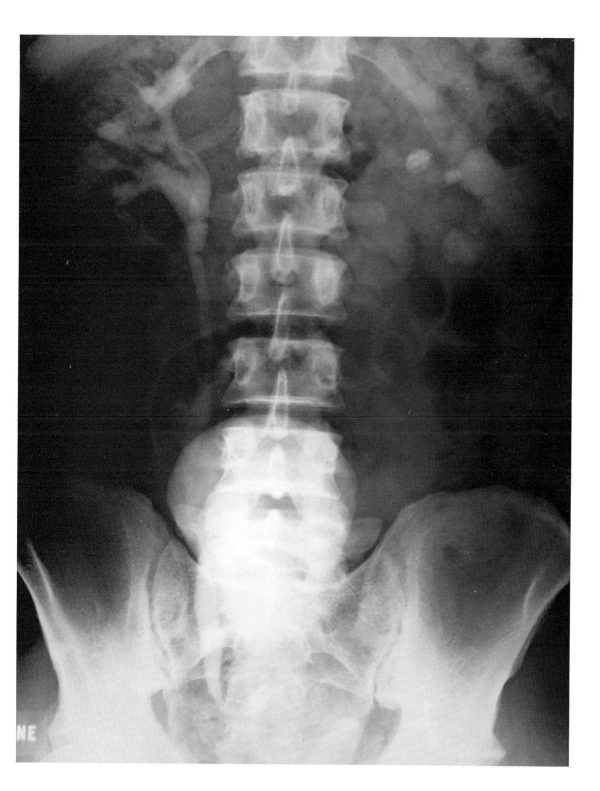

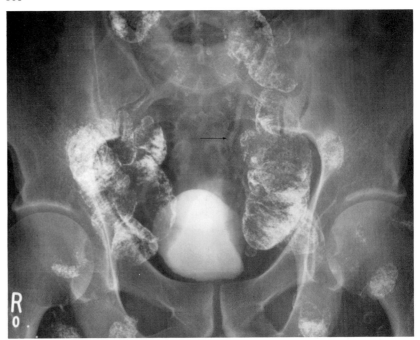

Fig. IV.3.E6 Lymphogram and IVU—
note bladder deformity and medial ureteric
displacement (arrow) because of enlarged
nodes in lymphoma.

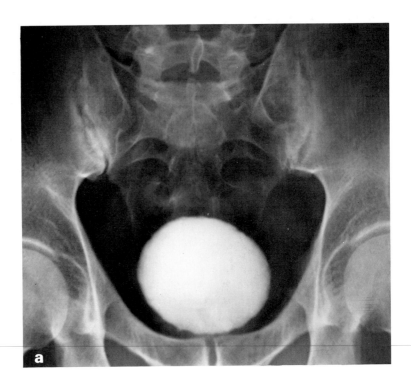

Fig. IV.3.E7a Normal bladder shape.

4. Neurofibromatosis

Mounds of neurofibromas may deform the bladder very considerably (Fig. IV.3.E8). This is a rare complication of the disease.

5. Trauma

Compression of the bladder into a pear shape by an extraperitoneal haematoma is considered in the next section.

F. TRAUMA

The victim falling off his horse, or astride a manhole cover, is a 19th century story: traffic accidents are now the commonest cause of injury to the bladder and urethra. In the Third World obstetric disasters (obstructed labour) remain an important topic.

Renal injuries have already been considered in Division 1 section J above. Lower urinary tract injuries may be in addition to such hurt, or seen on their own. Bleeding from the urethra is an obvious clinical pointer to such an injury. Fracture of the pelvis is the most helpful radiological sign, and should always raise the suspicion of lower urinary tract complications. Indeed, injury to the bladder or urethra in traffic accidents is uncommon in the absence of pelvic fracture.

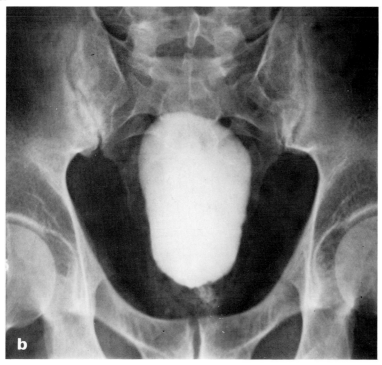

Fig. IV.3.E7b Two months later the bladder is squashed from side to side in this patient.

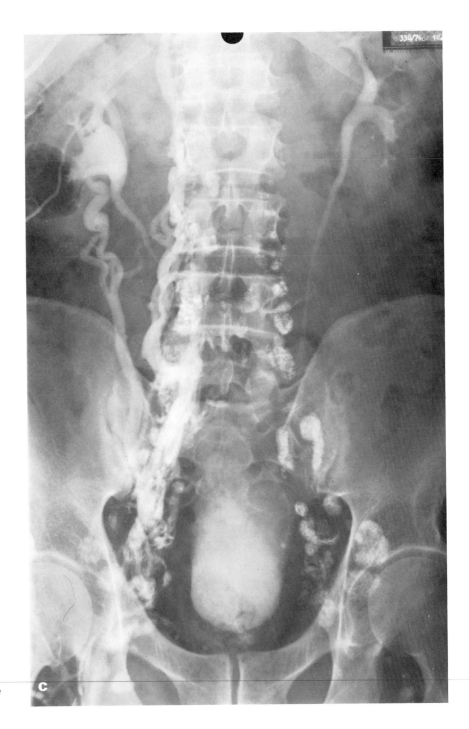

Fig. IV.3.E7c The cause is an obstructed vena cava—this venogram superimposed on a lymphogram shows the obstruction with collateral circulation.

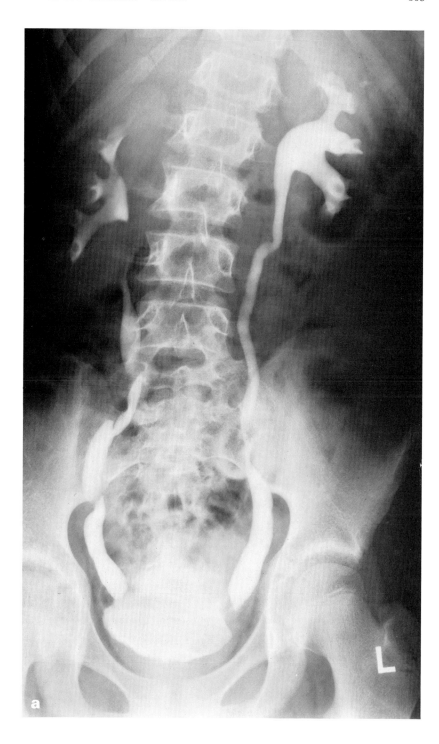

Fig. IV.3.E8a Neurofibromatosis involving the bladder—note bilateral ureteric hold up.

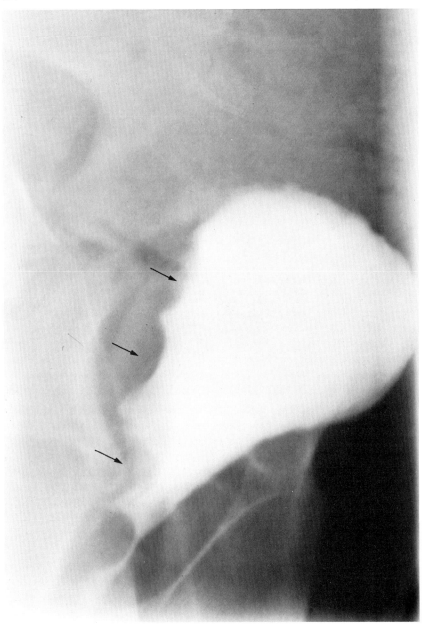

Fig. IV.3.E8b Arrows point to the
neurofibromas in the bladder wall on this
oblique projection.

As already emphasized in Division 1 section J, the IVU is an essential
investigation in trauma complicated by haematuria. It is also a good initial
examination for the lower urinary tract victim, so that the upper urinary tracts
can be assessed and the bladder seen. Occasionally the suspicion of lower
urinary tract injury is first raised by the IVU done very early on: the bladder is

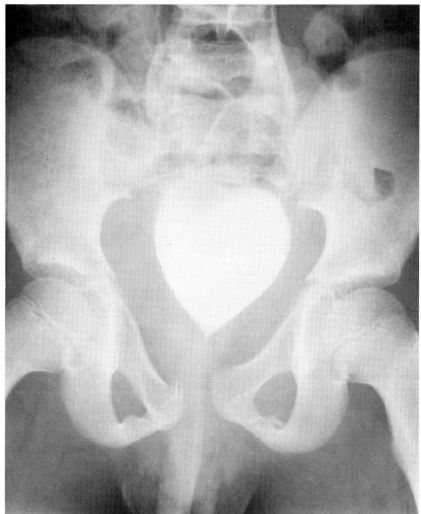

Fig. IV.3.F1 Pelvic fracture and perivesical haematoma—this boy has just been the victim of a road traffic accident. Note how his bladder is deformed and elevated.

deformed, or cannot be emptied. It may be found elevated with urethral rupture, or squashed by an extraperitoneal haematoma (Fig. IV.3.F1).

The next step is debatable. Conservative opinion would press for suprapubic drainage of the bladder, with later investigation at leisure of the precise site and extent of the injury. The school aiming at immediate specific diagnosis and management is gaining ground. These more active endeavours should not begin with attempts at catheterization, which may further damage the urethra. A retrograde urethrogram is done, using simple urographic contrast medium. The contrast jelly which is so useful for standard urethrograms is to be avoided—it contains various other substances which may set up an inflammatory reaction if they reach the tissues through a breach in the mucosa.

Once the extent of urethral damage has been gauged in this way, the decision can be taken whether it is safe to pass a catheter into the bladder for cystography.

Stricture formation and incontinence are the important late complications of urethral injury. Severe strictures will usually require surgery (Fig. IV.3.F2).

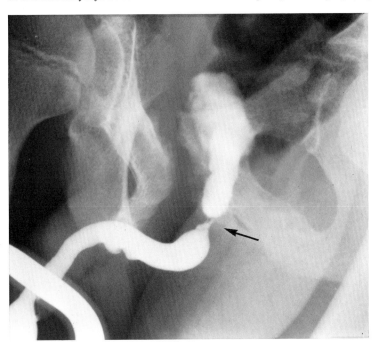

Fig. IV.3.F2 The same patient as in Fig. IV.3.F1, 5 months later. A urethrogram now shows his severe stricture at pelvic floor level (arrow).

REFERENCES

BARBARIC Z.L. (1976) Autonomic dysreflexia in patients with spinal cord lesions. *American Journal of Roentgenology* **127,** 293–295.

BRETLAND P.M. (1973) A device and technique for urethrography in the female. *British Journal of Radiology* **46,** 311–313.

HARRISON N.W., PARKS C. & SHERWOOD T. (1976) Ultrasound assessment of residual urine in children. *British Journal of Urology* **47,** 805–814.

MOSS A.A., CLARK R.E., GOLDBERG H.I. & PEPPER H.W. (1972) Pelvic lipomatosis. *American Journal of Roentgenology* **115,** 411–419.

PEPPER H.W., CLEMETT A.R. & DREW J.E. (1971) Pelvic lipomatosis causing urinary obstruction. *British Journal of Radiology* **44,** 313–315.

SHARR M.M., GARFIELD J.S. & JENKINS J.D. (1976) Lumbar spondylosis and neuropathic bladder. *British Medical Journal* **1,** 695–697.

SIMPSON W., DUNCAN A.W. & CLAYTON C.B. (1974) A useful sign in the diagnosis of bladder tumours on intravenous urograms. *British Journal of Radiology* **47,** 272–276.

TURNER WARWICK R.T. *et al* (1973a) A urodynamic view of prostatic obstruction and the results of prostatectomy. *British Journal of Urology* **45,** 631–645.

TURNER WARWICK R.T., WHITESIDE C.G., WORTH P.H.L., MILROY E.J.G. & BATES C.P. (1973b) A urodynamic view of the clinical problems associated with bladder neck dysfunction and its treatment by endoscopic incision and transtrigonal posterior prostatectomy. *British Journal of Urology* **45,** 44–59.

DIVISION 4. THE BLADDER AND URETHRA—CHILD

In the young child urinary tract infection often presents with unexplained fever, vomiting or failure to thrive. Pain, dysuria and frequency are highly specific adult symptoms—anyone waiting for them in early childhood will miss many urinary infections.

A. INCONTINENCE/INFECTION

Reflux and obstruction are the great mechanical themes running through childhood urinary infection. However, incontinence may appear as a complication. The establishment of urinary continence is a delicate process of physical maturation and of learning, and readily upset by an insult such as infection. Enuresis is the presenting symptom in 15% of children with urine infection, and their primary need is to have this diagnosed and set right (Meadow, 1976). Conversely incontinence may be the result of a urinary tract anomaly, e.g. ectopic ureter, which will itself be liable to infection. The double title of this section therefore emphasizes that this is a mixed topic.

The bedwetter

Children wetting their beds present a challenging but tractable problem to the paediatrician. Most children become dry at night during their third year, but there is a (normal) minority who do not achieve this accomplishment till later. A good history and physical examination are necessary for establishing a likely diagnosis and a plan of management. History and examination, not X-rays, are also the vital moves for excluding the structural causes that concern the radiologist.

The great majority of bedwetters do not need radiological studies. The paediatrician's concern is to pick out those few who do. Important pointers are:

1. History. If the child has even a few dry nights or days, the basic mechanism for continence appears intact. He/she is to be contrasted with the child who is always wet or just damp, day and night. This is highly suspicious of a structural abnormality, e.g. an ectopic ureter or neuropathic bladder.

2. Physical examination. This must include careful, informed examination of the genitalia (e.g. for epispadias) and of the back (e.g. for dimples etc. pointing to dysraphism).

3. Urine examination—obligatory in order to rule out infection.

If there are pointers to structural disease, the IVU is generally the most rewarding next investigation. Plain films of the spine are sometimes advocated

313

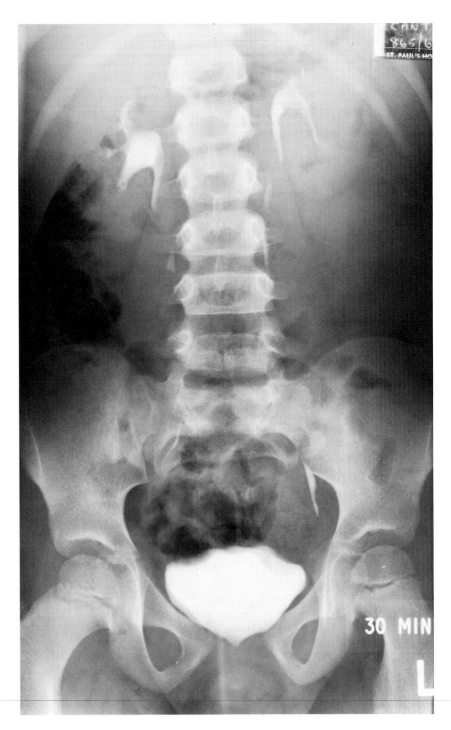

Fig. IV.4.A1 Epispadias—note the
widened symphysis but intact bladder.

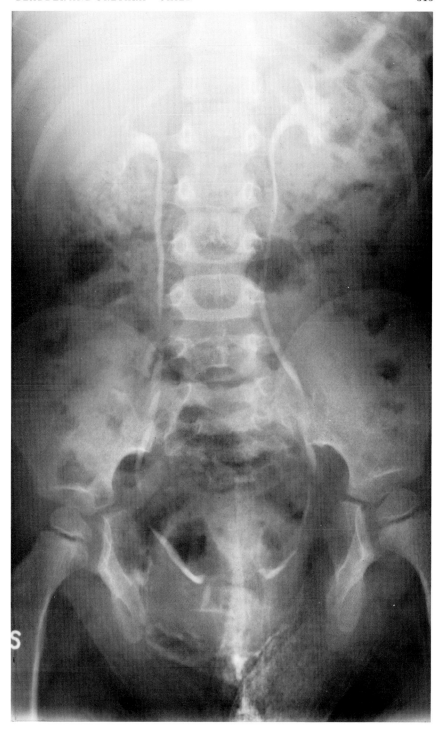

Fig. IV.4.A2 Exstrophy—widely separated symphysis, and bladder open on to the anterior abdominal wall.

first, but are really of no help on their own: if there is good reason for suspecting a neuropathic disorder, an IVU will be needed in any event. If there is not, radiological studies should not have been requested in the first place.

Epispadias/exstrophy

There is a range of disorders on the theme of a wide pubic symphysis and ventral defect of the lower urinary tract. The mildest of these is the 'pubic umbilicus', accompanied only by an open pelvic bony ring (Williams, 1974). It is worth noting that the normal range of pubic symphysis separation in children is 4–9 mm, so that a measurement above 1 cm is abnormal (Stannard & Lebowitz, 1978). *Epispadias* is a more severe disorder. It is a diagnosis to be made on clinical examination of the genitalia. In girls the inexpert may overlook the tell-tale bifid clitoris. The bladder is intact, and the IVU will therefore show the widened symphysis as the only abnormality (Fig. IV.4.A1). Girls with epispadias usually suffer from incontinence. In boys this is not invariable, and about a third may achieve continence (Williams, 1974).
Exstrophy. This term is much better than ectopia, since the bladder is turned inside out, not in the wrong place. The bladder presents on the anterior abdominal wall through a wide defect. There may be associated rectal prolapse and an umbilical hernia. The IVU is a key investigation to show the state of the upper urinary tracts, and the size of the bladder (Fig. IV.4.A2). The chances of reconstruction are very much influenced by the size assessment, and are small if the bladder is small. Complete reconstruction of the bony as well as the urinary and muscular abnormalities is sometimes attempted.

Ectopic ureter (see also Division 2 section A)

The ectopic ureter can drain within or without the urinary tract. *Within* the tract the opening may be at the bladder neck or into the urethra. If above the external sphincter, reflux may occur on voiding (Fig. IV.4.A3). A urethral opening is very likely to lead to incontinence in girls (Fig. IV.4.A4). This is not so in boys where the external sphincter is usually able to cope with the incontinence threat. With an opening *outside* the tract, the seminal vesicle may be involved in boys (see Fig. IV.2.A2). In girls the vagina is the likely site, and it is this which gives rise to most incontinence problems under this heading.

The great majority of ectopic ureters in girls are part of a duplication anomaly, and derive then from the upper renal moiety. The key to the diagnosis in a girl who is always damp, day and night, therefore lies in the upper urinary tracts. Such a child needs a first class IVU, not cystography.

The diagnosis on the IVU can sometimes be difficult, but the simple ground rules discussed in Division 2 section A generally make the diagnostic hunt straightforward and rewarding. It is important to give enough contrast medium, and to take delayed films if in doubt. A number of children still grow up with

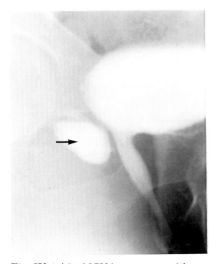

Fig. IV.4.A3 MCU in a woman with a long story of urinary infections and occasional dampness—note reflux into a cavity behind the urethra (arrow). This is the lower end of an ectopic ureter draining into the urethra.

unnecessarily wet pants where the diagnosis has been suspected, but missed because these rules have not been followed (Fig. IV.4.A5). The upper renal moiety giving rise to the ectopic ureter is always deformed. It may be rather

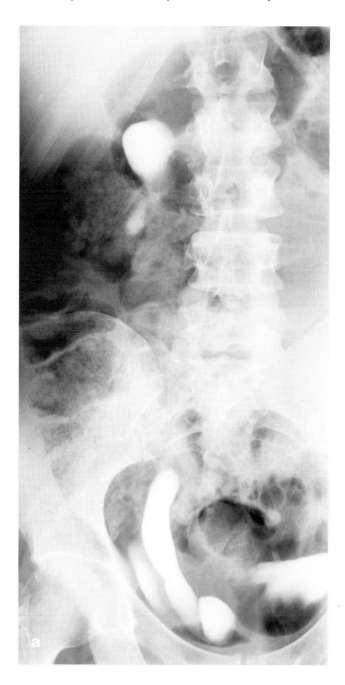

Fig. IV.4.A4a Same patient as Fig. IV.4.A3—the ectopic ureter has been filled by a retrograde study. Note distended upper renal moiety.

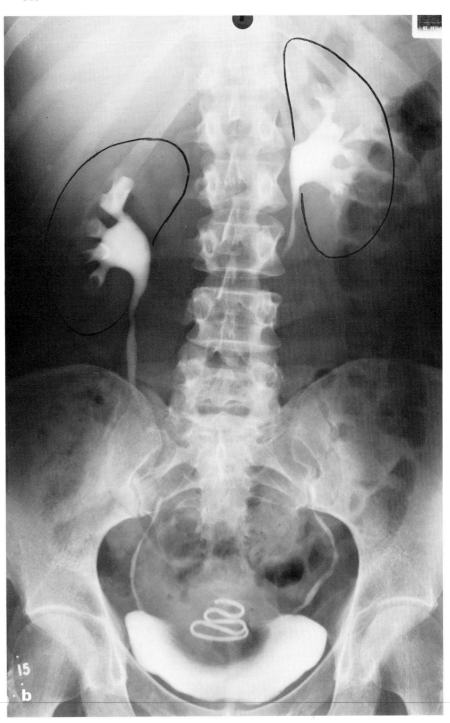

Fig. IV.4.A4b The renal outlines have been drawn in on this patient's IVU in order to highlight the non-excreting upper moiety of the right duplex kidney.

small. A sharp look-out is therefore to be kept on the nephrogram for any asymmetric depth of renal parenchyma not accounted for by neighbouring draining calices. Once the deformed pyelogram of the upper moiety is seen, the diagnosis is complete. Occasionally it will have to be inferred from the characteristic picture of the lower moiety alone. There is no point in searching for the precise entry of the ureter into the vagina: a thankless, usually unsuccessful task which will not alter management (heminephrectomy and ureterectomy).

It is a pity that the diagnosis of a readily treatable condition associated with much misery is sometimes not made till adult life (see Fig. IV.3.C2). The radiologist needs to be anxious on this score.

Summary comments

1. The ectopic ureter has an abnormal renal moiety above it: if a normal pyelogram is seen throughout a duplex kidney, the anomaly will *not* be on this side (Fig. IV.4.A6).

2. Bilateral ectopic ureters can occur with bilateral duplex kidneys.

3. Do not diagnose ectopic ureters on the strength of an unusual course of the lower ureter alone—you will probably be wrong (Fig. IV.4.A7).

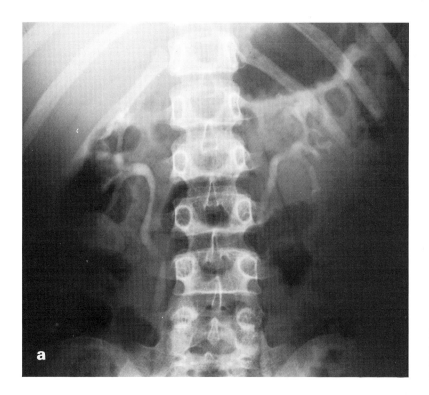

Fig. IV.4.A5a This girl has always been damp, and was thought to have a normal IVU. This is a fair example of several examinations.

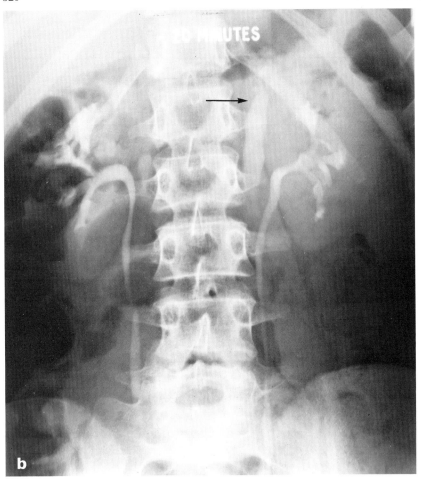

Fig. IV.4.A5b Three years later she has
an IVU with an adequate contrast
medium dose and a 20 min film. The
mis-shapen upper moiety of her left
kidney is now obvious (arrow). Ectopic
drainage into the vagina was the cause of
her symptoms, cured by
hemi-nephrectomy.

Wide bladder neck

This is a debatable entity (Williams, 1974). It is to be differentiated from a
well-defined but rare syndrome of the absent bladder neck, already mentioned in
Division 2 section A. This is better called bilateral single ectopic ureters, the
names emphasizing that the bladder neck will not develop normally when *both*
ureteric insertions are anomalous.

An open, wide bladder neck is occasionally seen at cystography and cystoscopy in young girls who present with stress incontinence. There are no abnormalities on dynamic studies, particularly no neuropathy and no obstruction.
The suspicion is naturally that a unilateral single ectopic ureter is responsible,
but this association is inconstant. It is particularly important not to confuse
these uncommon abnormalities with the widely open bladder neck often seen
during cystography in girls as the 'spinning top urethra'. This is a common

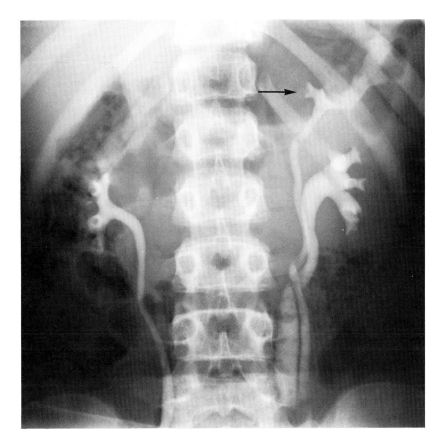

Fig. IV.4.A6 This girl also has a classical history pointing to an ectopic ureter. Although she has a duplex left kidney, it is clear that the perfectly made upper moiety on this side (arrow) cannot lead to an ectopic ureter. The presumed ectopic ureter must derive from a non-excreting upper moiety of the *right* kidney, not seen on this film (operative proof).

finding in girls voiding or about to void under the odd circumstances of this examination, and requires no action beyond recognizing it as normal.

Giggle incontinence

This interesting complaint of young girls has no radiological features, in particular no bladder instability. It disappears as the girl grows out of adolescence.

Vaginal reflux

Most female infants, examined in the horizontal position, reflux urine into the vagina during voiding cystography. It is important not to misdiagnose this

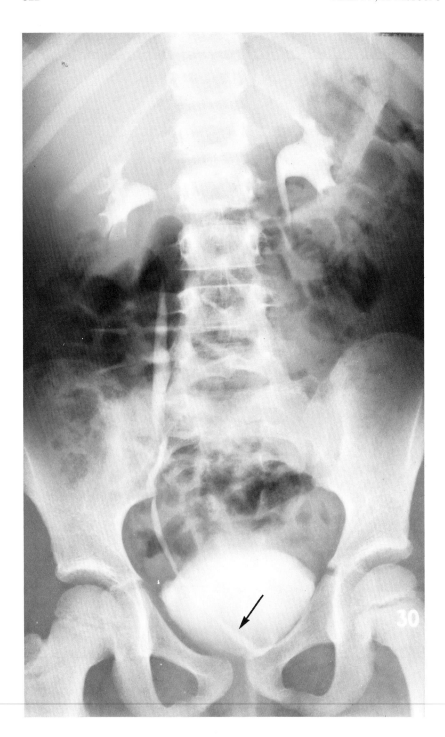

Fig. IV.4.A7   The arrow points to a splash of contrast medium just being propelled from a normally situated right ureteric orifice. This girl has normal kidneys, so she cannot have an ectopic ureter.

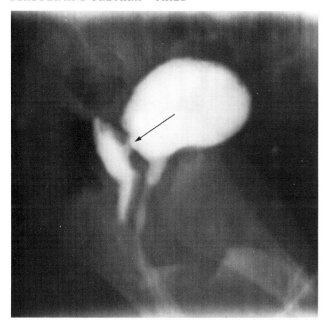

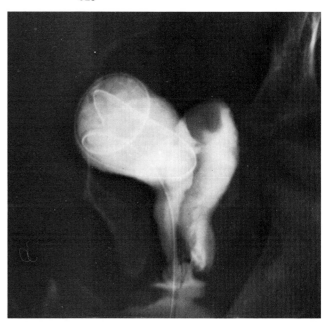

picture as a vesico-vaginal fistula (Fig. IV.4.A8). Older children may still experience vaginal reflux, even in the upright position. Rarely a troublesome puddle of urine may then be left after micturition, draining slowly and perhaps causing damp pants (Fig. IV.4.A9). The radiologist's main concern should be to recognize that this is a variant on the normal, not usually requiring action.

Fig. IV.4.A8 *(above left)* MCU in an infant girl—the vagina, situated behind the bladder, has filled by reflux. The arrow points to a vaginal fornix, *not* a fistula.

Fig. IV.4.A9 *(above right)* MCU in a girl complaining of dampness for some time after voiding. A coiled catheter is lying in the bladder whilst she is voiding, with reflux into the vagina. Slow dribbling from the vaginal collection later on is the cause of her complaint.

Neuropathic bladder

This is an important topic in childhood incontinence, but the essential features are similar to the adult problem (Fig. IV.4.A10). The reader is therefore referred to Division 3 section C above. Specific points to be made in childhood are:

1. Spina bifida occulta as a bony malfusion abnormality on its own is a frequent finding in children who are perfectly continent. It does not need further investigation. Widening of the spinal canal, vertebral deformity, or diastematomyelia are more helpful pointers to dysraphism. They will usually require myelography for complete diagnosis. Careful clinical examination of the back is of course essential in all children presenting with incontinence.

2. The absent sacrum as a cause of the neuropathic bladder usually presents in childhood, and is easy to miss (see Fig. IV.3.C6). *Rule-of-thumb.* If a child is having a cystogram for unexplained incontinence suspected to be neuropathic, the lateral film (or fluoroscopy) is a helpful prop for the radiologist.

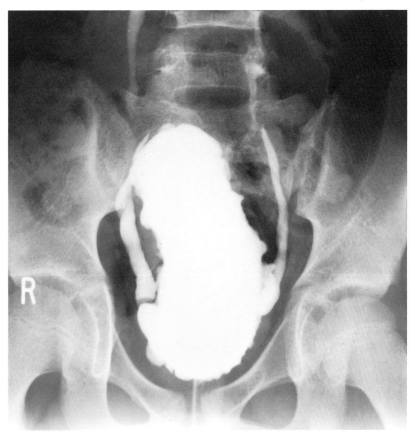

Fig. IV.4.A10 This boy's IVU might suggest a neuropathic bladder, with ureteric holdup, abnormal bladder shape and trabeculation. However, he has bladder outflow obstruction, emphasizing that this picture is *not* pathognomonic of neuropathy (see also Fig. IV.3.C4).

3. Occult neuropathic bladder. In a few children no abnormal neurological signs are found, but the bladder looks abnormal on cystography, and behaves abnormally on dynamic studies. It may then have to be given this rather unsatisfactory label, and treated expectantly as a neuropathic problem. As usual, a careful watch will have to be kept on the upper urinary tracts.

B. INFECTION/OBSTRUCTION

Interpreting the adult voiding cystogram is often more difficult than performing it. In the child these difficulties are reversed: the voiding cystogram may be a trial for patient and doctor, but it is a highly rewarding examination of vesical and urethral behaviour. The reason is of course that the questions asked are quite different. In children we want to know about vesico-ureteric reflux, major bladder disarrays (e.g. diverticula), and about urethral obstruction. In boys who have presented with a urinary infection, obstruction must always be excluded.

Indications for voiding cystography (see also Division 2 section C)

1. Children with a proven urinary tract infection should have an IVU. If this is abnormal, an MCU must also be done. Girls with a normal IVU after their first infection probably need no further investigation, given careful clinical follow-up. As explained in Division 2 section C, some refluxers will be missed. Boys should either be screened during voiding at the end of the IVU, or have a formal MCU if there is any doubt about possible obstruction.

2. Recurrent urinary tract infections.

3. Renal failure: the MCU is often the key investigation when infants present with renal failure, especially if the bladder is palpable. In distinction to adult practice, the MCU is then best done first, before an IVU.

Urethral valve

The singular for this lesion emphasizes that a single obstructing membrane is usually present, even though the origin is from a paired structure. In its usual form the valve is an exaggeration of the folds that normally run obliquely down to each side of the urethra from the verumontanum—the bifid lower end of the genital ridge.

Presentation

There is a wide range from the neonate in renal failure to the older child with an unexplained urinary infection. The diagnosis may even be delayed till adult life in mild cases (Fig. IV.4.B1). In the severely affected infant, the thick-walled bladder will usually be palpable. The IVU shows dilated upper urinary tracts (Fig. IV.4.B2).

Diagnosis

The MCU picture is characteristic, but good technique is essential (Fig. IV.4.B3). The important requirement is a good view of the urethra whilst the child is voiding, with no catheter in place at the time. If the examination is done via a urethral catheter, bladder filling is continued till the child begins to void past the catheter. This is then quickly withdrawn, and micturition carefully watched whilst the child is passing his best stream (Fig. IV.4.B4). It is important to catch this best stream picture: the posterior urethra above the obstructive valve will not distend during feeble micturition.

In making the diagnosis, the dynamic picture of obstruction reflected in the urethral calibre changes is more helpful than identifying the valve itself. There are a number of normal impressions on the urethra, and they can generally be discounted if there is no evidence of obstruction (Fig. IV.4.B5). Such impressions can be particularly deceptive if multiple—the 'corkscrew' urethra which

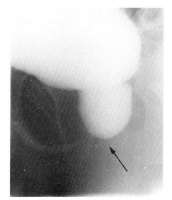

Fig. IV.4.B1 A young man with a urethral valve now discovered for the first time. Note the dilatation of the posterior urethra leading down to the valve (arrow).

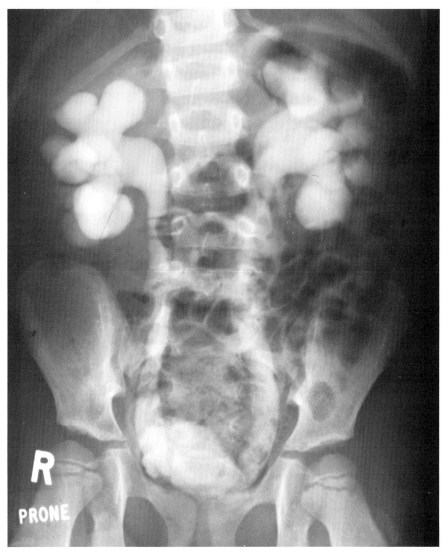

Fig. IV.4.B2 This boy has considerable dilatation of both upper urinary tracts, but note that the bladder is not distended, even though severely obstructed.

is a normal variant (Fig. IV.4.B6). The ascending urethrogram and MCU make up an instructive comparison in this condition, emphasizing the importance of functional interpretation of the MCU (Fig. IV.4.B7).

Sequelae of urethral valve

Unfortunately successful diagnosis and resection of the valve is not necessarily followed by a return to normal. Complication are:

1. Incontinence. Many boys, perhaps half (Whitaker *et al,* 1972), are left incontinent to some degree after surgery. The risk is greatest in those operated on earliest (i.e. neonatal presentation).

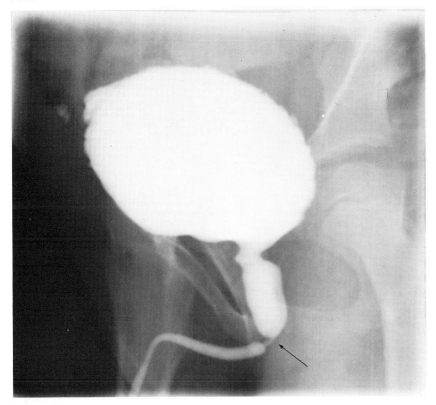

Fig. IV.4.B3 Same patient as Fig. IV.4.B2—the characteristic MCU of urethral valve. Note the distension of the obstructed posterior urethra down to the valve (arrow), situated at the lower end of the verumontanum.

Fig. IV.4.B4a This normal boy is voiding with the filling catheter in position during an MCU. It is not possible to assess the urethra under these conditions.
Fig. IV.4.B4b The bladder is filled again, and the catheter withdrawn as voiding begins. A normal urethra is now seen.

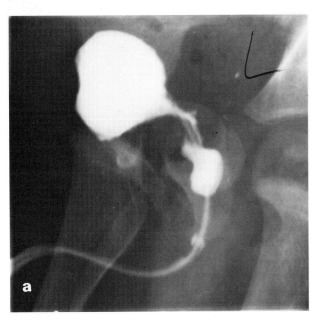

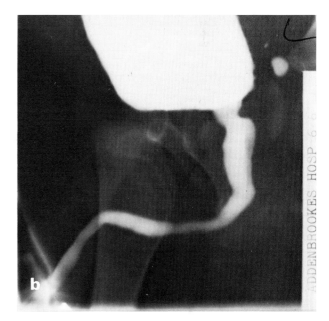

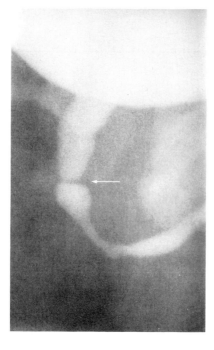

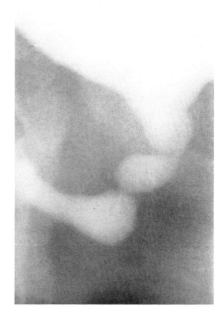

Fig. IV.4.B5 *(right)* Normal MCU—the arrow points to a transverse impression on the urethra which is of no functional importance, with no distension above.

Fig. IV.4.B6 *(far right)* 'Corkscrew urethra'—this looks rather odd, but is clearly of no functional moment in the presence of a good stream with no urethral distension.

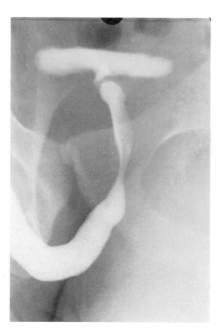

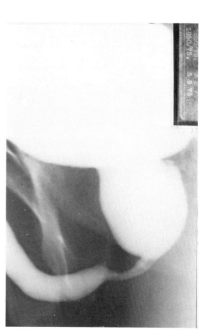

Fig. IV.4.B7 Retrograde urethrogram and antegrade voiding study in the same patient with an obstructed urethra—note that the ascending study gives no hint of the severe dynamic obstruction.

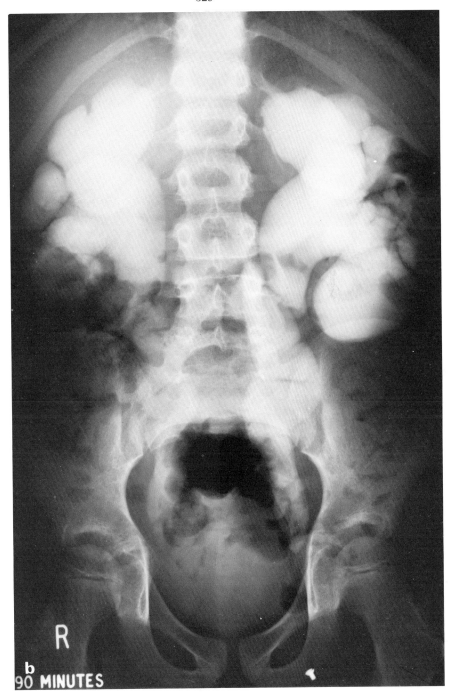

Fig. IV.4.B8a & b Same patient as in Fig. IV.4.B2 and IV.4.B3—his urethral valve has been successfully resected, and there is no residual urethral obstruction. However, 5 years later dilatation of his upper urinary tracts has advanced inexorably.

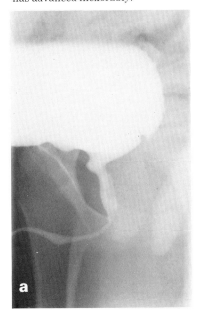

2. Thick-walled bladder. The changes of detrusor work hypertrophy induced by the obstructive valve do not regress when obstruction is relieved. They are sometimes important in the ureteric problems considered next.

3. Upper urinary tract dilatation. Calices and ureters may remain dilated following valve resection, or even deteriorate as the boy grows older (Fig. IV.4.B8). The suspicion then naturally arises that there is obstruction at the vesico-ureteric junction. The thickened bladder wall may be incriminated as the likely cause. However, pressure/flow studies are needed to resolve these very difficult problems (see Part I section D). The dilated upper urinary tract is not usually found obstructed in such studies. Abnormally high bladder pressure at rest may be discovered during the study. If not, the condition must be put down to ureteric failure. Because the wide ureter cannot appose its walls to propel a urine bolus effectively, surgery may still be indicated to narrow ('tailor') the faulty ureter. Surgical intervention is clearly much more pressing if obstruction has been diagnosed, demanding ureteric reimplantation.

4. Caliceal lacunae. These abnormal spaces are interesting remnants of severe caliceal distension, persisting into later life (Fig. IV.4.B9) (Ransley, 1976).

Misleading urethral pictures mimicking obstruction

1. Urinal. An anxious child or parent clutching the urinal used for voiding may press it hard into the perineum. Its neck then causes an extrinsic obstruction at the peno-scrotal junction, unseen on the X-ray because urinals are usually plastic (Fig. IV.4.B10). The radiologist should be quick to recognize this artefact.

Fig. IV.4.B9 *(below left)* The arrows point to caliceal lacunae, seen in a boy who has already had his urethral valve resected.

Fig. IV.4.B10 *(below centre)* MCU in a boy who might be thought to have a distal urethral obstruction, with dilatation of the proximal urethra. But this is simply pressure from a plastic urinal—the arrow points to the non-opaque neck of the urinal indenting the urethra during this study.

Fig. IV.4.B11 *(below right)* Late frame at the end of an MCU—this boy happens to blow out his foreskin like a balloon, but there is no obstruction.

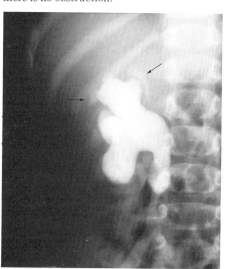

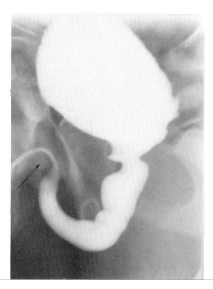

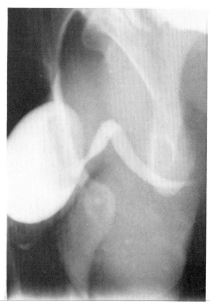

2. Foreskin balloon. In uncircumcized boys the foreskin may blow out as a small balloon during voiding (Fig. IV.4.B11). On its own this is an unremarkable finding, and does not spell a phimosis.

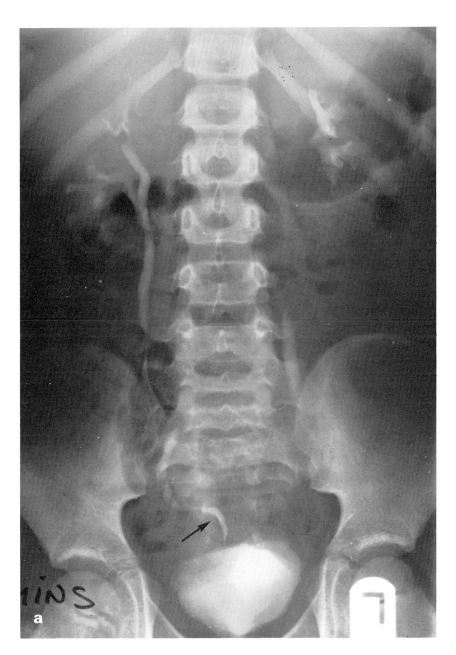

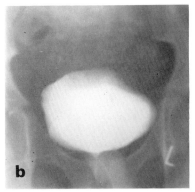

Fig. IV.4.B12a *(left)* Note the medial deviation of the lower right ureter (arrow) in this boy with urinary infections. See also Fig. IV.3.A16.

Fig. IV.4.B12b *(above)* The cause is a bladder diverticulum, but this is not apparent from the MCU during the filling stage.

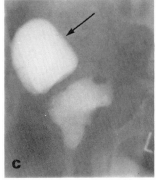

Fig. IV.4.B12c *(above)* It is only on voiding that the large right bladder diverticulum (arrow) is seen, and remains filled at the end of micturition.

Diverticula

1. Bladder diverticula. Bladder diverticula are usually congenital pouches in children, though they can be acquired in severe outflow obstruction (e.g. urethral valve). The congenital lesion may displace the ureter, and act as a reservoir of infection because of incomplete bladder emptying (Fig. IV.4.B12). It is worth surgical resection.

The small saccule often seen near the ureteric orifice when there is gross vesico-ureteric reflux is best regarded as a complication of the abnormal vesico-ureteric junction, not as a primary cause of reflux.

2. Congenital male urethral diverticula are of two main types:

A wide-mouthed shallow pouch, very easily missed on voiding or retrograde studies (Fig. IV.4.B13). The distal lip of such diverticula may float out across the urethra during voiding, forming an obstructive membrane. This is the common form of the misnamed 'anterior urethral valve'.

A narrow-necked bulbar pouch, presenting with infection, stone, or because of post-micturition dribbling (Fig. IV.4.B14).

3. Other male urethral pouches:

Traumatic (iatrogenic) diverticula are often anterior, arising after prolonged or repeated catheterization (Fig. IV.4.B15).

Prune belly urethra. The dilated posterior urethra characteristic of this condition may mimic a diverticulum, especially if there is also filling of the prostatic utricle (Fig. IV.4.B16). An obstruction is found on dynamic studies just below the dilatation, and bladder emptying can be improved by judicious endoscopic surgery here.

Male uterus is illustrated in Division 5 section D.

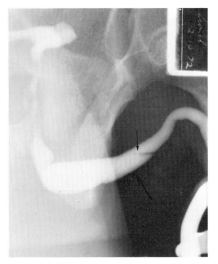

Fig. IV.4.B13 Retrograde urethrogram—the large arrow points to a shallow urethral diverticulum. Note how the distal lip lies free (small arrow) ready to act as an obstruction during voiding.

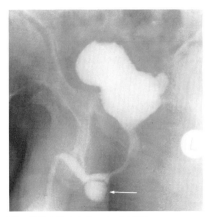

Fig. IV.4.B14 *(above)* MCU—an arrow points to a narrow-necked urethral diverticulum. A bladder diverticulum is also present.

Fig. IV.4.B15 *(right)* This boy has had prolonged catheter drainage of his bladder. An anterior urethral diverticulum (arrow) has developed as a complication.

Fig. IV.4.B16 *(far right)* MCU in a boy with the prune belly syndrome—note the apparent posterior urethral diverticulum.

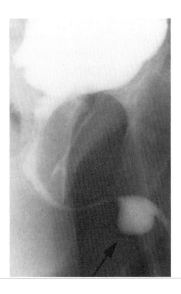

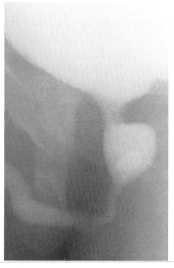

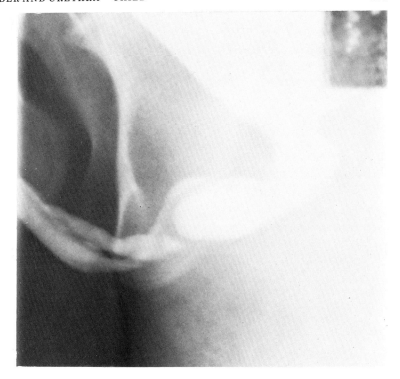

Fig. IV.4.B17 Double urethra—this MCU shows that one of the channels is obstructed.

Double urethra. Complete duplication is a rare anomaly (Fig. IV.4.B17). More frequently partial forms accompany hypospadias, with the small accessory duct lying distally and dorsally.

4. Congenital female urethral diverticula. These are uncommon childhood problems, raising the interesting question of whether they may be acquired when presenting in the adult. They are illustrated in Figs. IV.3.B3 and IV.3.B4.

C. DOUBLE MICTURITION

Severe vesico-ureteric reflux results in a large bolus of urine delivered upwards during voiding. The bladder will empty satisfactorily, only to refill almost at once from the ureteric reservoir. Double micturition can be encouraged to lessen this reservoir, and the radiological counterpart to these events can be seen during the voiding cystogram (Fig.IV.4.C1). Simple comparison of pre- and post-micturition films in such a child will falsely suggest a large vesical residue because of incomplete bladder emptying.

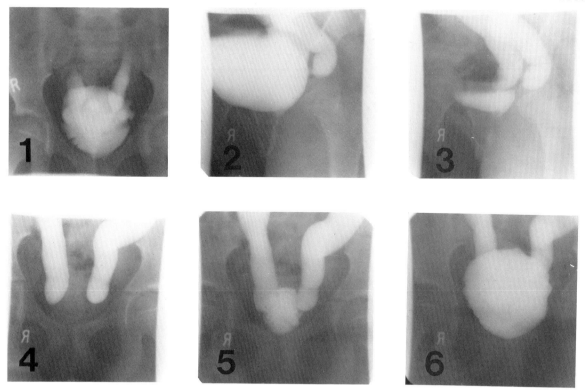

Fig. IV.4.C1 Voiding sequence in a girl with severe bilateral ureteric reflux. During micturition the ureteric reflux grows worse. Halfway through the sequence she comes to the end of voiding, and her bladder is then empty. As it relaxes it fills again at once from the distended ureters. The last view would be the 'post-micturition film' of her IVU, wholly misleading.

D. TRAUMA

Boys make up a large section of the victims of traffic accidents who suffer a fractured pelvis and urethral injury. The problems are unhappily similar to the adult ones considered in Division 3 section F above, with stricture formation and incontinence as frequent complications.

E. HAEMATURIA

Foreign bodies may be inserted up the urethra by children who then present with the respectable symptom of haematuria.

Acute cystitis is a rare cause of haematuria in this age group. Occasionally it may be induced by the drugs used to treat a sick child. The best known is *cyclophosphamide*. This can lead to a severe cystitis, with life threatening haematuria. The cystitis may advance to a chronic form, where gross bladder wall thickening and rigidity results, with much disability later, e.g. vesico-ureteric reflux (Fig. IV.4.E1).

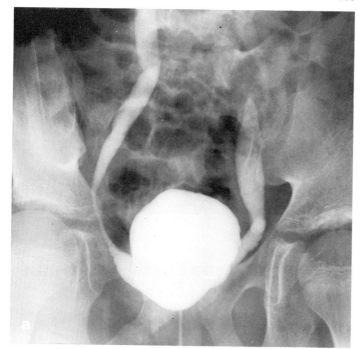

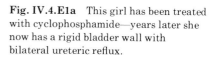

Fig. IV.4.E1a This girl has been treated with cyclophosphamide—years later she now has a rigid bladder wall with bilateral ureteric reflux.

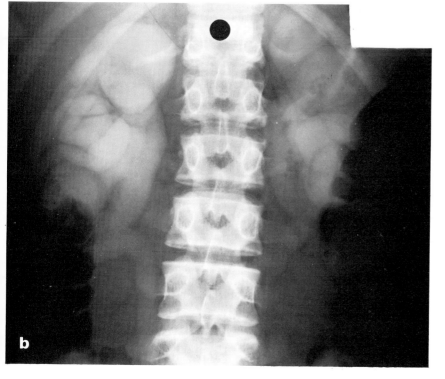

Fig. IV.4.E1b Four years later repeated attempts at ureteric reimplantation have failed because of the poor bladder wall, and she is in end-stage renal failure.

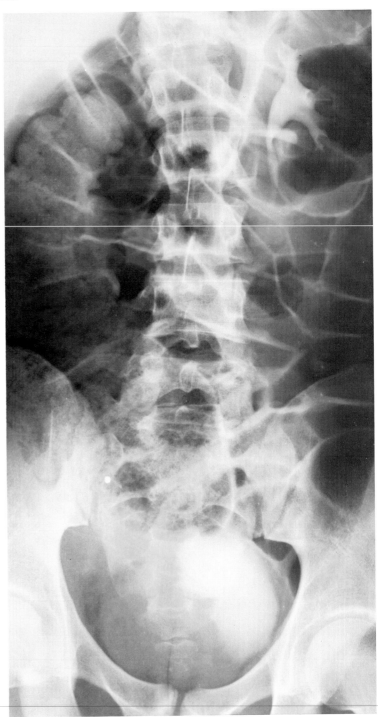

Fig. IV.4.E2 This boy with haematuria has a large bladder lesion obstructing his right kidney—it is a rhabdomyosarcoma.

Tumours

Rhabdomyosarcoma is the least uncommon of the rare childhood bladder tumours. It is sometimes known as sarcoma botryoides from its grape-like cluster. There is an obvious large filling defect, usually in a boy's bladder (Fig. IV.4.E2)—the prognosis is poor. Gross filling defects do not always spell bladder tumours in the child: cystitis (see Division 3 section D) and neurofibromatosis (see Division 3 section E) enter the differential diagnosis.

REFERENCES

MEADOW R. (1976) Disorders of micturition, abnormalities of urine, and urinary tract infection. *British Medical Journal* **1**, 1200–1202.

RANSLEY P.G. (1976) Opacification of the renal parenchyma in obstruction and reflux. *Pediatric Radiology* **4**, 226–232.

STANNARD M.W. & LEBOWITZ, R.L. (1978) Urography in the child who wets. *American Journal of Roentgenology* **130**, 959–962.

WHITAKER R.H., KEETON J.E. & WILLIAMS D.I (1972) Posterior urethral valves: a study of urinary control after operation. *Journal of Urology* **108**, 167–171.

WILLIAMS D. INNES (1974) Urology in childhood. *Encyclopedia of Urology,* Vol. 15, Supplement. Springer, Berlin.

DIVISION 5. THE MALE GENITAL TRACT

A. INFERTILITY

Sperm examination/analysis is the usual first step in the investigation of these problems. If abnormal, testicular biopsy may follow in order to look at the factory. However, it would appear sensible to consider not only the possibility of defective sperm production, but also that of faulty transport, e.g. blocked vasa. A vasogram may therefore be done at the same time, under the same general anaesthetic (Fig. IV.5.A1). This reasoning sounds sensible enough from the armchair, but does not stand up so well in the light of everyday practice: the pay-offs are uncertain and infrequent.

Many congenital and acquired structural abnormalities of vasa and seminal vesicles have been described on vasograms (Boreau, 1974). Close pathological corroboration of the various entities is often lacking. An association just worth remembering is cystic malformation of the seminal vesicle with an absent kidney (Blandy, 1976). The ectopic ureter draining into a seminal vesicle is illustrated in division 2 section A (Fig. IV.2.A2).

The range of successful surgical manoeuvres for correcting any deformities

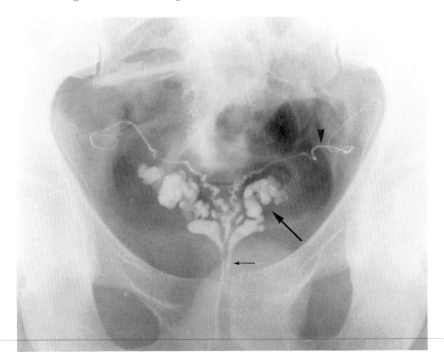

Fig. IV.5.A1 Normal vasogram—on one side the small arrow points to the ejaculatory duct, the large arrow to the seminal vesicle, and the arrowhead to the vas.

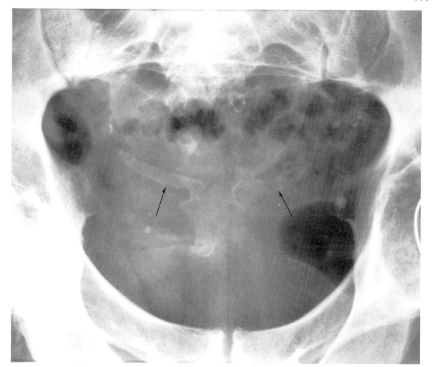

Fig. IV.5.A2 *(left)*   Calcified vasa in a diabetic man (arrows). (Courtesy of Dr H. Holland).

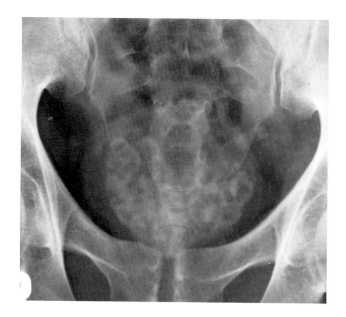

Fig. IV.5.A3 *(below left)*   Plain film in bilharzia—there is prominent calcification of the seminal vesicles, and more faintly of the bladder wall. (Courtesy of Dr A. A. Salem).

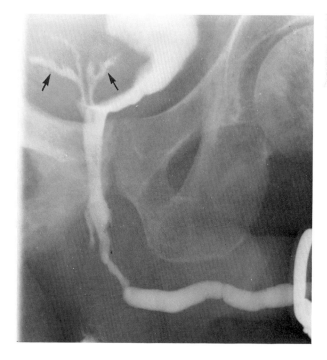

Fig. IV.5.A4 *(below right)*   Urethrogram done because of a urethral stricture—note reflux into both seminal vesicles (arrows).

found is very limited. For these various reasons the routine 'infertility vaso-gram' is not very rewarding and not widely practised. The combination of grossly defective sperm count and near-normal testicular biopsy is the obvious indication for the investigation.

Failure of ejaculation as the only abnormality in otherwise normal sexual performance, with sperm in the urine voided later, suggests an abnormality of bladder neck function. A voiding cystogram may be done to look at this, but is not usually very helpful.

Other genital tract oddities

Calcified vasa occur in this country most characteristically in diabetes as a symmetrical chance finding (Fig. IV.5.A2). Calcification of seminal vesicles is of course seen as part of the bilharzia picture (Fig. IV.5.A3). Grossly asymmetric, focal calcification of the genital tract is a possible complication of tuberculosis, but distinctly uncommon.

Urinary reflux into the genital tract may be seen in the presence of severe urethral strictures (Fig. IV.5.A4). Minor prostatic reflux is common in older men, but gross reflux opacifying the whole prostate generally denotes abnormal urethral urodynamics, e.g. stricture (Fig. IV.5.A5 and IV.5.A6).

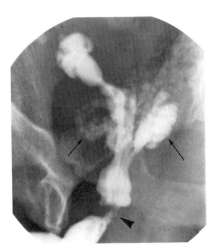

Fig. IV.5.A5 *(above)* Reflux is seen into prostatic ducts (small arrows), associated with a urethral stricture (arrowhead).

Fig. IV.5.A6 *(right)* This patient also has urethral strictures, with prostatic reflux dense enough to produce a 'prostatogram'.

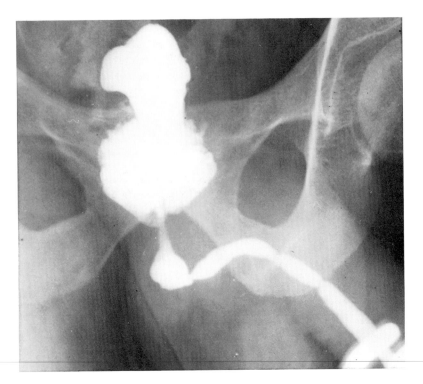

B. DEFORMITY

Chordee denotes curvature of the penis. Ventral chordee is commonly associated with hypospadias, but may exist on its own. The dorsal deformity is rare: it may be found with a double urethra. Radiological studies of these lesions are needed for the urethral and genital tract problems that may accompany them, not for the deformity itself.

Peyronie's disease

In this interesting disease of unknown origin, fibrous plaques form in the corpora cavernosa. They give rise to penile deformity, and to pain on erection. The natural history is not inexorably downhill, so that spontaneous resolution may occur, bedevilling the assessment of various treatments tried for the condition.

A minority of the plaques calcify. Soft tissue radiography is therefore helpful if active therapeutic measures are to be undertaken. If calcified, the extent of the plaque (often underestimated on palpation) can be documented, and gauged against treatment (Fig. IV.5.B1).

The technique of cavernography (see Part I section I) has also been used to this end, but is not practised widely (Fig. IV.5.B2).

Fig. IV.5.B1 Peyronie's disease—arrows point to calcified plaques in the corpora cavernosa.

Priapism

There are few radiological features to this urological emergency (the chances of avoiding impotence are small if treatment is delayed beyond 24 h). Anastomosis between one or other corpus cavernosum and the saphenous vein is generally performed if the patient is seen early enough—it is only the corpora cavernosa that are involved in the abnormal erection, not the corpus spongiosum. The patency of the anastomosis can then be checked by venography via the corpus cavernosum (see above). Calcification in the thickened useless corpora remaining after untreated priapism is a rare finding (Fig. IV.5.B3).

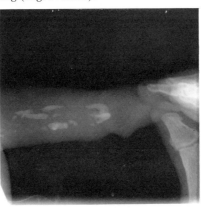

Fig. IV.5.B3 *(right)* Calcification in corpora cavernosa as a late complication of priapism.

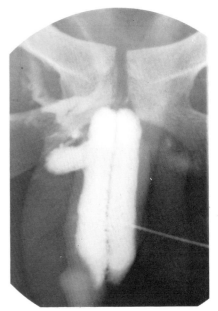

Fig. IV.5.B2 *(above)* Normal cavernogram—note symmetry of the two corpora cavernosa.

C. TUMOURS

Penile carcinoma is worth mention in a radiological text in order to emphasize that lymphography has little to offer these patients. The regional nodes are almost always 'involved' with filling defects on lymphograms, because of the infection associated with the lesion. Interpretation and staging accuracy are therefore poor.

Testicular tumours

Lymphography plays an important part in assessing testicular seminomas and teratomas. The investigation stages the demonstrable extent of the disease, so that treatment can be given as appropriate. Radiotherapy is often carried forward prophylactically one stage beyond this, i.e. if the para-aortic nodes are shown to be involved, the mediastinum is irradiated. It might be thought then that lymphography was inappropriate in two circumstances: if lung metastases are already present, or if surgical para-aortic node dissection is to be done. However, present practices veer toward aggressive attack on the highly responsive seminoma in particular, reducing tumour node bulk by surgery, followed by irradiation. To this end preoperative lymphography is useful for demonstrating the site and extent of even advanced disease. There are the usual reservations about sending oil emboli to the lungs if respiratory function is already compromised (see Part I section H).

Interpretation of the testicular tumour lymphogram depends on the usual criteria of filling defects, node enlargement, or unusual filling patterns. Follow-up films can be very helpful in doubtful cases. Two important points:

1. The lymphatic drainage path of the testis is of course upwards to the renal hilum, and then to the para-aortic nodes at renal level. The first node in the renal hilum will not necessarily be opacified by the contrast medium injected into the feet, and ureteric deviation can be an important clue to the renal hilum nodes (Fig. IV.5.C1).

2. Iliac nodes may be involved if there is direct invasion of the whole spermatic cord (Fig. IV.5.C1).

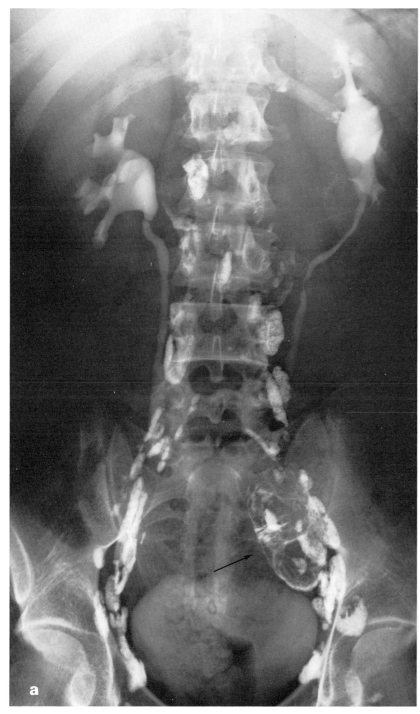

Fig. IV.5.C1a Lymphogram in a patient
with a seminoma—note rotation of the
left kidney and displacement of the left
upper ureter by the enlarged nodes lying
in the renal hilum. The arrow points to an
involved iliac node, implying invasion
through the spermatic cord.

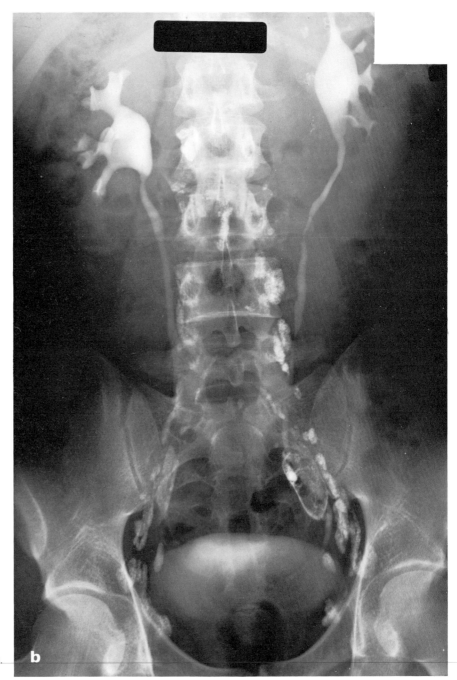

Fig. IV.5.C1b One month later
following irradiation there is
improvement in all the abnormal features.
(Courtesy of Dr N. Bowley).

D. INTERSEX STATES

For these patients skilled clinical and laboratory help is needed to make an accurate diagnosis, vital for assigning a manageable and consistent sexual status at an early age. Cremin (1974) has stressed the radiological contribution toward this by the technique of genitography. The genital tract is outlined by simple injection of water-soluble contrast medium. Depending on the severity of the malformation this will be either into an obvious urogenital sinus, or in the case of a boy with hypospadias into the abnormal urethral opening. In complex cases the genitogram may provide a very helpful assessment of the internal anatomy, showing for instance a vagina or uterus in the boy with hypospadias (Fig. IV.5.D1).

E. SCROTUM

A *haematocoele,* a collection of blood in the layers of the tunica vaginalis, usually traumatic, may advance to calcification, so producing the only radiological sign of interest at this site (Fig. IV.5.E1). *Vale!*

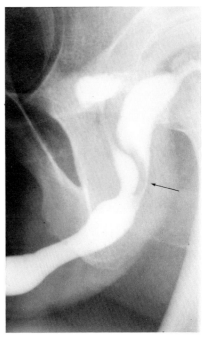

Fig. IV.5.D1 *(above)* This boy's urethrogram shows a posterior channel (arrow) leading to a uterine cavity behind the bladder.

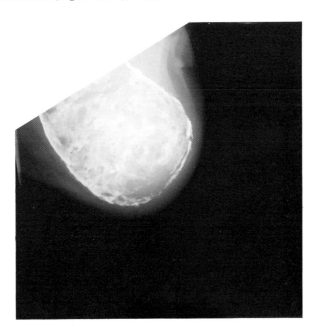

Fig. IV.5.E1 *(left)* Calcified haematocoele following scrotal trauma.

REFERENCES

BLANDY J.P. (1976) *Urology,* Chapter 47. Blackwell Scientific Publications, Oxford.

BOREAU J. (1974) *Images of the Seminal Tracts.* S. Karger, Basel.

CREMIN B.J. (1974) Intersex states in young children: the importance of radiology in making a correct diagnosis. *Clinical Radiology* **25,** 63–73.

INDEX

Angiomyolipoma   195
Antegrade pyelogram   15
Arteriogram   21, 78
  adrenalin   26
  complications   24, 80
  contrast medium   25
  embolization   26, 195
  hypertension   78
  renal artery stenosis   79
  renal failure   97, 115, 139

Bilharzia   234
  bladder   296
  genital tract   298, 340
Bladder
  —see also Obstruction (lower urinary
    tract)
  cystitis—q.v.
  diverticulum   240, 268, 332
  double micturition   333
  dynamic studies   12, 262
  exstrophy   316
  fistula   276
  infection   272
  instability   265, 281, 283
  lipomatosis   72, 301
  neurofibromatosis   307
  neuropathy   286, 323
  odd shapes   301
  rhabdomyosarcoma   337
  stone   268, 296
  trauma   307
  tumour   291
    CT   71
    IVU   291
    ultrasound   31
Bladder neck
  absent   213, 320
  obstruction   266
  wide   320
Blood in upper urinary tract   121, 227

Calix   141
  crescent sign   116, 174
  diverticulum   163
  extrinsic impression   155
  hydrocalicosis   157
  lacunae   330
  megacalices   162
  polycalicosis   162
  stricture   154
Cavernogram   36
Chordee   341
Chyluria   164

Contrast medium (IVU)   1
  compounds   1, 5
  dose   2, 107
  excretion   2
  reactions   6
  renal failure   107
CT   59
  accuracy   64
  bladder   71
  kidney   60
  pelvis   70
  perirenal   66
  prostate   71
  renal cyst   62
  renal failure   65
  renal mass   61
  retroperitoneum   67
  technique   59
Cystitis
  acute   275, 294
  children   313
  chronic   296
  cyclophosphamide   296, 334
  men   275
  women   272
Cystogram   10
  double contrast   12
  dynamic   12, 262, 281
  radionuclide   55

Diverticulum
  bladder   240, 268, 332
  calix   163
  urethra   272, 275, 332
Duplex kidney   211
  ectopic drainage   212, 283, 316
  renal mass   173
  vesico-ureteric reflux   220
  yo-yo reflux   212
Dynamic cystogram   12, 262, 281
Dynamic upper tract studies   20, 116, 244

EMG syndrome   132, 164
Epispadias   316
ERPF   41
Exstrophy   316

Filariasis   164
Fistula
  arterio-venous   204
  bladder   276
  ureter   283

Genitogram   345

GFR   41
Goodpasture's syndrome   103

Horseshoe kidney   88
Hydrocalicosis   157
Hydronephrosis   100, 116
Hyperparathyroidism
    nephrocalcinosis   133
    renal failure   103
Hypertension   75
    arteriogram   78
    IVU   76
    renal vein sampling   83
    renography   44, 78

Incontinence   281
    children   313
    giggle incontinence   321
    prostatic   283
    stress   281
Infertility   338
Intersex   345
IVU   1
    children   37, 241
    compression   8
    contrast media   1
    contrast medium dose   2, 107
    contrast medium excretion   2
    contrast medium reactions   6
    dehydration   4, 108
    diuresis   242
    hypertension   76
    renal failure   103
    technique   8, 108, 169

Kidney
    —see also Renal
    abscess   52, 96, 195
    absent   31, 93
    angiomyolipoma   195
    Ask-Upmark   145
    carcinoma   101, 182
        arteriogram   191
        CT   61
        diagnosis   183, 193
        embolization   195
        puncture   188
        ultrasound   31
    compression   102
    cyst   180, 197
        arteriogram   181
        CT   62
        diagnosis   183
        puncture   186

Kidney—cont.
    cyst—cont.
        ultrasound   31
    duplex
        —see Duplex kidney
    dysplasia   163
    ectopic   88
    failure (unilateral)   87
        absence   93
        compression   102
        CT   65
        ectopia   88
        infection   96
        obstruction   100
        renal artery stenosis   97
        renal size   88
        renal vein obstruction   98
        tumour   101
    horseshoe   88
    hydronephrosis   100, 116
    infarct   53, 97, 164
    infection
        abscess   52, 96, 195
        acute suppurative pyelonephritis   96
        chronic atrophic pyelonephritis   141,
            238
        gallium scans   51
        xanthogranuloma   196
    island   49, 166
    malrotation   93
    mass
        adult   176
        childhood   170
        ultrasound   32
    medullary sponge   129
    multicystic   100, 174
    nephrocalcinosis   128
    polyarteritis nodosa   115, 202
    polycystic
        —see Polycystic disease
    post-obstructive atrophy   157
    rupture   8
    size   87
        renal failure   108
        small kidneys   112
    stones   124
        nephrocalcinosis   128
        obstruction   100, 222
        site   125
    trauma   199
        arteriogram   200
        IVU   200
        radionuclide scanning   50
    Wilms' tumour   170

Lipomatosis (pelvis) 72, 301
Lipomatosis (renal sinus) 168
Loin pain and haematuria syndrome 202
Lymphogram 33
    complications 34
    contraindications 34
    filariasis 164
    prostatic tumours 34
    technique 34
    testicular tumours 342

MCU 10
    children 37
Medullary sponge kidney 129
Megacalices 162
Megaureter 228, 245
Multicystic kidney 100, 174

Nephrocalcinosis 128
Nephrogram
    mechanism 2
    radiolucent masses 175
    renal failure 109
Nephroma (infantile) 172
Nephrostomy (antegrade) 16
Neuroblastoma 173
Neurofibromatosis 307
Nuclear medicine 41
    bone scans 55
    cystograms 55
    gallium scans 50
    perfusion studies 45
    radionuclides for scanning 48
    renogram—q.v.
    residual urine 47
    scintillation scans 47
    split renal function 43, 50
    total renal function 41

Obstruction (lower urinary tract) 255,
        324
    bladder neck 266
    bladder neuropathy 290
    bladder stone 268
    dynamic studies 12, 262, 281
    mimicking neuropathy 286, 323
    prostate 255
    urethral stricture 267, 312
    urethral valve 325, 332
    urinal 330
Obstruction (upper urinary tract) 100,
        222, 244
    bladder neuropathy 289
    dynamic studies 20, 116, 244

Obstruction (upper urinary tract)—cont.
    hydronephrosis 116
    kidney failure (unilateral) 100
    renal failure 109
    renogram 43
    stone 223
    ultrasound 31
Osteitis pubis 262

Paediatric work 36
Papillary necrosis
    —see Renal papillary necrosis
Pelvi-ureteritis cystica 120
Penis
    carcinoma 342
    chordee 341
    deformity 341
    epispadias 316
    hypospadias 333, 341
    Peyronie's disease 341
    priapism 36, 341
Perirenal haematoma 102, 200
Peyronie's disease 341
Pneumaturia 276
Polyarteritis nodosa 115, 202
Polycalicosis 162
Polycystic disease 175
    adult 176
    infantile 132, 176
    medullary 176
    renal failure 112
Post-obstructive atrophy 157
Priapism 36, 341
Prostate
    bladder outflow obstruction 255
    carcinoma 255, 278
    CT 71
    incontinence 283
    IVU 255, 262
    lymphogram 34
    reflux 340
    ultrasound 32
Prune belly syndrome 245, 332
Pyelogram
    —see Antegrade, Dynamic, Retrograde
        etc
Pyelonephritis,
    acute suppurative 96
    chronic atrophic 141, 238
    xanthogranulomatous 196

Reflux
    prostatic 340
    vaginal 321

Reflux—*cont.*
  vesico-ureteric 238
    bladder neuropathy 289
    chronic atrophic pyelonephritis 141,
      240
    double micturition 333
    duplex kidney 220
Renal
  —*see also* Kidney
  arteritis 202
  artery
    aneurysm 78, 97, 205
    arteritis 202
    dissection 24, 45, 97
    fistula 47, 204
    multiple 23
    occlusion 45, 97
    stenosis—*q.v.*
  artery stenosis 79, 97
    atheroma 79
    fibromuscular disease 79
    kidney failure (unilateral) 97
    pharmacoangiogram 81
    radionuclide scanning 44
    renal failure 45, 109
    renal vein sampling 83
  cortical necrosis 138
  failure 102
    CT 65
    initial radiographs 102
    IVU 103
    large kidneys 108
    obstruction 109
    renal artery occlusion 45, 97
    renal size 108
    renal vein obstruction 98, 108
    renography 44
    retrograde pyelogram 111
    small kidneys 112
    ultrasound 31, 110
  papillary necrosis 103, 137, 146
    causes 147
  sinus fat 87, 168
  transplant 42, 45, 47
  tubular acidosis 137
  vein 24
    obstruction 27, 98, 108
    renin ratio 86
    sampling 83
Renogram 42
  hypertension 44
  obstruction 43
Residual urine 255
  bladder neuropathy 291

Residual urine—*cont.*
  nuclear medicine studies 47
  ultrasound 31
Retrograde pyelogram 20
  renal failure 111
Retrograde ureterogram 20
Retroperitoneal fibrosis 234
  CT 69
Retroperitoneum
  CT 67
  ultrasound 31

Schistosomiasis
  —*see* Bilharzia
Scrotum 345
Scintillation scans 47
Stone 124
  bladder 268, 296
  renal 122
  ureteric 223

Testis
  tumours 342
  ultrasound 32
Tuberculosis 149, 154

Ultrasound 29
  bladder 31
  kidney 30, 32
  prostate 32
  renal failure 31, 94, 110
  retroperitoneum 31
  technique 32
  testis 32
Ureter
  dilatation 222, 330
    without obstruction 242
  diversion 241, 249, 279
  dynamic studies 244
  ectopic 212, 283, 316
  fistula 283
  megaureter 228, 245
  obstruction 222
  polyp 231
  prune belly syndrome 245
  reflux 238
  retrocaval 237
  retroperitoneal fibrosis 234
  stone 223
  stricture 231
  tumour 119, 231
  ureteritis 228
Ureterocele 213
  diagnosis 221

Ureterocele—*cont.*
  ectopic 215
  orthotopic 215
Urethra
  carcinoma 298
  diverticulum 272, 275, 332
  double 333, 341
  epispadias 316
  hypospadias 333, 341
  obstruction by urinal 330
  prune belly syndrome 332
  stricture 267, 312
  trauma 307, 332
  valve 325, 332
  warts 298
Urethrogram 13
Urinary infection
  —*see also* Kidney infection *and* Cystitis

Urinary infection—*cont.*
  adults 272
  children 241, 313, 324
Urinoma 196
Urothelial tumours 119, 123, 192, 249, 291
  differential diagnosis 119
Uterus, male 345

Vas deferens calcification 340
Vasogram 35, 338
Vena cava (inferior)
  obstruction 303
  venogram 27
Venogram 26

Wilms' tumour 170

Xanthogranuloma 196